Ultrasound: Clinical Techniques and Technical Advances

Ultrasound: Clinical Techniques and Technical Advances

Editor: Michelle Skinner

AMERICAN
MEDICAL PUBLISHERS
www.americanmedicalpublishers.com

AMERICAN
MEDICAL PUBLISHERS
www.americanmedicalpublishers.com

Cataloging-in-Publication Data

Ultrasound : clinical techniques and technical advances / edited by Michelle Skinner.
p. cm.
Includes bibliographical references and index.
ISBN 978-1-63927-084-2
1. Ultrasonic imaging. 2. Ultrasonics in medicine. 3. Diagnostic ultrasonic imaging.
4. Diagnostic imaging. 5. Imaging systems in medicine. I. Skinner, Michelle.
RC78.7.U4 U48 2022
616.075 43--dc23

American Medical Publishers,
41 Flatbush Avenue,
1st Floor, New York,
NY 11217, USA

ISBN 978-1-63927-084-2 (Hardback)

Contents

Preface

Every book is a source of knowledge and this one is no exception. The idea that led to the conceptualization of this book was the fact that the world is advancing rapidly; which makes it crucial to document the progress in every field. I am aware that a lot of data is already available, yet, there is a lot more to learn. Hence, I accepted the responsibility of editing this book and contributing my knowledge to the community.

Ultrasound is the sound wave that is above the range of sound audible to humans. It is used in many different fields. In a clinical perspective, ultrasound is used to produce images of structures within the human body. Medical sonography is used to visualize, tendons, muscles, and many other internal organs. It captures their size, structure and any pathological lesions with real time tomographic images. It is also used to visualize fetuses during routine and emergency prenatal care and detection of pelvic abnormalities. It plays a crucial role in trauma and first aid cases. This book unravels the recent studies in the field of ultrasonography. It strives to provide a fair idea about this discipline and to help develop a better understanding of the latest advances within this field. This book is appropriate for students seeking detailed information in this area as well as for experts.

While editing this book, I had multiple visions for it. Then I finally narrowed down to make every chapter a sole standing text explaining a particular topic, so that they can be used independently. However, the umbrella subject sinews them into a common theme. This makes the book a unique platform of knowledge.

I would like to give the major credit of this book to the experts from every corner of the world, who took the time to share their expertise with us. Also, I owe the completion of this book to the never-ending support of my family, who supported me throughout the project.

Editor

1

Non-opaque soft tissue foreign body: sonographic findings

Afshin Mohammadi[1*], Mohammad Ghasemi-Rad[2] and Maryam Khodabakhsh[3]

Abstract

Background: Soft tissue foreign bodies are a common cause of orthopedic consultation in emergency departments. It is difficult to confirm their existence because conventional radiology only detects radio-opaque foreign bodies. Sonography can be a useful diagnostic method. The aim of this study is to evaluate diagnostic accuracy of sonography in detection and localization of non-opaque foreign bodies.

Methods: We evaluated 47 patients with suspected foreign body retention in soft tissues by 10 MHz linear array transducer. A single radiologist performed all examinations with 6 years' experience in musculoskeletal Sonography. We detected and localized the presence of the foreign body in the soft tissue as guidance for facilitating the surgery.

Results: We detected soft tissue foreign body in 45 cases as hyperechoic foci. Posterior acoustic shadowing was seen in 36 cases and halo sign was seen in 5 cases due to abscess or granulation tissue formation. Surgery was performed in 39 patients and 44 foreign bodies were removed.

Conclusion: Sonography is a useful modality in detection and localization of radiolucent foreign bodies in soft tissue which can avoid misdiagnosis during primary emergency evaluation.

Background

Penetrating object injuries are a common problem in the emergency department, and retained foreign bodies in soft tissues complicate many such injuries. Because a retained foreign body may cause severe infection or inflammatory reaction, detection and removal of foreign bodies are necessary [1].

Punctured wounds and soft tissue lacerations are inspected, palpated and explored to rule out the presence of a foreign body, and radiographic evaluations are routinely obtained to confirm radio-opaque foreign bodies such as glass, metal, and stone within the soft tissue [2,3], However 38% of such foreign bodies are overlooked at initial examination in the emergency room [4].

A radiolucent foreign body such as wood frequently remains undetected [3]. In such situations, other imaging modalities are needed for diagnosis. Sonography plays an important role in the evaluation of these patients [5].

* Correspondence: mohamadi_afshin@yahoo.com
[1]Radiology Department, Urmia University of Medical Sciences, Urmia, Iran
Full list of author information is available at the end of the article

Sonography has a reported sensitivity of 95% for detection of foreign bodies [6,7].

In previous reports the positive predictive value of Conventional Radiography (CR) and Sonography (US) were 100% and 95% respectively and for Computed Tomography (CT) and Magnetic Resonance Imaging (MRI) were 95% and 93.8% respectively. CT had a negative predictive value of 78.3%, while US, MRI, and CR had 73.7%, 70.1%, and 53.7%, respectively [8].

Non-opaque foreign bodies are visualized as hyperechoic foci with accompanying acoustic shadows [5]. This shadow may be either complete or partial depending on the angle of insonation and the composition of the foreign body [4]. A hypoechoic halo surrounding the foreign body is sometimes seen, which represents edema, abscess or granulation tissue [9].

The purpose of the study was to determine effectiveness of Sonography for detection of radiolucent foreign bodies and to summarize all clinical experiences using Sonography in the management of patients with a suspected retained foreign body.

Methods

Forty-seven patients were referred for Sonographic examination because of possible retention of soft tissue foreign bodies in the upper or lower extremities during a 3-year period (January 2006 to January 2009). General physicians of the emergency department of Imam Khomeini University Hospital, Urmia, Iran, referred 44 male patients and 3 female patients. All patients had undergone plain X-rays that were negative for foreign bodies. Mean age was 26 years (Range 12 to 44). Those patients having X-rays negative for foreign bodies were referred for Sonographic evaluation.

We evaluated the site of penetrating trauma and location of the patients' chief complaint both longitudinally and transversely by high frequency Sonographic scanning.

A radiologist with 6 years experience in musculoskeletal system obtained all Sonography (Esaote MyLab 50, Genova, Italy).

For obtaining a good soft tissue resolution, we need a high frequency linear transducer which has been shown to be helpful in detecting small foreign bodies [10].

In all patients, the contra-lateral extremity was examined as a comparison. Whenever a foreign body was localized, its length and depth beneath the skin was measured with computerized calipers.

We evaluated the Sonographic findings of various soft tissue foreign bodies, such as posterior acoustic shadowing, posterior comet tail, and a halo sign in all patients.

The University research and ethics committee approved the study protocol; written informed consent was obtained from all patients.

Results

We detected and localized the foreign bodies in 45 of the 47 patients by Sonography. The sensitivity and specificity of Sonography in comparison with surgery in diagnosis of soft tissue foreign bodies was 100%.

Surgery revealed that 20 objects were wooden particles and date rose thorns; 6 objects were fish bones in fishmonger and 18 objects were broken glass particles (39 patients with 44 objects).

Thirty-nine foreign bodies that were diagnosed by Sonography under local anesthesia were surgically removed. All patients were symptom free during follow-up with no further complications recorded during observation.

Six patients had small foreign bodies with minor symptoms and without impairment of limb function. All 6 patients opted for regular follow-ups instead of surgical removal. The patients were symptom free after 3 months of follow-up. Two patients had negative Sonographic findings that were followed-up with non-surgical conservative treatment.

The smallest foreign body was a glass object detected in the forearm which measured 3 mm in length. The mean ± SD length of detected foreign body was 7.9 ± 0.6 mm. Wooden objects were the most common type.

We detected foreign bodies in toes (6 patients), forearms (7 patients), fingers (13 patients), soles of the foot (16 patients) and calves (3 patients) by Sonography.

One of the patients had 4 pieces of foreign body in his foot and one patient had 3 pieces of foreign body in his finger.

Surgery was performed in 39 patients and 44 foreign bodies were removed.

Sonography revealed the foreign body as hyper-echoic objects with or without posterior acoustic shadowing in all 45 patients. (Figures 1, 2 & 3)

Sonography revealed the foreign body as the late complication of previous penetrating trauma with sustained pain and tenderness on trauma site in 5 patients with hypo-echoic mass surrounding the foreign objects due to abscess and granulation tissue formation. (Figure 4).

We detected posterior acoustic shadowing in 15 cases of wooden objects; Rose thorns in 21 patients with wooden foreign bodies. Posterior acoustic shadowing or comet tail sign was not seen in 6 patients. The mean ± SD length of detected wooden foreign bodies with posterior acoustic shadowing was 9.8 ± 0.4 mm and 4.6 ± 0.3 mm without posterior acoustic shadowing.

We detected posterior acoustic shadowing in 15 out of 18 patients with broken glass objects and posterior comet tail sign in 2 patients (50 mm and 9 mm foreign bodies in length respectively). Posterior acoustic shadowing or posterior comet tail sign was not detected in one patient (4 mm foreign body in length).

We detected posterior acoustic shadowing in all fish bone foreign bodies (6 patients). The mean ± SD length of detected fish bones with posterior acoustic shadowing was 6.9 ± 0.6 mm.

The type of foreign body, its mean ± SD measure, and the body locations are expressed in table 1.

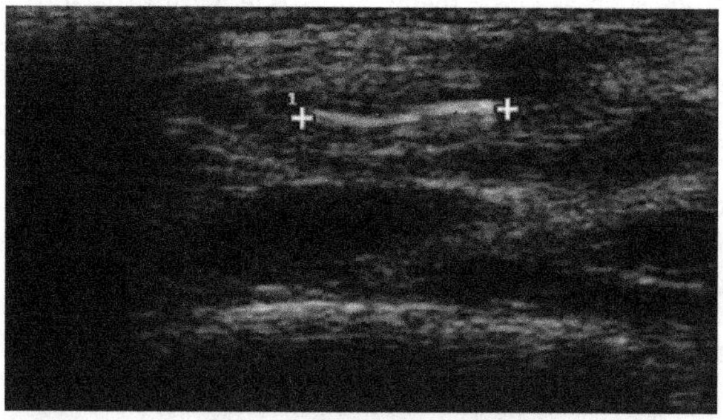

Figure 1 Longitudinal sonogram shows a hyperechoic 4 mm long broken glass (long arrow) without posterior acoustic shadowing in the forearm of a 24 years old man.

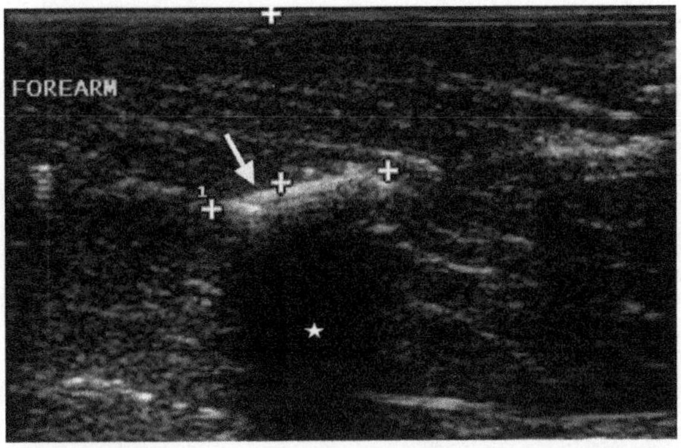

Figure 2 **Longitudinal sonogram shows a hyperechoic 2 cm long wooden foreign body (long arrow) with posterior acoustic shadowing (satellites) forearm of 21 years old man.**

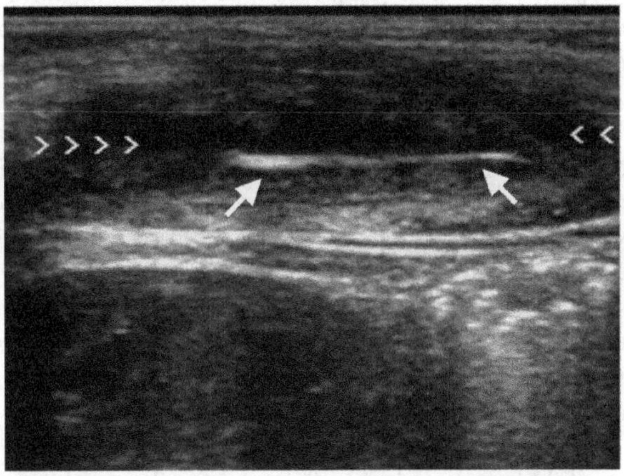

Figure 4 **Longitudinal sonogram shows a hyperechoic 6 mm wooden foreign body (long arrow) without posterior acoustic but with surrounding halo sign (arrowhead) due to soft tissue abscess in the forearm.**

Discussion

A retained foreign body in the soft tissues of extremities is not very common. Diagnosis requires high index of suspicion. Exclusion of its presence is important, given the possible allergic, inflammatory, and infectious complications associated with a retained foreign body [1].

Conventional radiographs should be obtained to rule out the presence of radio-opaque foreign objects. Plain radiographs will depict approximately 80% of all foreign bodies, but several types of radiolucent foreign bodies such as wood remain undetected [11]. Plain radiographs of wooden FB are negative in 86% of such patients [4]. In these patients Sonography is the modality of choice for identification of such radiolucent FB.

The identification of wooden foreign bodies may be difficult on MRI, especially when foreign bodies are small and there is no associated abscess, granulation tissue, or fluid collection. In such cases, the foreign body may appear as a signal void with surrounding nonspecific granulation tissue. Wooden foreign bodies may be seen signal void in all sequences, but after water absorption it could be seen hypo-intense on T1 and hyper-intense on T2 images [5].

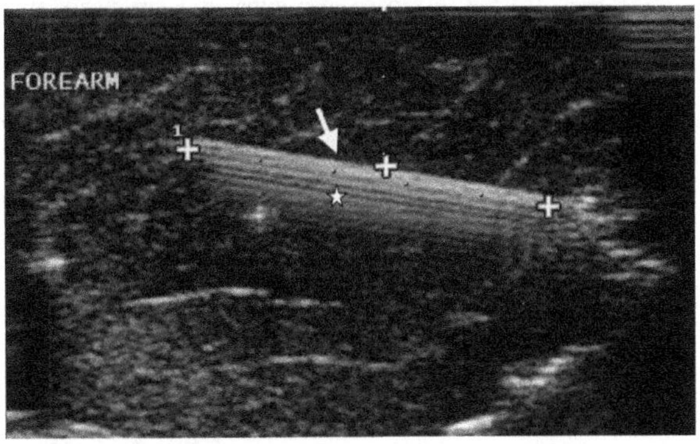

Figure 3 **Longitudinal sonogram shows a hyperechoic 5 cm long broken glass foreign body (long arrow) with posterior comet tail (satellites) in forearm of 21 years old man.**

When compared with Sonography, MRI is more expensive, less readily available, and has less value in the detection of small wooden foreign bodies. Likewise, MRI has obvious limitations for the evaluation of patients in the emergency room.

Sonographic evaluation provides important information on the depth, size and anatomical relationship with surrounding structure [6,9], and [12]. Although CT has sensitivity 5-15 times greater than that of plain X -ray, it is not as sensitive as US, or MRI [2]. Additionally, the expense, use of radiation, and availability make the use of CT less than optimal in the clinical setting.

Surgical dissection is facilitated by accurate knowledge of location of the FB related to muscles, tendons and vessels. Detection of foreign body is difficult in interphalangeal space and in air contaminated tissue after a penetrating trauma. FB must be distinguished from hyper-echoic body tissue such as ossified cartilage sesamoid bones, scar tissue, gas bubble, intermuscular fascia etc. Acoustic shadowing is an important clue in the

Table 1 Summerized the type of foreign body, its mean measurements and the location

	Type of FB		
Site of FB	*Wooden FB MD: 7.2 mm*	*Glass MD: 9.4 mm*	*Fish bone MD: 6.9 mm*
Sole of Foot	10	5	-
Finger	1	8	4
Forearm	4	1	2
Toe	3	3	-
Calves	2	1	-
All	20	18	6

FB: Foreign Body, MD:Mean Diameter.

differential diagnosis [6,9]. Acoustic shadowing can differentiate foreign body from scar tissue, gas bubble and normal intermuscular fascia, because they are void of acoustic shadowing.

Our results demonstrate the effectiveness of Sonography for detection of radiolucent FB. It is therefore an important modality that facilitates removal of the object by enabling a shorter exploration with less iatrogenic tissue damage.

Peterson JJ et al [5] showed that Sonography is the modality of choice in patients who present with a history of antecedent skin puncture or when a penetrating injury is suspected.

We detected the posterior acoustic shadowing in 15 out of 20 wooden objects that was similar to the previous study [13] that demonstrated posterior acoustic shadowing in only 11 out of 17 cases of wooden FB. This is perhaps because of the orientation of the FB relative to the sound bean and chronicity of the retained FB. Retained wooden FB absorbs fluid, which alters its imaging characteristics [1].

Fornage BD et al [14] showed that retained wooden foreign bodies are easily identified, with the leading edge of the echogenic wood resulting in marked acoustic shadowing.

Jacobson JA [15] showed that Sonography could be used effectively to locate wooden foreign bodies as small as 2.5 mm in length.

Dumarey A et al [16] showed that CT gave a good anatomic overview, but was not able to show the smaller fragments. Performing Sonography is mandatory in patients with penetrating injuries by foreign bodies because it is very sensitive.

We detected the posterior comet tail sign in only 2 out of 18 patients with broken glass objects in soft tissue.

The depth of all foreign bodies was smaller than 4 cm, because all of them were embedded in the distal part of upper and lower limbs.

We believe that all foreign bodies were seen during Sonographic examination as echogenic objects and most of them (wooden, glass, and etc...) may also show similar Sonographic findings. Most of them show posterior acoustic shadowing.

Conclusion

In conclusion, Sonography can be used effectively to locate radiolucent FB with high certainty, and should be considered for patients suspected of having a FB in the setting of negative X-rays. US can be used as a modality of choice in the emergency department to avoid missed, or under diagnosis of retained foreign bodies.

Acknowledgements

We would like to thank Dr Ahmadreza Afshar orthopedic surgeons and all nurses of Imam Khomaini Hospital, Urmia University of medical sciences for their kind help.

We would like to thank Dr Faisal Tawwab Gulf medical university for English editing.

Author details

[1]Radiology Department, Urmia University of Medical Sciences, Urmia, Iran. [2]Student research committee, School of Medicine, Urmia University of Medical Sciences, Urmia, Iran. [3]School of Medicine, Urmia University of Medical Sciences, Urmia, Iran.

Authors' contributions

AM participated in the idea, planning, data analysis and interpretation, statistical analysis, and writing the report.

MG participated in data collection; follow up, analysis and drafting.

MK participated in the data analysis and interpretation, statistical analysis. All authors read and approved the final manuscript.

Competing interests

The authors declare that they have no competing interests.

References

1. Mohamadi A, Kodabakhsh M: **Wooden foreign body in lung parenchyma, a case report.** *Turkish Journal of trauma and emergency surgery* 2010, **16(5)**:480-482.
2. Flom LL, Ellis GL: **Radiologic evaluation of foreign bodies.** *Emerg Med Clin North Am* 1992, **10**:163-176.
3. Graham DD Jr: **Ultrasound in the emergency department: detection of wooden foreign bodies in the soft tissues.** *J Emerg Med* 2002, **22(1)**:75-9.
4. Anderson MA, Newmeyer WL, Kilgore ES: **Diagnosis and treatment of retained foreign bodies in the hand.** *Am J Surg* 1982, **144**:63-67.
5. Peterson JJ, Bancroft LW, Kransdorf MJ: **Wooden foreign bodies: imaging appearance.** *AJR Am J Roentgenol* 2002, **178(3)**:557-62.
6. Crowford R, Matheson AB: **Clinical value of ultrasonography in detection and removal of radiolucent foreign bodies.** *Injury* 1989, **20**:341-343.
7. Ober CP, Jones JC, Larson MM, Lanz OI, Werre SR: **Comparison of ultrasound, computed tomography, and magnetic resonance imaging in detection of acute wooden foreign bodies in the canine manus.** *Vet Radiol Ultrasound* 2008, **49(5)**:411-8.
8. Venter NG, Jamel N, Marques RG, Djahjah F, Mendonça Lde S: **Evaluation of radiological methods for detection of wood foreign body in animal model.** *Acta Cir Bras* 2005, **20(Suppl 1)**:34-41.
9. Little CM, Parker MG, Callowich MC, Sartori JC: **The ultrasonic detection soft tissue foreign bodies.** *Invest Radiol* 1986, **21**:275-7.
10. Walter JP: **Physics of high resolution -practical aspect.** *Radiol Clin North Am* 1985, **23**:3-11.
11. Donaldson J: **Radiographic imaging of foreign bodies in the hand.** *Hand Clin* 1991, **7**:125-134.
12. Conti RJ, Shinder M: **Soft tissue calcification induced by local corticosteroid injection.** *J Foot Surg* 1991, **30**:34-7.
13. Gilbert FJ, Campbel RSD, Bayliss AP: **The role of ultrasound in detection of non- opaque foreign bodies.** *Clin Radiol* 1990, **40**:109-112.
14. Fornage BD, Schernberg FL: **Sonographic diagnosis of foreign bodies of the distal extremities.** *AJR* 1986, **147**:567-569.
15. Jacobson JA, Powell A, Craig JG, Bouffard JA, van Holsbeeck MT: **Wooden foreign bodies in soft tissue: detection at US.** *Radiology* 1998, **206(1)**:45-8.
16. Dumarey A, De Maeseneer M, Ernst C: **Large wooden foreign body in the hand: recognition of occult fragments with ultrasound.** *Emerg Radiol* 2004, **10(6)**:337-9.

2

In vivo thyroid vibro-acoustography

Azra Alizad[1,2*], Matthew W Urban[1], John C Morris[3], Carl C Reading[4], Randall R Kinnick[1], James F Greenleaf[1] and Mostafa Fatemi[1]

Abstract

Background: The purpose of this study was to evaluate the utility of a noninvasive ultrasound-based method, vibro-acoustography (VA), for thyroid imaging and determine the feasibility and challenges of VA in detecting nodules in thyroid.

Methods: Our study included two parts. First, in an *in vitro* study, experiments were conducted on a number of excised thyroid specimens randomly taken from autopsy. Three types of images were acquired from most of the specimens: X-ray, B-mode ultrasound, and vibro-acoustography. The second and main part of the study includes results from performing VA and B-mode ultrasound imaging on 24 human subjects with thyroid nodules. The results were evaluated and compared qualitatively.

Results: *In vitro* vibro-acoustography images displayed soft tissue structures, microcalcifications, cysts and nodules with high contrast and no speckle. In this group, all of US proven nodules and all of X-ray proven calcifications of thyroid tissues were detected by VA. *In vivo* results showed 100% of US proven calcifications and 91% of the US detected nodules were identified by VA, however, some artifacts were present in some cases.

Conclusions: *In vitro* and *in vivo* VA images show promising results for delineating the detailed structure of the thyroid, finding nodules and in particular calcifications with greater clarity compare to US. Our findings suggest that, with further development, VA may be a suitable imaging modality for clinical thyroid imaging.

Keywords: Elasticity imaging techniques, Vibro-acoustography, Thyroid neoplasm, Thyroid nodule, Ultrasound, Imaging

Background

The clinical practice of thyroidology has been revolutionized over the last decade by the inclusion of real-time ultrasound (US) in the evaluation of nodular thyroid disease. Ultrasonography can accurately determine the number and the size of thyroid nodules. US imaging is extremely useful in guiding fine needle aspiration biopsy (FNAB); however, its role in predicting malignancy is limited such that ultrasound-guided FNAB is carried out routinely in the evaluation of thyroid nodules [1]. Conventional ultrasound characteristics of thyroid nodules are not sufficiently specific to reliably determine the malignant potential of thyroid nodules [2]. Thus, despite the obvious utility of conventional ultrasound, the gold standard for diagnosis of benign versus malignant thyroid nodules is the FNAB [2,3].

FNAB is an invasive procedure and technique accuracy depends largely on the skill of the aspirator, the expertise of the cytologist, and the difficulty in distinguishing some benign cellular adenomas from their malignant counterparts and wide variability in interpretative skill regarding cytopathology of the thyroid nodule. Because of these limitations, the results are indeterminate in approximately 15-20% of cases. Analysis of recent data from some series suggests a false-negative rate of up to 11%, a false-positive rate of up to 8%, with a sensitivity of about 80%, and a specificity of 73% [4-8].

Thyroid magnetic resonance imaging (MRI) and X-ray computed tomography (CT) scans are not as sensitive as US in detecting thyroid nodules, however, they are helpful in staging of the thyroid cancer [9,10].

Another major area of uncertainty in the management of thyroid nodules is the issue of follicular neoplasm of

* Correspondence: Alizad.azra@mayo.edu
[1]Department of Physiology and Biomedical Engineering, Mayo Clinic, 200 First Street SW, Rochester, MN 55905, USA
[2]Department of Internal Medicine, Mayo Clinic, 200 First Street SW, Rochester, MN 55905, USA
Full list of author information is available at the end of the article

the thyroid. Approximately 5% of all thyroid nodules are follicular neoplasm, most of which are benign follicular adenomas, but 10-20% are follicular thyroid cancers. Neither conventional ultrasound appearance nor FNAB is sufficient to distinguish between these two lesions largely because the cytology of follicular adenoma is not sufficiently different from that of follicular carcinomas [3,11,12]. Currently, most of patients with FNAB cytology indicating "follicular neoplasm" or "suspicious for follicular neoplasm" are sent for thyroidectomy in order to make a definitive diagnosis. Thus, this issue represents a major area of clinical practice that requires new and innovative technological approaches for resolution.

Improved methods for thyroid nodule differentiation are required to effectively and appropriately select biopsy candidates in suspected nodules within the thyroid. Elasticity imaging is an emerging field of medical imaging for noninvasive and objective evaluation of tissue viscoelasticity. Magnetic resonance elastography (MRE) can be used to differentiate normal and pathological thyroid gland [13], however, this method is based on expensive MRI technology and thus less likely to see wide clinical application. Thyroid static ultrasound elastography has been developed to obtain tissue stiffness information [14,15]. The resulting image is typically the strain distribution after a stress has been applied by the user which reflects the elastic characteristics of tissues. There are very promising reports in clinical applications in thyroid nodules [16-22]. However, it has not been proven that real-time elastography alone is useful in differentiation of thyroid nodules and the technique needs additional quantitative information [23].

Acoustic radiation force impulse (ARFI) imaging and supersonic imaging (SSI) use ultrasound radiation force to generate shear waves and quantify tissue elasticity from measured propagation speed of shear wave. Studies using ARFI and SSI for thyroid nodule screening provide quantitative tissue elasticity information and preliminary results have been very promising [24-31]. However, the sensitivity of SSI and ARFI in differentiation of thyroid nodules is not high as a stand-alone diagnostic tool [32]. Thus, the role of imaging in thyroid cancer detection continues to evolve. In this paper, we present the *in vitro* and *in vivo* results of an imaging modality called vibro-acoustography on human thyroid.

Vibro-acoustography (VA) is a methodology based on the dynamic radiation force of ultrasound [33,34]. In this technique, the ultrasound energy is converted into a low-frequency vibration, which in turn produces a sound that is used to construct the image. Hence, a VA image is sensitive not only to the ultrasound properties of the object but also to the dynamic behavior of the object at low frequencies, which means that VA offers information that is not available with conventional ultrasound. We researched and evaluated the use of VA for thyroid imaging. In particular, we focused on studying images of the tissue structures and various lesions in excised thyroid samples as well as human thyroid *in vivo*. The goal of this study was to understand the properties of thyroid images and to pave the way for a larger *in vivo* thyroid imaging study by VA.

Materials and methods

Principles of VA

The VA technique is based on the radiation force of ultrasound, which is a nonlinear phenomenon in acoustic wave propagation [33,34]. The general principle of VA is illustrated in Figure 1.

VA uses two ultrasound beams at slightly different frequencies (f_1 and f_2). The ultrasound energy is transmitted in the form of two tonebursts. The beams are oriented so that they intersect at their mutual focal point. At this point, the two beams mix to produce an ultrasound field with intensity that varies at the difference frequency, Δf, where, $\Delta f = f_2 - f_1$. The ultrasound field produces a radiation force [33,34] on the object at the focus of the combined beams. This force is proportional to the intensity of the ultrasound field; hence, it varies in time at the Δf. As a result, a sound field at the Δf is produced and is detected by the hydrophone. The hydrophone signal represents the object's dynamic response to the force exerted at one point in the object. The hydrophone signal is used to modulate the brightness of a point on the display that corresponds to the position of the focal point on the object. As the ultrasound beams are scanned across the object, the VA image of the object is constructed on the display. Although the image is constructed from a low-frequency signal at Δf, which is often in the kilohertz range, the spatial resolution of the image is determined by the focal spot size, which is typically in submillimeter to millimeter range—a range very suitable for clinical imaging. Figure 1 demonstrates a diagram of the experimental vibro-acoustography system for thyroid imaging.

We note that VA images are in the C-plane, i.e., the plane perpendicular to the ultrasound beam, which is also perpendicular to the B-plane used in B-mode ultrasound imaging. This C-plane is a constant distance from the surface of the transducer. Therefore, VA and B-mode present two perpendicular cross-sections of tissue.

A VA image depicts two types of information about the object. First, the image represents the ultrasonic properties of the object, such as its scattering and power absorption characteristics. These properties are also present in traditional ultrasonography [35]. The second type of information is the dynamic characteristics of the object at the Δf, which describes how the object responds

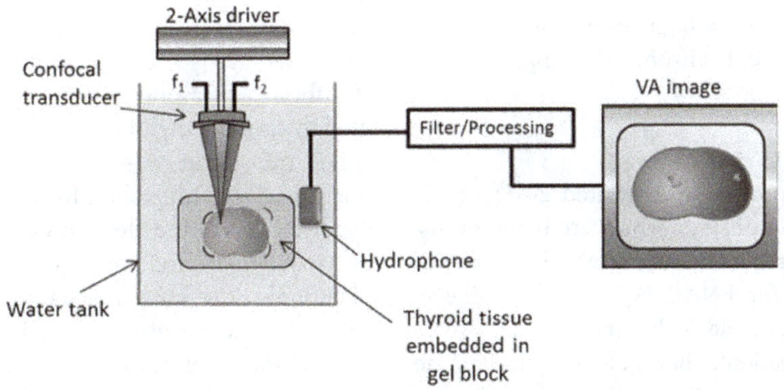

Figure 1 Diagram of the experimental vibro-acoustography system for *in vitro* thyroid imaging. The thyroid sample in the gel block is placed inside a water tank and is then scanned by the dual-beam ultrasound from the confocal transducer focused at the desired depth inside the sample. The difference frequency (Δf) between the two ultrasound beams (f_2 and f_1) is represented as $\Delta f = f_2 - f_1$. The hydrophone receives the acoustic field at the Δf from the sample. This signal is then processed and mapped into an image.

to a vibrating force at low frequencies [35]. This information is not available from conventional ultrasound imaging. Because VA images are formed using the acoustic signal at a low frequency, the resulting images are speckle free, which is an important advantage over traditional ultrasound imaging [36].

VA has been tested in numerous potential clinical applications, including *in vitro* experiments on heart valves [37], *in vitro* human vessels [38], *in vivo* animal arteries [39], breast tissue [40,41], liver tissue [42], bone [43], and, more recently, *in vivo* human breast [44-46]. Recent reports on prostate applications of VA include evaluation of VA for imaging prostate brachytherapy seeds [47] and for monitoring prostate cryotherapy [48]. It should be noted that VA in its present form is not intended for quantitative imaging. Diagnostic information from VA is based on image contrast, which is also the case in most other imaging modalities.

Imaging in vitro thyroid tissues

In an *in vitro* study, after obtaining the approval of the Mayo Clinic Institutional Review Board (IRB) for tissue specimens, experiments were conducted on a number of whole excised human thyroids from autopsy. The specimens were randomly taken and there was no previous knowledge of the presence of nodules inside these thyroid tissues. Tissue samples were fixed in 10% formaldehyde for 1 hour to prevent potential contamination, after which they were thoroughly rinsed in water to remove residual formaldehyde before embedding [42]. Tissues were embedded in a tissue mimicking gel block (~10 x 10 x 3 cm). To make the gel block, gelatin powder (G2500, Sigma-Aldrich, St. Louis, MO) was first dissolved in water in a 60 g/L ratio and heated to 50°C. Once the gelatin was fully dissolved, glycerol (G7757, Sigma-Aldrich, St. Louis, MO) was added at 10% by volume. The solution was then cooled to 42°C and the tissue specimen was placed in the liquid gel. The tissue and liquid were degassed under vacuum to remove air from both the tissue and liquid. After degassing, the liquid and tissue specimen were carefully poured into a square mold and refrigerated overnight before scanning.

The VA experiment was conducted in a water tank; the diagram of the experimental VA for *in vitro* imaging is shown in Figure 1, where the tissue is scanned by a dual-beam confocal ultrasound transducer focused at the desired depth inside the sample. VA images were acquired from each specimen. VA images, 50 × 50 mm, were acquired at several Δf frequencies normally ranging over 30–90 kHz. In addition to performing VA with tonebursts of length 100 μs, we also used two intersecting continuous wave (CW) focused ultrasound beams of different frequencies to generate a localized oscillatory stress field for imaging. Figure 2 shows a photograph of an excised thyroid embedded in a gel block

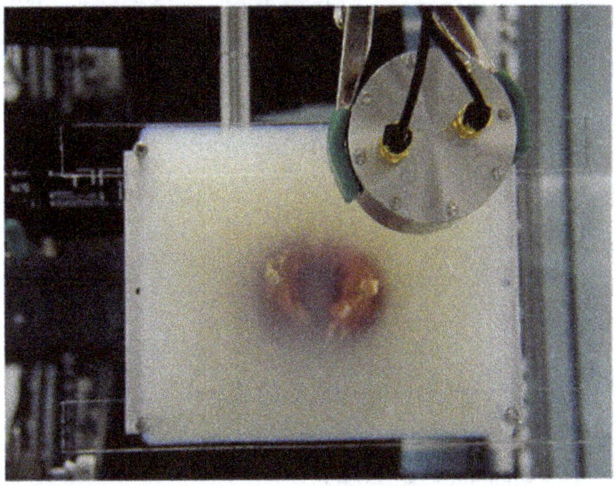

Figure 2 Experimental setup for *in vitro* thyroid imaging by vibro-acoustography. The excised thyroid is embedded in a gel block.

being scanned by a dual-beam confocal transducer. Specimens were also imaged with a high-resolution specimen radiography machine (M50; Faxitron, Wheeling, IL), dedicated for research.

Imaging human thyroid in vivo

After obtaining IRB approval, we recruited 24 (10 male and 14 female) patient volunteers, who were being evaluated for thyroid nodularity and were referred to the Department of Radiology for FNAB. Ages of the subjects ranged from 37 to 82 years old with a mean of 57.8 years old. Normally, these patients have already undergone diagnostic ultrasound examinations. Because the biopsy needle may alter tissue characteristics, VA was performed before FNAB to avoid these possible errors. B-mode ultrasound and VA images of thyroid were obtained from 20 patients. The patient had his/her clinical FNAB after this step as part of his or her health care. The nodule or nodules selected for FNAs were marked as a region of interest on thyroid ultrasound by our radiologist (C.C.R.), which later was used for VA nodule detection. The results of biopsy were analyzed and evaluated by a pathologist.

The diagram of the dual modality system for *in vivo* VA and B-mode imaging is shown in Figure 3. For B/C-mode and VA imaging we used a modified General Electric ultrasound scanner (Vivid 7, GE Healthcare Ultrasound Cardiology, Horton, Norway), which was described by Urban, *et al.* [49] A linear array transducer (7 L, GE Healthcare Ultrasound Cardiology, Horton, Norway) was used to scan the thyroid.

The transducer was mounted on a linear translation stage that was controlled by an external PC. The transducer moved in the elevation direction of the transducer to acquire B-mode images at consecutive parallel planes; also the same mechanism is used to acquire VA data from consecutive parallel lines of the VA image. The C-mode images are formed by summing the backscattered ultrasound signal from the B-mode images using a window that was centered at a specified depth and had a length of 2.5 mm.

For VA, the scanner produced two ultrasound beams with different frequencies both focused at a joint focal point. Electronic focusing delays are used to focus at different focal depths. The two beams were electronically steered together across the object along the length of the array (also called azimuthal direction). Comparing to the system used for *in vitro* experiments, the steering function of the array probe along the azimuthal direction replaces the similar scanning motion that was performed for the *in vitro* VA imaging by mechanical means. The ultrasound frequencies were around 3 MHz and Δf was

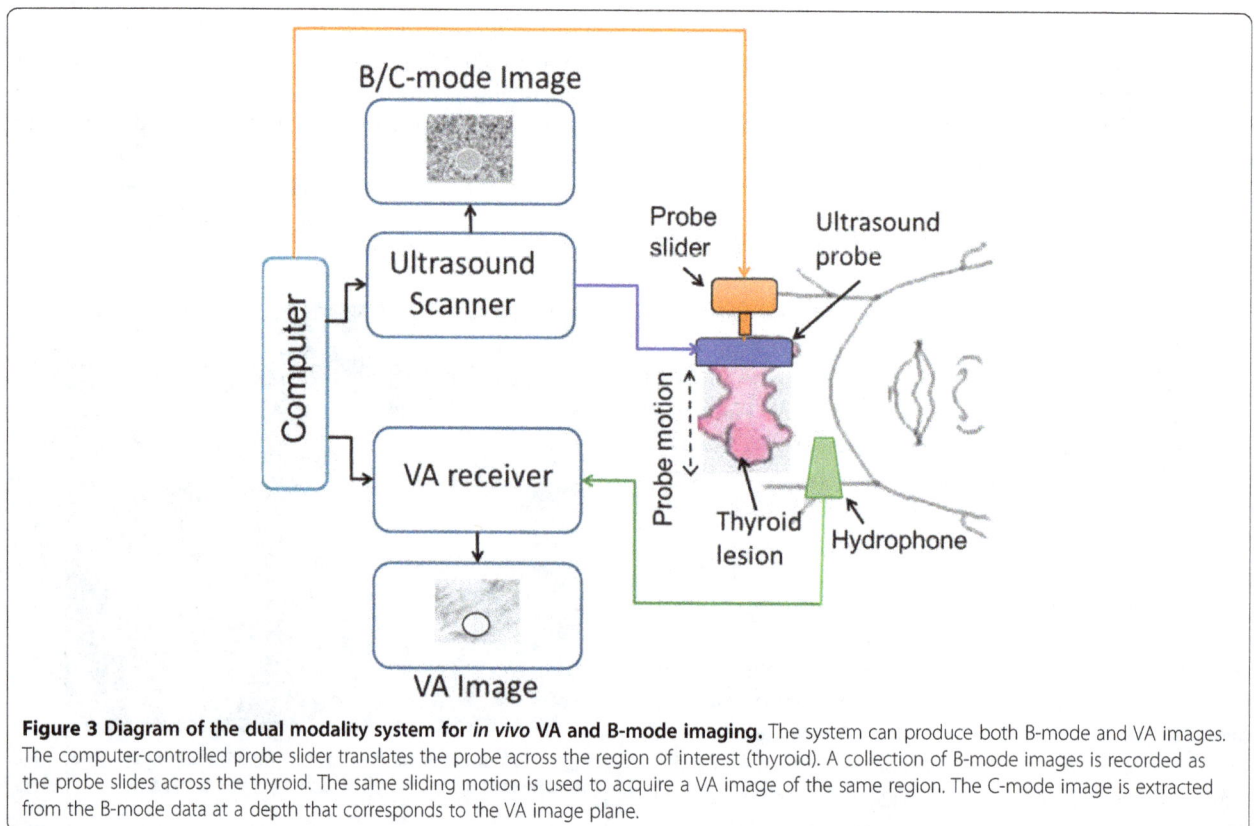

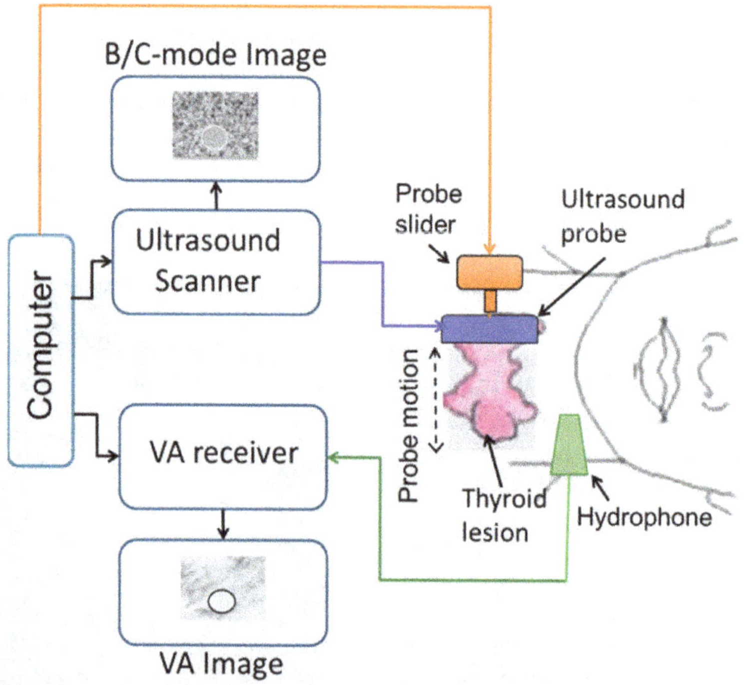

Figure 3 Diagram of the dual modality system for *in vivo* VA and B-mode imaging. The system can produce both B-mode and VA images. The computer-controlled probe slider translates the probe across the region of interest (thyroid). A collection of B-mode images is recorded as the probe slides across the thyroid. The same sliding motion is used to acquire a VA image of the same region. The C-mode image is extracted from the B-mode data at a depth that corresponds to the VA image plane.

around 50 kHz. In most cases, the ultrasound beams had frequencies $f_1 = 3.64$ MHz and $f_2 = 3.58$ MHz making $\Delta f = 54$ kHz. The beams were constructed using an aperture with 64 elements which were assigned a signal with frequency f_1 adjacent to a group of 64 elements, which were assigned a signal with frequency f_2. This aperture was translated across the transducer array as described by Urban, *et al.* [49].

The hydrophone was placed on the neck of the subject and the acoustic emission signal was recorded during the VA scanning procedure. Multiple planes in depth were investigated during each scanning session. All the VA images were 50 × 47 mm.

Results

In vitro study results

To optimize the VA system for *in vivo* human studies, we initially tested the system on 20 excised human whole thyroid tissues. Vibro-acoustography images of excised thyroids displayed calcifications and nodules. Thyroid nodules and cysts were detectable. Image contrast was significantly higher than ultrasound images. The VA appearance of a normal excised human thyroid tissue with no nodules is seen in Figure 4. In Figure 5, a large calcification, about 2.5 mm in diameter, is seen in VA and US images of an excised human thyroid from a cadaver.

X-ray, C-mode US and VA images of an excised thyroid tissue are shown in Figure 6. Three lesions, one of which is calcified, are seen in all VA images. In the X-ray image only the calcified lesion is seen, but the other two are not visible. In the C-mode ultrasound image (tissue was cut in 2 pieces) the nodules can be seen. In general, image contrast in the VA images was substantially higher than that in the ultrasound images in VA tissue experiments.

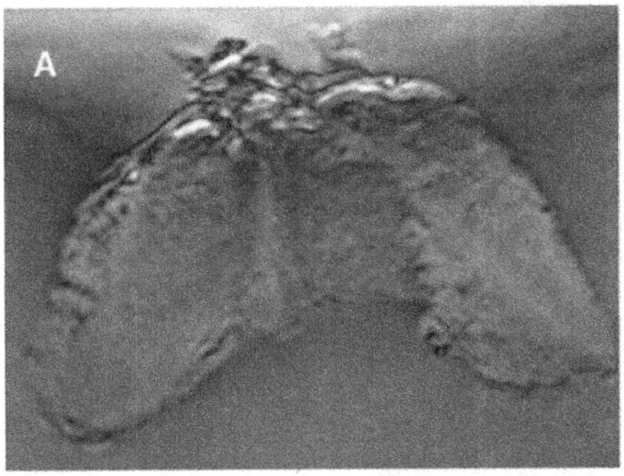

Figure 4 VA image of an excised human healthy thyroid tissue. The image size is 55 × 75 mm. The image is taken at 6 mm depth and shows normal thyroid tissue structure with no nodule and calcifications.

In the *in vitro* study, we assessed the appearance of calcifications (CAs) and nodules in vibro-acoustography by classifying each image into one of these three categories: (A) Positive (clearly identified calcifications at locations indicated in the corresponding X-ray image or nodules at the locations indicated in the corresponding C-mode US); (B) Suspicious (image showed some indication of calcifications that could not be clearly differentiated from the background tissue and in case of nodules the border was not clearly defined); and (C) Negative (no calcification could be distinguished at locations indicated in the corresponding X-ray image and no nodules could be distinguished at locations indicated in the corresponding C-mode US image).

VA was able to detect all (3/3) of X-ray proven calcifications and all (2/2) of ultrasound proven nodules within thyroid tissues (Table 1). The measurements of the top right calcified nodule were 8.8 mm × 7.9 mm in X-ray; 7.9 mm × 7.2 mm in C-mode; and 10.3 mm × 8.7 mm in VA images. Since the goal of this *in vitro* study was to optimize the system for our *in vivo* imaging, tissue samples were randomly chosen from human cadavers regardless of pathology.

In vivo study results

We performed thyroid VA and US imaging on 24 adult patients on one side and on two lobes in one patient. All the VA scans were 50 × 47 mm. The results from six patients are shown in Figures 7, 8, 9, 10, 11, 12.

Ultrasound data are depicted in B-mode and C-mode. C-mode image plane corresponds to VA image plane, where this plane is perpendicular to the B-mode image plane. To clarify image orientation, we use a three-axis Cartesian coordinate system of x, y, and z, where x represents the scan direction in B-mode image (also known as azimuth direction), y represents the probe motion (also known as elevation direction), and z representing the depth. Ultrasound B-mode images are presented in the x-z plane, while C-mode and VA images are in the x-y plane.

Figure 7 demonstrates US and VA images of the left thyroid lobe of a 48-year-old female patient with a benign thyroid nodule. B-mode ultrasound identifies a large nodule measuring about 47 × 27 mm (x-z dimensions) with small cystic appearance. The nodule appears on C-mode US, taken at 2 cm depth, measuring about 44.2 mm × 30.5 mm (x-y dimensions). The VA image taken at 2.0 cm depth identifies the large nodule with distinct margin measuring about 30.5 mm in the y-direction and more than 47 mm in the x-direction, with its side margins extending out of VA image window. Its shape and location correlates to the US C-scan at 2 cm depth. Note that the resolution cell of the VA system in the depth direction was around 2–3 mm, which is similar to that of C-mode images.

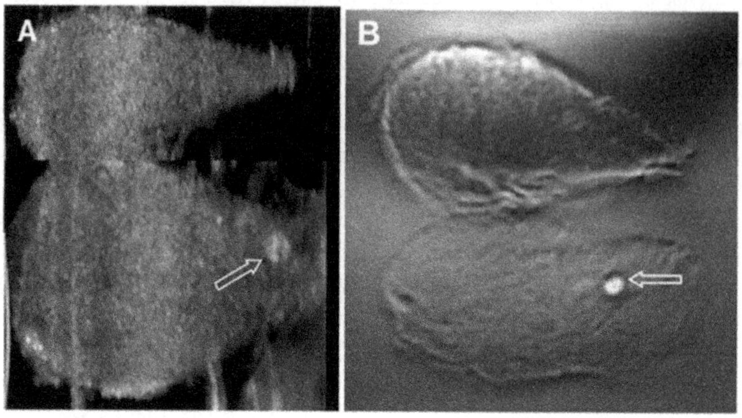

Figure 5 Excised Human Thyroid. A) C-mode ultrasound of an excised human thyroid from a cadaver, **B**) VA image of this tissue in 60 × 60 mm scan dimension. The arrow shows a 2.5 x 2.5 mm calcification in VA image with more contrast than shown in the US image.

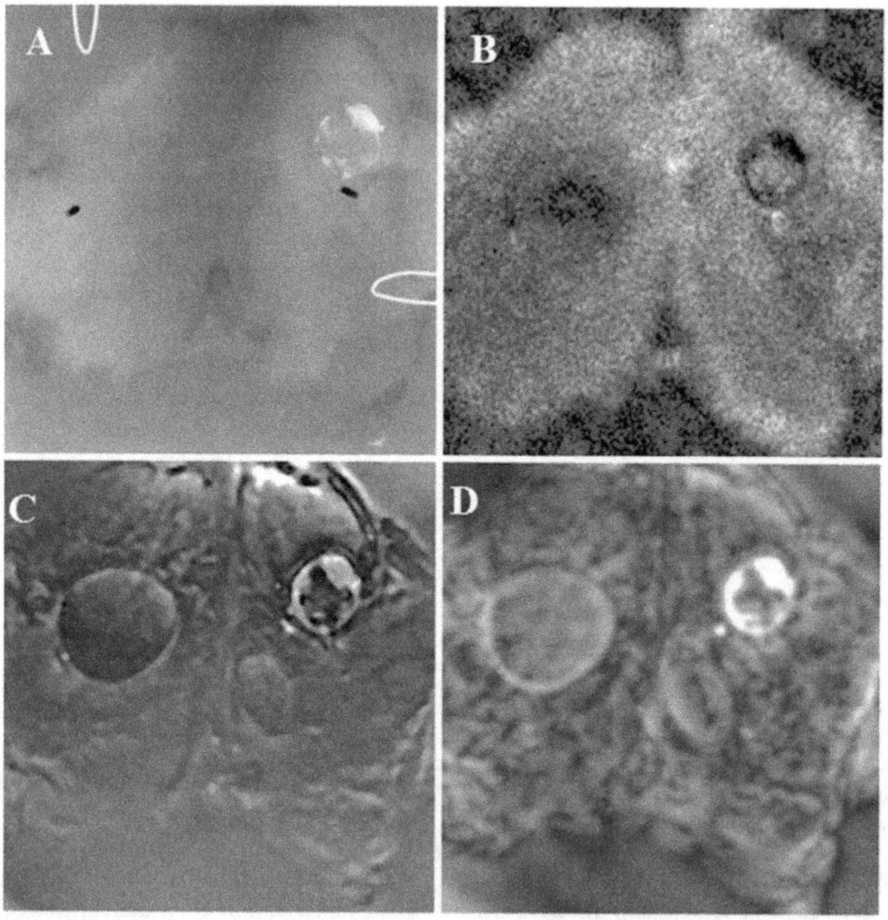

Figure 6 Excised Human Thyroid. A) X-ray of an excised thyroid tissue from cadaver; **B**) US C-scan of the same tissue at 5 MHz; **C**) VA image using toneburst excitation with $\Delta f = 50$ kHz. The image is 50 × 50 mm. **D**) VA image using CW excitation with $\Delta f = 16.3$ kHz. VA images were taken in water tank. All VA images are 50 × 50 mm.

Table 1 Summary of VA experimental results on 20 *ex vivo* thyroid samples

	Positive	Suspicious	Negative
Presence of X-ray proven calcification in VA	3/3	0	0
Presence of ultrasound proven Nodules in VA	2/2	0	0

Figure 8 demonstrates US and VA images of a 71 year old man with a nodule on the left side of his thyroid. The nodule on B-mode US measures about 29 × 42 × 40 mm. On the VA scan at 1.75 cm depth, the nodule appears larger and almost covers most of the scan image with little normal tissue around, as denoted by arrows. It should be noted that the VA scan depth was set to be where the largest dimension of the nodule was observed in the B-mode US image. The histology of the nodule revealed benign appearance with degenerative changes.

Figure 9 demonstrates US and VA images of the left side of the thyroid of a 56 year old female with a benign adenoma. The nodule appears on B-mode and C-mode US, taken at a depth of 1.25 cm, as an isoechoic nodule protruding from the lower pole of the left thyroid lobe measuring 12.5 mm × 12.0 mm in C-mode. The VA scan at 2.25 cm depth identifies the nodule at the same location seen in C-mode US but larger, measuring about 11.6 × 23.8 mm.

Figure 10 demonstrates US and VA images of the right side thyroid of 37 year old male with papillary thyroid carcinoma. On B-mode US, a cystic nodule appears measuring about 1.0 × 1.3 × 1.4 cm in the upper right lobe of the thyroid with peripheral calcifications, characteristic of a papillary carcinoma. The VA scan at 2.5 cm depth identifies the nodule with a cystic appearance and slightly larger dimensions plus some peripheral calcifications, denoted by arrows, with greater clarity than shown in the US image. It is difficult to measure the size of the nodule in both the US and VA images reliably due to indistinct margins.

Figure 11 presents US and VA images of a 41-year-old woman with a thyroid nodule in the left lobe. On B-mode US, two nodules appear, a cystic nodule measuring 2.6 × 2.9 × 3.7 cm and an almost solid nodule about 2.1 cm in greatest dimension with the coarse calcifications in the inferior left lobe. The VA scan with the array probe at 2 cm depth identifies the ill-defined nodules denoted by the circle. The VA scan is taken at the largest dimension of nodule of its B-mode image. For this reason, the nodule appears larger and covered most of the image. Coarse calcifications appear on the VA image with greater clarity as shown by arrows. The VA and US appearance were suggestive for malignancy and the pathology of FNA sample from the inferior left thyroid nodule containing coarse calcifications revealed papillary thyroid carcinoma.

Figure 12 demonstrates US and VA images of the left side thyroid of an 82-year-old male patient with benign thyroid nodule with degenerative changes. In the inferior aspect of the left thyroid lobe there is an oval well defined heterogeneously echogenic nodule that measures 2.0 × 1.5 × 1.5 cm on B-mode ultrasound. The VA scan at 2.0 cm depth identifies the nodule slightly larger, as denoted by circle.

To assess the appearance of clinical ultrasound proven nodules and CAs in B-mode and or C- mode, we classified each B/ C-mode image into one of the following

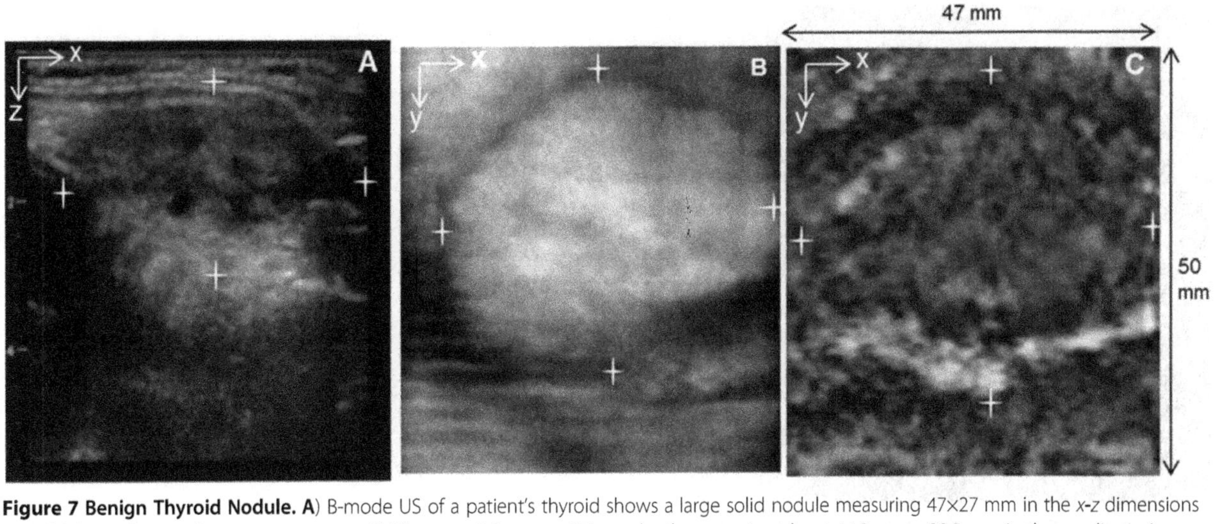

Figure 7 Benign Thyroid Nodule. A) B-mode US of a patient's thyroid shows a large solid nodule measuring 47×27 mm in the *x-z* dimensions on left lobe with a small cystic component, **B**) Ultrasound C-scan at 2.0 cm depth measuring about 44.2 mm x 30.5 mm in the x-y dimensions, and **C**) *In vivo* VA image of thyroid (with 7 L array probe, f_1 = 3.64 MHz and Δf = 54.27 kHz) at 2.0 cm depth which correlates to the one of C-scan plane, measuring more than 47 mm in the *x*-direction and 30.5 mm in the *y*-direction and the star shows the dimensions. The VA image is 47 ×50 mm.

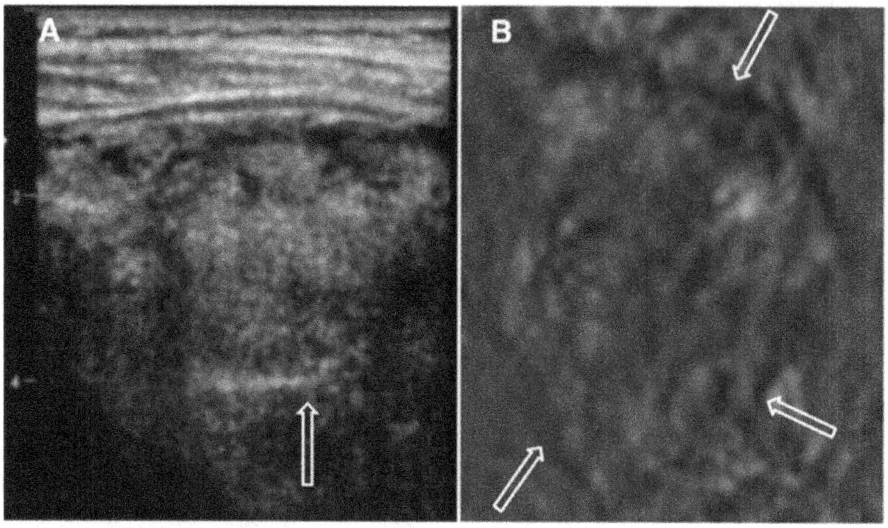

Figure 8 Benign Thyroid Nodule with Degenerative Changes. A) B-mode US of 71 year old patient's thyroid on left side. The arrow points to a nodule measuring 2.9 × 4.2 × 4.0 cm, **B**) VA image at 2.25 cm depth, the arrows point a large nodule covering most of image. The pathology result was a benign nodule with degenerative changes. The VA image is 47 × 50 mm. Orientations of the images are similar to those as Figure 7.

categories: A) Good (nodules and CAs were clearly seen at locations indicated in the corresponding clinical US, B) Fair (image showed some indication of calcifications that could not be clearly differentiated from the background tissue and in case of nodules part of the border could not be identified. C) Inconclusive (no calcification and nodules could be distinguished at locations indicated in the corresponding clinical US). The same classification criteria were used for presence of CAs and nodules in VA images were compared to the corresponding B/C mode US.

In summary, as shown in Table 2, VA was able to detect 20 nodules out of 22 nodules that were detected in the corresponding B/C-mode images, where 12 images were classified as Good and 8 were classified as Fair, because VA images were affected by some types of artifacts but the lesion was still detectable. In 2 cases the VA image was classified as inconclusive.

VA was able to detect the US-detected calcifications (CAs) with greater clarity though they appeared larger than in US. In a number of experiments, some levels of either system artifact or body motion artifact, mainly

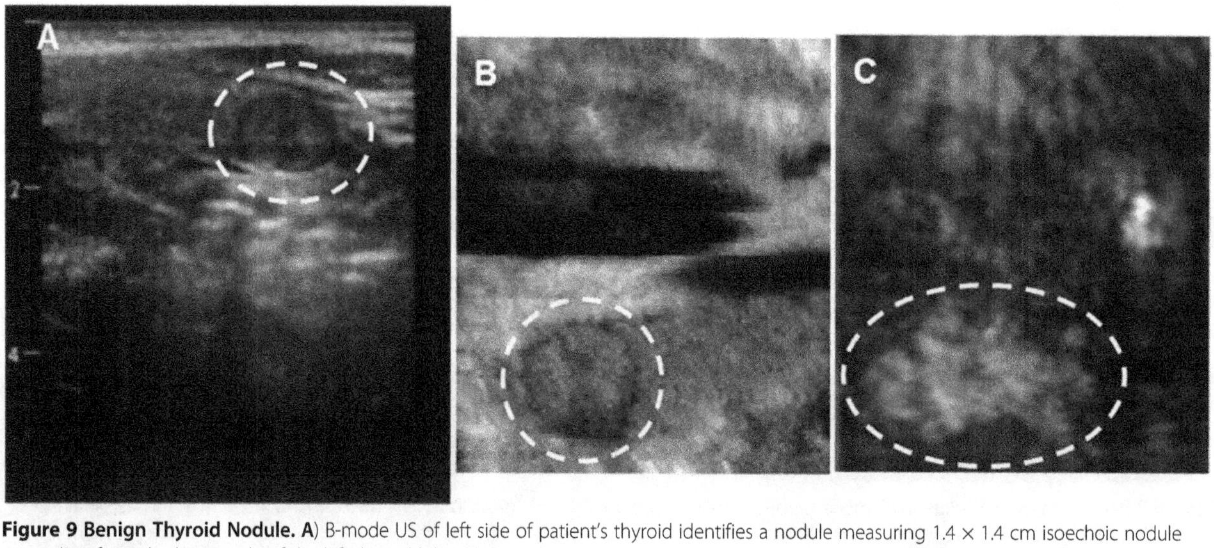

Figure 9 Benign Thyroid Nodule. A) B-mode US of left side of patient's thyroid identifies a nodule measuring 1.4 × 1.4 cm isoechoic nodule protruding from the lower pole of the left thyroid lobe, **B**) C-mode US at 2.25 cm depth shows the nodule, **C**) VA scan at 2.25 cm depth shows nodule at the same location as seen in C-mode but larger, measuring about 1.0 × 1.5 × 3.4 cm. Orientations of the images are similar to those as Figure 7.

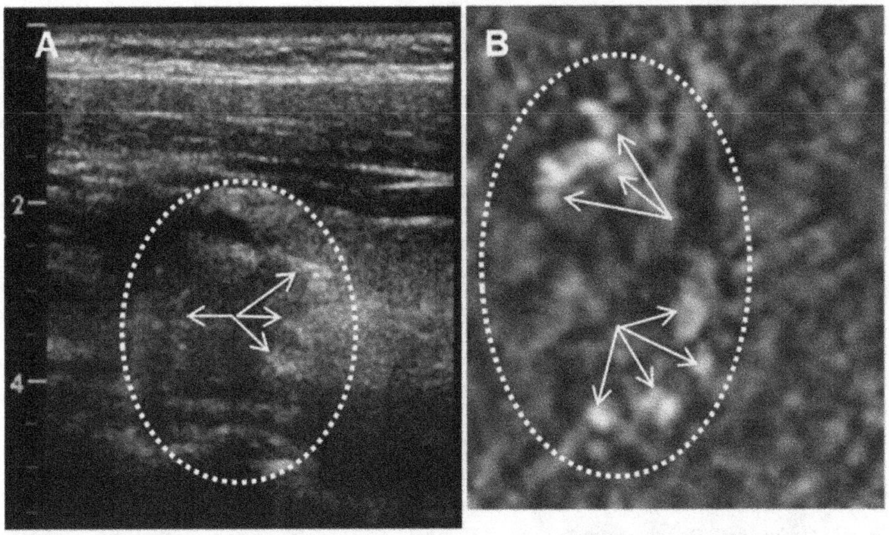

Figure 10 Papillary Thyroid Cancer. A) B-mode US shows a cystic nodule measuring 1.0 × 1.3 × 1.4 cm in the upper right lobe of the thyroid with peripheral calcifications as denoted by arrows. VA scan at 2.5 cm depth shows the nodule with cystic appearance slightly larger dimensions plus some coarse peripheral calcifications. Orientations of the images are similar to those as Figure 7.

due to breathing, were present. In two cases the artifacts were dominant and masked the nodules. The pathology revealed papillary thyroid carcinoma in two cases of VA-detected nodules and the rest were benign. The two papillary carcinomas had pathology-proven calcifications that could be seen in US as well as VA images.

Discussion

In the *in vitro* study, the VA images could visualize normal tissue structures and lesions free of the speckle associated with conventional B-mode ultrasound as demonstrated in Figures 4, 5 and 6. Figure 6 demonstrates that the X-ray was only sensitive to one of the lesions that were present and US revealed two nodules with no apparent calcifications, whereas the VA images could detect all three nodules and calcifications in the thyroid tissue. Additionally, the contrast and the edge detail were enhanced in the VA images as compared to the US images. It should be noted that, VA in the present form is not intended as a quantitative imaging. Similar to most other medical imaging modalities, diagnostic information in VA is based on image contrast.

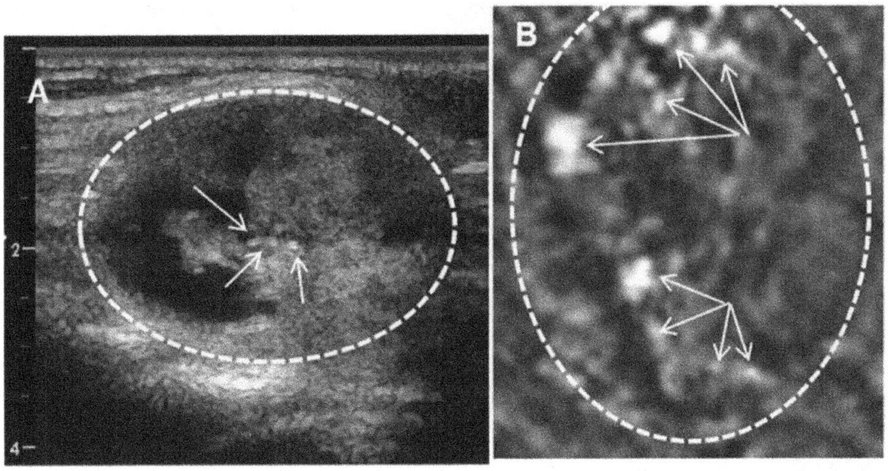

Figure 11 Papillary Thyroid Cancer. A) B-mode US shows a cystic nodule measuring 2.6 cm × 2.9 cm × 3.7 cm and a solid nodule about 2.1 cm in greatest dimension with peripheral coarse calcifications in the inferior left lobe. **B**) VA scan with array probe at 2.0 cm depth shows the ill-defined nodules, and partial cystic appearance. The VA scan is taken at the largest diameter of nodule of shown at B-mode and appears larger covering most of the image, (shown by circle) with arrows pointing to the calcifications. Orientations of the images are similar to those as Figure 7.

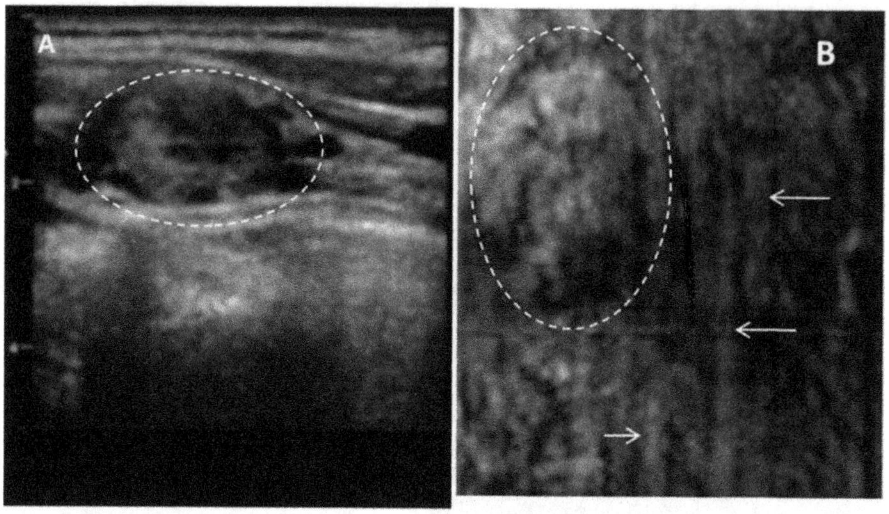

Figure 12 Benign Thyroid Nodule with Degenerative Changes. (**A**) B-mode US of left lobe of a patient's thyroid, circle points to an oval nodule measures 2.0 cm × 1.5 cm × 1.5 cm and (**B**) VA image at 2 cm depth (with 7 L array probe, f_1 = 3.64 MHz and Δf = 54.27 kHz) show a large nodule in a human thyroid marked by circle. The vertical bands marked by the arrows are system artifacts. The pathology analysis revealed that this was a benign nodule. Orientations of the images are similar to those as Figure 7.

It is important to note that formaldehyde can significantly change tissue properties; particularly it increases tissue stiffness. However, we also note that the study on excised tissue will have the benefit of providing valuable information and allowing us to optimize our system before moving to *in vivo* studies. Although short term fixing with formaldehyde somewhat alters the stiffness of the thyroid tissue, such changes affect both healthy and diseased areas. Hence, tissue fixation should not have a major effect on the capability of VA imaging to detect a contrast between normal and diseased tissue [42].

The confocal transducer used in this study was mechanically scanned in a water tank for the *in vitro* portion of this study. With this experimental setup the scan time could take 6–8 minutes. In order to translate this method for clinical use and improve the scan times, the modified scanner equipped with the linear array was used for the *in vivo* study. This system acquires images of similar size in about 2 minutes. It should be noted since the beamforming technique used for *in vivo* imaging is significantly different from that used for in vitro imaging; the resulting image quality is not the same. One reason for such difference is the fact that the confocal transducer used in the *in vitro* experiments has a large circular aperture that is capable of producing high-resolution images with symmetric resolution cells. Such images are typically smooth and clear. The beamforming with linear array used for the *in vivo* study has a much smaller aperture thus resulting in lower resolution images and non-symmetric resolution cell. This is a limitation of the ultrasound scanner – not the VA technique – because the ultrasound scanner can only support linear (rectangular) arrays with relatively small apertures.

Table 2 Results summary of 24 *in vivo* thyroid VA experiments

	Detctable	Inconclusive
Appearance of nodules by B-mode	22/24	2/24
Appearance of B-mode US proven nodules in VA	20/22	2/22
Appearance of Calcifications on B-mode	2	4/6
Appearance of Calcifications in VA	6	0/6
	Malignant PTC	**Benign nodules**
Histology of 20 VA detected nodules	2	18

The results from the *in vivo* study show that nodules could be detected by in the VA images and the edges could be defined. Size of nodules appeared larger in most of VA images than in the corresponding B-mode and C-mode images. The difference may be attributed to the fact that the information content of VA and B-mode are different; that is, VA is sensitive to properties of tissue at ultrasound as well as low (Δf) frequencies, whereas B-mode and C-mode images are sensitive only to the ultrasound properties of tissue. VA was able to detect all the calcifications, in the form of micro- and coarse calcifications, within the nodules with greater clarity than those of seen in US. The histology of nodules proved the presence of calcifications including in two papillary carcinomas. It is known that the presence of calcification within solitary thyroid nodule is highly associated with thyroid malignancy [50-54]. VA is sensitive to calcifications and to our experience [37,41,45,46], it shows calcifications better than ultrasound. In US calcifications are often detected by their shadow, but in VA we can directly see and identify calcifications.

There were a few difficulties that were encountered in the *in vivo* study. First, we have identified a system artifact associated with steering the VA beams across the aperture which creates streaks in the resulting image. These types of artifacts were observed in Figure 12B as marked by arrows. We have developed an algorithm to correct for these streaks [49], but this algorithm can, in some instances, diminish image details and we are working on alternatives to correct this artifact.

Additionally, during the *in vivo* scanning, there is an artifact associated with motion due to patient breathing. This breathing artifact is manifested as jagged image details. A mild case of this artifact is shown in Figure 7C with jagged edges in the horizontal direction when comparing adjacent vertical rows. When the patient breathes, the thyroid can move in and out of the VA focal plane, so the same tissue is not necessarily excited. Because the scan takes about 2 minutes, we could not ask the subject to simply hold their breath. We did ask the patient to breath shallowly to avoid large excursions. We also placed the transducer on a spring mounted assembly so that the transducer would move with the patient during breathing as well as conform to the neck of the subject. Another limitation of this study is the limited sample size. It should be noted that the goal of this paper is to report the results of a pilot study conducted on a small number of thyroids and provide the basis for future studies. We did not intend or claim to have sufficient number of samples for a complete statistical analysis. For this reason we have not presented a sample size calculation. Results of this study may be used to determine the sample size for future studies. A larger study would provide a more accurate assessment of the sensitivity and specificity of thyroid nodule detection by VA. Results of this paper suggest that VA may be used as an additional thyroid imaging tool, however, this method is not meant to replace B-mode US or FNAB at present time.

Conclusion

Herein, we have reported on our examination of the use of VA for *in vitro* and *in vivo* imaging of the thyroid. This study was a prerequisite for a larger population of thyroid patients. Our experiments on excised and *in vivo* thyroids demonstrate the capability of VA for the detection of thyroid nodules and calcifications. These results suggest that VA may be a useful clinical tool in thyroid imaging; however, at present VA is not intended to replace B-mode US or FNAB. In conclusion, our pilot study has shown that thyroid vibro-acoustography is feasible. However, larger studies are needed to determine sensitivity and specificity of this imaging tool in thyroid cancer detection and differentiation.

Consent section

Written informed consent was obtained from the patient(s) for publication of this manuscript and accompanying images.

Abbreviations

f_1: frequency 1; f_2: frequency 2; VA: Vibro-acoustography; Δf: Difference frequency; MRI: Magnetic resonance imaging/image; US: Ultrasonographic, ultrasonography, ultrasound; VA: Vibro-acoustography; PTC: Papillary thyroid carcinoma.

Competing interests

Disclosure: Drs Greenleaf, Fatemi, and Alizad disclose Mayo Clinic's patents on the vibro-acoustography technology (discussed in this manuscript) as a potential financial conflict of interest.

Authors' contributions

AA: conducting human study, writing most of the manuscript. MWU: image processing, writing some of discussion section, manuscript editing. JCM: patient selection, image interpretation, manuscript editing. CCR: patient selection, image interpretation manuscript editing, RRK: system technician, operating the vibro-acoustography system, some of method section. JFG: technique development, vibro-acoustography system design, manuscript editing. MF: technique development, vibro-acoustography system design, writing the technical section of the paper, supervising data acquisition and signal processing. All authors read and approved the final manuscript.

Acknowledgments

The authors acknowledge Thomas M. Kinter for software support. This described study was supported by Grant Number: 2–2008 from AIUM-EER.

Disclosure of conflict of interest

Some of the authors (Greenleaf and Fatemi) and Mayo Clinic have financial interests associated with the technology used in this research and that technology has been licensed in part to industry.

Author details

[1]Department of Physiology and Biomedical Engineering, Mayo Clinic, 200 First Street SW, Rochester, MN 55905, USA. [2]Department of Internal Medicine, Mayo Clinic, 200 First Street SW, Rochester, MN 55905, USA. [3]Division of Endocrinology, Department of Internal Medicine, Mayo Clinic, 200 First Street SW, Rochester, MN 55905, USA. [4]Department of Radiology, Mayo Clinic, 200 First Street SW, Rochester, MN 55905, USA.

References

1. Davies LWH: **Increasing incidence of thyroid cancer in the united states, 1973–2002.** *JAMA* 2006, **295**(18):2164–2167.
2. Papini E, Guglielmi R, Bianchini A, Crescenzi A, Taccogna S, Nardi F, Panunzi C, Rinaldi R, Toscano V, Pacella CM: **Risk of malignancy in nonpalpable thyroid nodules: Predictive value of ultrasound and color-Doppler features.** *J ClinEndocrinol Metab* 2002, **87**(5):1941–1946.
3. Castro MR, Gharib H: **Continuing controversies in the management of thyroid nodules.** *Ann Intern Med* 2005, **142**(11):926–931.
4. Gharib H, Goellner JR: **Fine-needle aspiration biopsy of the thyroid: an appraisal.** *Ann Intern Med* 1993, **118**(4):282–289.
5. Burch HB, Burman KD, Reed HL, Buckner L, Raber T, Ownbey JL: **Fine needle aspiration of thyroid nodules. Determinants of insufficiency rate and malignancy yield at thyroidectomy.** *Acta Cytol* 1996, 40(6):1176–1183.

6. Goellner: *Fine needle aspiration of the thyroid gland.* Philadelphia: Lippincott-Raven Publishers; 1996.
7. Alexander EK: **Approach to the patient with a cytologically indeterminate thyroid nodule.** *J Clin Endocrinol Metab* 2008, **93**(11):4175–4182.
8. Raab SS, Vrbin CM, Grzybicki DM, Sudilovsky D, Balassanian R, Zarbo RJ, Meier FA: **Errors in thyroid gland fine-needle aspiration.** *Am J Clin Pathol* 2006, **125**(6):873–882.
9. Hopkins CR, Reading CC: **Thyroid and parathyroid imaging.** *Seminars in Ultrasound, CT and MRI* 1995, **16**(4):279–295.
10. Imanishi Y, Ehara N, Mori J, Shimokawa M, Sakuyama K, Ishikawa T, Shinagawa T, Hirose C, Tsujino D: **Measurement of thyroid iodine by CT.** *J Comput Assist Tomogr* 1991, **15**(2):287–290.
11. Haas S, Trujillo A, Kunstle J: **Fine needle aspiration of thyroid nodules in a rural setting.** *Am J Med* 1993, **94**(4):357–361.
12. Cap J, Ryska A, Rehorkova P, Hovorkova E, Kerekes Z, Pohnetalova D: **Sensitivity and specificity of the fine needle aspiration biopsy of the thyroid: clinical point of view.** *Clin Endocrinol (Oxf)* 1999, **51**(4):509–515.
13. Bahn MM, Brennan MD, Bahn RS, Dean DS, Kugel JL, Ehman RL: **Development and application of magnetic resonance elastography of the normal and pathological thyroid gland in vivo.** *J Magn Reson Imaging* 2009, **30**(5):1151–1154.
14. Lyshchik A, Higashi T, Asato R, Tanaka S, Ito J, Hiraoka M, Brill AB, Saga T, Togashi K: **Elastic moduli of thyroid tissues under compression.** *Ultrason Imaging* 2005, **27**(2):101–110.
15. Rago T, Santini F, Scutari M, Pinchera A, Vitti P: **Elastography: new developments in ultrasound for predicting malignancy in thyroid nodules.** *J Clin Endocrinol Metab* 2007, **92**(8):2917–2922.
16. Lyshchik A, Higashi T, Asato R, Tanaka S, Ito J, Mai JJ, Pellot-Barakat C, Insana MF, Brill AB, Saga T, *et al*: **Thyroid gland tumor diagnosis at US elastography.** *Radiology* 2005, **237**(1):202–211.
17. Bojunga J, Herrmann E, Meyer G, Weber S, Zeuzem S, Friedrich-Rust M: **Real-time elastography for the differentiation of benign and malignant thyroid nodules: a meta-analysis.** *Thyroid* 2010, **20**(10):1145–1150.
18. Xing P, Wu L, Zhang C, Li S, Liu C, Wu C: **Differentiation of Benign From Malignant Thyroid Lesions Calculation of the Strain Ratio on Thyroid Sonoelastography.** *J Ultrasound Med* 2011, **30**(5):663–669.
19. Hong Y, Liu X, Li Z, Zhang X, Chen M, Luo Z: **Real-time ultrasound elastography in the differential diagnosis of benign and malignant thyroid nodules.** *J Ultrasound Med* 2009, **28**(7):861–867.
20. Bae U, Dighe M, Dubinsky T, Minoshima S, Shamdasani V, Kim Y: **Ultrasound thyroid elastography using carotid artery pulsation: preliminary study.** *J Ultrasound Med* 2007, **26**(6):797–805.
21. Dighe M, Bae U, Richardson ML, Dubinsky TJ, Minoshima S, Kim Y: **Differential diagnosis of thyroid nodules with US elastography using carotid artery pulsation.** *Radiology* 2008, **248**(2):662–669.
22. Ragazzoni F, Deandrea M, Mormile A, Ramunni MJ, Garino F, Magliona G, Motta M, Torchio B, Garberoglio R, Limone P: **High Diagnostic Accuracy and Interobserver Reliability of Real-Time Elastography in the Evaluation of Thyroid Nodules.** *Ultrasound Med Biol* 2012.
23. Lippolis PV, Tognini S, Materazzi G, Polini A, Mancini R, Ambrosini CE, Dardano A, Basolo F, Seccia M, Miccoli P, *et al*: **Is elastography actually useful in the presurgical selection of thyroid nodules with indeterminate cytology?** *J Clin Endocrinol Metab* 2011, **96**(11):E1826–1830.
24. Friedrich-Rust M, Romenski O, Meyer G, Dauth N, Holzer K, Grünwald F, Kriener S, Herrmann E, Zeuzem S, Bojunga J: **Acoustic Radiation Force Impulse-Imaging for the evaluation of the thyroid gland: a limited patient feasibility study.** *Ultrasonics* 2012, **52**(1):69–74.
25. Bojunga J, Dauth N, Berner C, Meyer G, Holzer K, Voelkl L, Herrmann E, Schroeter H, Zeuzem S, Friedrich-Rust M: **Acoustic radiation force impulse imaging for differentiation of thyroid nodules.** *PLoS One* 2012, **7**(8):e42735.
26. Gu J, Du L, Bai M, Chen H, Jia X, Zhao J, Zhang X: **Preliminary Study on the Diagnostic Value of Acoustic Radiation Force Impulse Technology for Differentiating Between Benign and Malignant Thyroid Nodules.** *Jl Ultrasound Med* 2012, **31**(5):763–771.
27. Sebag F, Vaillant-Lombard J, Berbis J, Griset V, Henry J, Petit P, Oliver C: **Shear wave elastography: a new ultrasound imaging mode for the differential diagnosis of benign and malignant thyroid nodules.** *J Clin EndocrinolMetab* 2010, **95**(12):5281–5288.
28. Ruchala M, Szczepanek-Parulska E, Zybek A, Moczko J, Czarnywojtek A, Kaminski G, Sowinski J: **The role of sonoelastography in acute, subacute and chronic thyroiditis: a novel application of the method.** *Eur J Endocrinol* 2012, **166**(3):425–432.
29. Bercoff J, Tanter M, Fink M: **Supersonic shear imaging: a new technique for soft tissue elasticity mapping.** *IEEE Trans Ultrason Ferroelectr Freq Control* 2004, **51**(4):396–409.
30. Arda K, Ciledag N, Aktas E, Aribas BK, Kose K: **Quantitative assessment of normal soft-tissue elasticity using shear-wave ultrasound elastography.** *Am J Roentgenol* 2011, **197**(3):532–536.
31. Slapa RZ, Piwowonski A, Jakubowski WS, Bierca J, Szopinski KT, Slowinska-Srzednicka J, Migda B, Mlosek RK: **Shear Wave Elastography May Add a New Dimension to Ultrasound Evaluation of Thyroid Nodules: Case Series with Comparative Evaluation.** *J Thyroid Res* 2012.
32. Sebag F, Vaillant-Lombard J, Berbis J, Griset V, Henry JF, Petit P, Oliver C: **Shear wave elastography: a new ultrasound imaging mode for the differential diagnosis of benign and malignant thyroid nodules.** *J Clin Endocrinol Metab* 2010, **95**(12):5281–5288.
33. Fatemi M, Greenleaf JF: **Ultrasound-stimulated vibro-acoustic spectrography.** *Science* 1998, **280**(5360):82–85.
34. Fatemi M, Greenleaf JF: **Vibro-acoustography: An imaging modality based on ultrasound-stimulated acoustic emission.** *Proc Natl Acad SciUSA* 1999, **96**(12):6603–6608.
35. Alizad A: **Breast vibro-acoustography.** In *Emerging Technologies in Breast Imaging and Mammography. Volume 1.* 2008th edition. Edited by Suri RR. Valencia, California: American Scientific Publishers; 2006:197–205.
36. Urban MW, Alizad A, Aquino W, Greenleaf JF, Fatemi M: **A Review of Vibro-acoustography and its Applications in Medicine.** *Current medical imaging reviews* 2011, **7**(4):350–359.
37. Alizad A, Fatemi M, Nishimura RA, Kinnick RR, Rambod E, Greenleaf JF: **Detection of calcium deposits on heart valve leaflets by vibro-acoustography: An in vitro study.** *J Am Soc Echocardiogr* 2002, **15**(11): 1391–1395.
38. Fatemi M, Greenleaf JF: **Probing the dynamics of tissue at low frequencies with the radiation force of ultrasound.** *Phys Med Biol* 2000, **45**(6):1449–1464.
39. Pislaru C, Kantor B, Kinnick RR, Anderson JL, Aubry MC, Urban MW, Fatemi M, Greenleaf JF: **In vivo vibroacoustography of large peripheral arteries.** *Invest Radiol* 2008, **43**(4):243–252.
40. Fatemi M, Wold LE, Alizad A, Greenleaf JF: **Vibro-acoustic tissue mammography.** *IEEE Trans Med Imaging* 2002, **21**(1):1–8.
41. Alizad A, Fatemi M, Wold LE, Greenleaf JF: **Performance of vibro-acoustography in detecting microcalcifications in excised human breast tissue: A study of 74 tissue samples.** *IEEE Trans Med Imaging* 2004, **23**(3):307–312.
42. Alizad A, Wold LE, Greenleaf JF, Fatemi M: **Imaging mass lesions by vibro-acoustography: modeling and experiments.** *IEEE Trans Med Imaging* 2004, **23**(9):1087–1093.
43. Alizad A, Walch M, Greenleaf JF, Fatemi M: **Vibrational characteristics of bone fracture and fracture repair: application to excised rat femur.** *J Biomech Eng* 2006, **128**(3):300–308.
44. Alizad A, Whaley D, Greenleaf J, Fatemi M: **Potential applications of vibro-acoustography in breast imaging.** *Technol Cancer Res Treat* 2005, **4**(2):151–157.
45. Alizad A, Whaley DH, Greenleaf JF, Fatemi M: **Critical issues in breast imaging by vibro-acoustography.** *Ultrasonics* 2006, **44**:e217–e220.
46. Alizad A, Whaley DH, Urban MW, Carter RE, Kinnick RR, Greenleaf JF, Fatemi M: **Breast vibro-acoustography: initial results show promise.** *Breast Cancer Re* 2012, **14**(5):R128.
47. Mitri FG, Davis BJ, Urban MW, Alizad A, Greenleaf JF, Lischer GH, Wilson TM, Fatemi M: **Vibro-acoustography imaging of permanent prostate brachytherapy seeds in an excised human prostate–preliminary results and technical feasibility.** *Ultrasonics* 2009, **49**(3):389–394.
48. Mitri FG, Davis BJ, Alizad A, Greenleaf JF, Wilson TM, Mynderse LA, Fatemi M: **Prostate cryotherapy monitoring using vibroacoustography: preliminary results of an ex vivo study and technical feasibility.** *IEEE Trans Biomed Eng* 2008, **55**(11):2584–2592.
49. Urban MW, Chalek C, Kinnick RR, Kinter TM, Haider B, Greenleaf JF, Thomenius KE, Fatemi M: **Implementation of vibro-acoustography on a clinical ultrasound system.** *IEEE TransUltrason, Ferroelectr, FreqControl* 2011, **58**(6):1169–1181.
50. Reading CC, Charboneau JW, Hay ID, Sebo TJ: **Sonography of thyroid nodules: a "classic pattern" diagnostic approach.** *Ultrasound Q* 2005, **21**(3):157–165.

51. Khoo MLC, Asa SL, Witterick IJ, Freeman JL: **Thyroid calcification and its association with thyroid carcinoma.** *Head Neck* 2002, **24**(7):651–655.
52. Yoon DY, Lee JW, Chang SK, Choi CS, Yun EJ, Seo YL, Kim KH, Hwang HS: **Peripheral Calcification in Thyroid Nodules Ultrasonographic Features and Prediction of Malignancy.** *J Ultrasound Med* 2007, **26**(10):1349–1355.
53. Moon WJ, Jung SL, Lee JH, Na DG, Baek JH, Lee YH, Kim J, Kim HS, Byun JS, Lee DH: **Benign and Malignant Thyroid Nodules: US Differentiation—Multicenter Retrospective Study1.** *Radiology* 2008, **247**(3):762–770.
54. Taki S, Terahata S, Yamashita R, Kinuya K, Nobata K, Kakuda K, Kodama Y, Yamamoto I: **Thyroid calcifications: sonographic patterns and incidence of cancer.** *ClinImaging* 2004, **28**(5):368–371.

3

An assessment of the vulnerability of carotid plaques: a comparative study between intraplaque neovascularization and plaque echogenicity

Yangyang Zhou[1†], Yingqi Xing[3†], Yan Li[2], Yang Bai[2], Ying Chen[3], Xiaofeng Sun[2], Yingqiao Zhu[2] and Jiang Wu[1*]

Abstract

Background: Carotid plaque echolucency as detected by Color Doppler ultrasonography (CDUS) has been used as a potential marker of plaque vulnerability. However, contrast-enhanced ultrasound (CEUS) has recently been shown to be a valuable method to evaluate the vulnerability and neovascularization within carotid atherosclerotic plaques. The aim of this study was to compare CEUS and CDUS in the assessment of plaque vulnerability using transcranial color Doppler (TCD) monitoring of microembolic signals (MES) as a reference technique.

Methods: A total of 46 subjects with arterial stenosis (≥ 50%) underwent a carotid duplex ultrasound, TCD monitoring of MES and CEUS (SonoVue doses of 2.0 mL) within a span of 3 days. The agreement between the CEUS, CDUS, and MES findings was assessed with a chi-square test. A *p*-value less than 0.05 was considered statistically significant.

Results: Neovascularization was observed in 30 lesions (44.4%). The vascular risk factors for stroke were similar and there were no age or gender differences between the 2 groups. Using CEUS, MES were identified in 2 patients (12.5%) within class 1 (non-neovascularization) as opposed to 15 patients (50.0%) within class 2 (neovascularization) ($p = 0.023$). CDUS revealed no significant differences in the appearance of the MES between the 2 groups (hyperechoic and hypoechoic) ($p = 0.237$).

Conclusion: This study provides preliminary evidence to suggest that intraplaque neovascularization detected by CEUS is associated with the presence of MESs, where as plaque echogenicity on traditional CDUS does not. These findings argue that CEUS may better identify high-risk plaques.

Keywords: Contrast-enhanced ultrasound (CEUS), Plaque vulnerability, Monitoring of microembolic signals (MES), Color Doppler ultrasonography (CDUS)

Background

Internal carotid artery (ICA) disease is frequently observed in ischemic stroke patients. Histological and imaging studies [1-3] have demonstrated that stroke is dependent on the degree of stenosis and the morphological features of the plaque, such as ulcers or fissures. These morphological features can cause a rupture [4] of the plaque and result in embolization, which is known as "vulnerability". All of these factors should be considered when developing an accurate diagnostic and preventive approach aimed at risk stratification and treatment planning to reduce the incidence and severity of acute cerebrovascular disease. Color Doppler ultrasonography (CDUS) has been the the screening test of choice for assessing carotid atherosclerosis. Echolucency of the Carotid plaque is a valuable marker of the plaque vulnerability [5-7].

However, recently several studies have confirmed the feasibility of using contrast-enhanced ultrasound (CEUS) for the evaluation of neovascularization within carotid

* Correspondence: yyangyangzhou@gmail.com
†Equal contributors
[1]Department of Neurology, The First Norman Bethune Hospital of Jilin University, Xinmin Street 71#, 130021, Chang Chun, China
Full list of author information is available at the end of the article

atherosclerotic plaques. Furthermore, this technique may also be used to assess the vulnerability of carotid plaques [8-11]. Levovist is an ultrasound contrast agent (BR1; Bracco SpA, Milan, Italy; Definity, Lantheus Medical Imaging) that enables the optimization of technically difficult explorations using a Doppler signal of sufficient intensity and improves the detection of minimal flow rates and slow velocities in severe cases of stenosis.

Previous studies [12,13] demonstrate that echolucent plaques tend to have greater contrast enhancement compared to echogenic plaques. Echolucent plaques are known to exhibit a larger number of vulnerable pathological features and correlate with a higher risk of cerebrovascular events [14]. However, studies to determine the most accurate technique for assessing plaque vulnerability have been limited. The aim of our study was to compare CEUS-detected neovascularization with plaque morphology on CDUS with regards to their correlation with MESs.

Materials and methods

Patient group and informed consent

This study was approved by the local ethics committee and written informed consent was obtained from all patients. The following data was recorded from the patient: age, sex, previous symptoms (Transient ischemic attacks (TIA), dysphasia, single limb paresis and amaurosis fugax) and co-morbid risk factors (hypertension, hyperlipidemia, diabetes and smoking habits) (Table 1 and Table 2). Both asymptomatic and symptomatic patients were included.

Between March 2011 and March 2012, 54 subjects with arterial stenosis (≥50%) underwent CDUS ($PSV_{ICA} \geq 125$ cm/s and visible plaque [15]) at the First Norman Bethune Hospital of Jilin University. In addition, TCD monitoring of MES and CEUS examinations were performed within 3 days by two independent researchers (Y.L. and Y.B.). MES monitoring was performed by two neuroradiologists (Y-Q.X and Y.C.). Patients with any of the following conditions were excluded: [1] complete ICA occlusion or <50% stenosis based on CDUS; [2] evidence of cardioembolism, such as atrial fibrillation, mechanical valve replacement, left atrial or left ventricular thrombus, bacterial endocarditis, or recent myocardial infarction; [3] ipsilateral stenosis of the middle cerebral artery (MCA) or intracranial internal carotid artery in the TCD; [4] a poor temporal window; or [5] poor image quality of the vessel wall or lumen. Therefore, data from remaining 46 patients (43 male and 3 women) with satisfactory image quality were analyzed.

Table 1 Differences in the clinical characteristics of class 1 (non-neovascularization) and class 2 (neovascularization) determined by CEUS

	Class 1 (n = 16)	Class 2 (n = 30)	P-value
Age (years), mean ± SD	64.38 ± 11.32	61.50 ± 6.26	0.186
Men, n (%)	16 (100%)	27 (90%)	0.542
Neurological symptoms*, n (%)	6 (37.5%)	18 (60%)	0.217
Hypertension, n (%)	9 (56.3%)	13 (43.3%)	0.538
Diabetes mellitus, n (%)	3 (18.8%)	9 (30.0%)	0.498
Hypercholesterolemia, n (%)	9 (56.3%)	18 (60.0%)	1.000
Current smoker, n (%)	8 (50.5%)	19 (63.3%)	0.531

*Neurological symptoms include previous transient ischemic attacks (TIA), dysphasia, single limb paresis, and amaurosis fugax.

Table 2 Differences in the clinical characteristics of group 1 (hyperechoic) and group 2 (hypoechoic) determined by CDUS

	Group 1 (n = 28)	Group 2 (n = 18)	P-value
Age (years), mean ± SD	62.22 ± 6.31	62.96 ± 9.54	0.456
Men, n (%)	26 (92.9%)	17 (94.4%)	1.000
Neurological symptoms*, n (%)	16 (57.1%)	8 (44.4%)	0.295
Hypertension, n (%)	17 (60.7%)	10 (55.6%)	0.767
Diabetes mellitus, n (%)	8 (28.5%)	5 (27.8%)	1.000
Hypercholesterolemia, n (%)	15 (53.6%)	12 (66.7%)	0.541
Current smoker, n (%)	18 (64.3%)	13 (72.2%)	0.749

*Neurological symptoms include previous transient ischemic attacks (TIA), dysphasia, single limb paresis, and amaurosis fugax.

Color Doppler ultrasonography (CDUS)

We used an ultrasound Philips iU22 system (Philips Healthcare Solutions, Bothell, WA, USA) equipped with an L-9-3 linear-array transducer. The instrument was operated by 2 experienced readers (Y-YZ and YC), who were blinded to all of the clinical laboratory findings and other imaging data.

The maximal thickness of the lesion located at the bifurcation and proximal to the bifurcation was assessed as a continuous variable and measured from the anterior, lateral and cross-sectional scanning plane using a longitudinal image from the media-adventitia to the intima-lumen boundaries. The B-mode settings were adjusted to optimize the quality of the gray-scale images and the pulse repetition frequency (PRF) used with the color Doppler flow imaging was adjusted according to the flow velocity.

The characteristics of the plaques were described according to the modified Gray Weale classification [16]. The lesion echogenicity was classified into group 1 (uniformly hyperechoic or predominantly (>50%) hyperechoic) or group 2 (uniformly hypoechoic or predominantly (>50%) hypoechoic). All results were agreed upon by at least two experienced neuroradiologists.

Contrast-enhanced ultrasound (CEUS)

A contrast-enhanced ultrasound examination was performed using an Acuson Sequoia 512 imaging system (Siemens, Mountain View, CA, USA) with a 2-MHz transducer by 2 experienced readers (Y.B. and Y.L.), who were blinded to all of the clinical laboratory findings and other imaging data. Disagreements between the readers were settled by a consensus reading. The patients were placed in a supine position. A 5-mL solution was prepared from 1 mL of the activated contrast agent (BR1; Bracco SpA, Milan, Italy; Definity, Lantheus Medical Imaging) diluted in 4 mL of saline. An initial bolus injection was quickly performed. The second injection was performed slowly and was followed by 5 mL of normal saline to flush out the contrast from the vein. The time gap between the injections was approximately 3 minutes. The contrast-enhanced ultrasound imaging application included a low mechanical index (0.07) to avoid early bubble destruction and harmonics with pulse inversion to optimize the depiction of the IV contrast agent and minimize echoes from the surrounding tissues. Cine loops were recorded for 5 heart cycles, starting from the time in which the contrast agent could be observed in the carotid lumen. Following the infusion of the ultrasound contrast agent, the lumen of the carotid artery was enhanced, resulting in visualization of enhanced plaque luminal morphology. The presence of blood flow "activity" was identified on the basis of the dynamic movement of the echogenic reflectors (microspheres) in the intraplaque microvessels.

Intraplaque neovascularization (contrast agent enhancement) was categorized using a modified grading scale and classified as class 1 (non-neovascularization) or class 2 (neovascularization).

TCD ultrasound examination

MES monitoring was performed by two experienced neuroradiologists (Y-YZ and YC) with a TCD machine (EME TC8080; Nicolet, Madison, WI, USA) with a 2-MHz transducer. The patients were placed in the supine position and bilateral MCA recordings were obtained for 30 minutes at a depth of 44–60 mm. The MES were identified on the basis of Doppler waves obtained from the MCA ipsilateral to the side of the ICA stenosis. The following definitions for emboli signals were used: typical, visible, and audible (click, chirp, whistle). Short-duration, high-intensity signals within the Doppler flow spectrum occurred at random intervals during the cardiac cycle. Signals were defined at 6 dB above the background threshold on the basis of standard consensus criteria described in previous studies. The presence of MES was assessed by an independent expert reader (Y-QX), who was blinded to all of the clinical laboratory findings and other imaging data.

Database and statistical analysis

All of the data were analyzed with SPSS 17.0. The results are expressed as the mean value and standard deviation (SD) for each measurement. Categorical variables were assessed using the chi-square test. A p-value of less than 0.05 was considered statistically significant.

Results

Forty-six patients (43 men and 3 women) with satisfactory image quality were analyzed. The differences in the clinical characteristics are reported in Table 1 and Table 2.

CEUS revealed neovascularization in 30 patients (44.4%). The stroke vascular risk factors were similar between groups, and there were no age or gender differences between the 2 classes (Table 1). MES were observed in 2 patients (12.5%) within class 1 (non-neovascularization) and in 15 patients (50.0%) within class 2 (neovascularization) ($p = 0.0230$) (Table 3, Figure 1).

Using CDUS, 28 patients were identified in group 1 (hyperechoic), and 18 were identified in group 2 (hypoechoic). Stroke vascular risk factors, age and gender were similar between the 2 groups (Table 2). Moreover, no significant differences were observed in the appearance of the MES between the 2 groups ($p = 0.2368$) (Table 4).

Discussion

In this study, we examined the relationship between CEUS and CDUS characteristics of the carotid plaque with special reference to MES. We found an association between MES monitoring and the degree of contrast-agent enhancement using ultrasound imaging ($p=0.0230$). However, we did not observe a significant association between the MES results and CDUS properties ($p = 0.2368$). Although plaque echolucency is a marker of high-risk lesions (rupture prone plaques), our findings indicate that CEUS appears to be more accurate at assessing plaque vulnerability.

CDUS has replaced digital subtraction angiograph for the diagnosis of carotid stenosis, in part because CDUS provides enhanced definition of plaque morphology [17,18]. Several studies [5,14,19-21] have demonstrated that echogenic plaques are well-established markers of high-risk lesions and are associated with the presence of neurological symptoms and the development of future strokes in previously symptomatic individuals. Furthermore, echogenic plaques also coincide with the occurrence of acute coronary syndromes. Several studies have

Table 3 Comparison of the MES measurements (mean D) of class 1 (non-neovascularization) and class 2 (neovascularization) determined by CEUS

	Class 1 (n = 16)	Class 2 (n = 30)	P-value
MES (z), n (%)	2 (12.5)	15 (50.0)	0.023

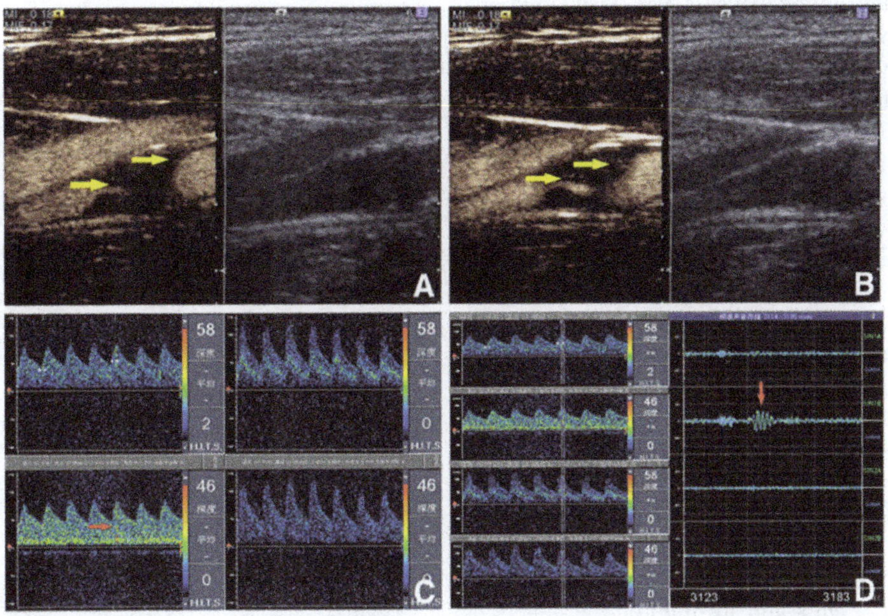

Figure 1 A 56 year-old female patient with TIA. CEUS (**A** and **B**) detected 2 consecutive frames of intra-plaque neovascularization (yellow arrow). MES (red arrow) was detected in the ipsilateral middle cerebral artery (**C** and **D**).

reported [22-26] that echogenic plaques are prone to rupture due to their increased lipid content and macrophage density as well as intraplaque hemorrhage; in addition, increased plasma and low-density lipoprotein cholesterol levels make them vulnerable and prone to ulceration and embolization.

Neovascularization is considered an important feature in plaque development and vulnerability and is triggered by inflammation and hemorrhage [8,27,28]. The vulnerability of the neovasculature to rupture increases the risk of cerebral emboli. Several pathological studies [28-30] have confirmed that plaque rupture is strongly associated with the presence and degree of neovascularization within the plaque.

Intraplaque microvessels (angiogenesis) within the atherosclerotic lesions arise mainly from the adventitial vasa vasorum. Extension of the vasa vasorum to the full thickness of the media and intima of atherosclerotic segments represents pathological neovascularization, which is stimulated by plaque hypoxia, reactive oxygen species, hypoxia-inducible factor signaling and inflammation [31,32].

Feinstein et al. [33] and Assaf Hoogi et al. [11] compared the results of CEUS with histological characteristics. Their findings revealed that contrast enhancement within the plaque is correlated with a higher number of microvessels. The studies of Staub *et al.* [10] and Faggioli *et al.* [34] have indicated the feasibility of using CEUS to depict neovascularization within the carotid plaque to facilitate the further stratification of the risk of rupture of carotid artery lesions. Thus, CEUS has been proposed as a method to preoperatively identify vulnerable plaques.

Table 4 Comparison of the MES measurements (mean D) of group 1 (hyperechoic) and group 2 (hypoechoic) determined by CDUS

	Group 1(n = 28)	Group 2 (n = 18)	P-value
MES (z), n (%)	12 (42.9)	5 (27.8)	0.237

Consistent with the data obtained in previous reports [12,13], neovascularization visualized using CEUS is correlated with the morphological features of plaque vulnerability, including echogenic plaques, as a marker of high risk lesions.

Coli *et al.* [12] reported that carotid plaque contrast agent enhancement correlated with echogenic plaques ($p = 0.001$) and is associated with the histological density of neovessels. Interestingly, intraplaque neovascularization in CEUS images correlated well with histological microvessel density rather than plaque echolucency suggesting that low echo intensity is not correlated with the histological density of the vasa vasorum. Thus CEUS is a more specific imaging modality to identify highly vascularized and inflamed vulnerable lesions as compared to standard CDUS in isolation.

Our observations strongly indicate a positive relationship between neovascularization in plaques and MES while there is a poor correlation between plaque echolucency and MES. Embolism is an important mechanism of cerebral infarcts in patients with ICA stenosis [35]. The detection of cerebral microembolisms by transcranial Doppler sonography may permit the definition of a high-risk subgroup among patients with asymptomatic high-grade internal carotid artery stenosis [36]. To the best of our knowledge, this is the first study to explore neovascularization in stroke patients with ICA stenosis using MES and CEUS.

There were some limitations in this study. The first limitation was that the pilot study was conducted with a small sample size. Second, we used a semi-quantitative approach to evaluate the contrast-agent enhancement; however, this limitation does not alter our observations or conclusions. This quantitative method needs to be further investigated. Finally, several patients could not be examined because of an inadequate insonation window during the TCD monitoring that prevented further analysis. Future studies in larger populations are required to validate the results of the present study. Moreover, prospective clinical studies are also needed to evaluate the use of contrast-enhanced ultrasound imaging of plaque neovascularization to assess the risk of cerebrovascular events and to monitor the effects of anti-atherosclerotic therapies.

Conclusions

Intraplaque neovascularization detected by CEUS but not plaque echolucency is correlated with MES, suggesting that CEUS may provide valuable information about plaque risk stratification and may be an accurate method for assessing vulnerable plaques beyond the echogenicity of CDUS.

Competing interests

The authors declare that there are no competing interests.

Authors' contributions

YZ and YX participated in the design of the study, performed the statistical analysis, participated in the sequence alignment, CDUS, and MES studies, and drafted the manuscript. YL, YB, XS, and YZ performed the CEUS studies. YC participated in the CDUS and MES studies. YX and JW developed the concept of the study and participated in its design and coordination. All authors have read and approved the final manuscript.

Acknowledgements

This work was performed at First Norman Bethune Hospital of Jilin University and was funded by the Jilin Provincial Health Department of China. The authors declare that they have no competing interests. Unrelated to this study, Dr. Xing receives/received research funding from the National Natural Science Foundation of China (Grant No. 81100855 and 81000490).
The Medical Ethical Committee of Jilin University gave the approval for the study.

Author details

[1]Department of Neurology, The First Norman Bethune Hospital of Jilin University, Xinmin Street 71#, 130021, Chang Chun, China. [2]Center for Abdominal Ultrasound, The First Norman Bethune Hospital of Jilin University, Chang Chun, China. [3]Center for Neurovascular Ultrasound, The First Norman Bethune Hospital of Jilin University, Chang Chun, China.

References

1. Fisher M, Paganini-Hill A, Martin A, Cosgrove M, Toole JF, Barnett HJ, Norris J: **Carotid plaque pathology: thrombosis, ulceration, and stroke pathogenesis.** *Stroke* 2005, **36:**253–257.
2. Kolodgie FD, Gold HK, Burke AP, Fowler DR, Kruth HS, Weber DK, Farb A, Guerrero LJ, Hayase M, Kutys R, Narula J, Finn AV, Virmani R: **Intraplaque hemorrhage and progression of coronary atheroma.** *N Engl J Med* 2003, **349:**2316–2325.
3. Nandalur KR, Baskurt E, Hagspiel KD, Phillips CD, Kramer CM: **Calcified carotid atherosclerotic plaque is associated less with ischemic symptoms than is noncalcified plaque on MDCT.** *AJR Am J Roentgenol* 2005, **184:**295–298.
4. Naghavi M, Libby P, Falk E, Casscells SW, Litovsky S, Rumberger J, Badimon JJ, Stefanadis C, Moreno P, Pasterkamp G, Fayad Z, Stone PH, Waxman S, Raggi P, Madjid M, Zarrabi A, Burke A, Yuan C, Fitzgerald PJ, Siscovick DS, de Korte CL, Aikawa M, Juhani Airaksinen KE, Assmann G, Becker CR, Chesebro JH, Farb A, Galis ZS, Jackson C, Jang IK, Koenig W, Lodder RA, March K, Demirovic J, Navab M, Priori SG, Rekhter MD, Bahr R, Grundy SM, Mehran R, Colombo A, Boerwinkle E, Ballantyne C, Insull W Jr, Schwartz RS, Vogel R, Serruys PW, Hansson GK, Faxon DP, Kaul S, Drexler H, Greenland P, Muller JE, Virmani R, Ridker PM, Zipes DP, Shah PK, Willerson JT: **From vulnerable plaque to vulnerable patient: a call for new definitions and risk assessment strategies: Part I.** *Circulation* 2003, **108:**1664–1672.
5. Seo Y, Watanabe S, Ishizu T, Moriyama N, Takeyasu N, Maeda H, Ishimitsu T, Aonuma K, Yamaguchi I: **Echolucent carotid plaques as a feature in patients with acute coronary syndrome.** *Circ J* 2006, **70:**1629–1634.
6. Gronholdt ML, Nordestgaard BG, Schroeder TV, Vorstrup S, Sillesen H: **Ultrasonic echolucent carotid plaques predict future strokes.** *Circulation* 2001, **104:**68–73.
7. Ogata T, Yasaka M, Wakugawa Y, Kitazono T, Okada Y: **Morphological classification of mobile plaques and their association with early recurrence of stroke.** *Cerebrovasc Dis* 2010, **30:**606–611.
8. Huang PT, Chen CC, Aronow WS, Wang XT, Nair CK, Xue NY, Shen X, Li SY, Huang FG, Cosgrove D: **Assessment of neovascularization within carotid plaques in patients with ischemic stroke.** *World J Cardiol* 2010, **2:**89–97.
9. Caplice NM, Martin K: **Contrast-enhanced ultrasound and the enigma of plaque neovascularization.** *JACC Cardiovasc Imaging* 2010, **3:**1273–1275.
10. Staub D, Patel MB, Tibrewala A, Ludden D, Johnson M, Espinosa P, Coll B, Jaeger KA, Feinstein SB: **Vasa vasorum and plaque neovascularization on contrast-enhanced carotid ultrasound imaging correlates with cardiovascular disease and past cardiovascular events.** *Stroke* 2010, **41:**41–47.
11. Hoogi A, Adam D, Hoffman A, Kerner H, Reisner S, Gaitini D: **Carotid plaque vulnerability: quantification of neovascularization on contrast-enhanced ultrasound with histopathologic correlation.** *AJR Am J Roentgenol* 2011, **196:**431–436.
12. Coli S, Magnoni M, Sangiorgi G, Marrocco-Trischitta MM, Melisurgo G, Mauriello A, Spagnoli L, Chiesa R, Cianflone D, Maseri A: **Contrast-enhanced ultrasound imaging of intraplaque neovascularization in carotid arteries: correlation with histology and plaque echogenicity.** *J Am Coll Cardiol* 2008, **52:**223–230.
13. Staub D, Partovi S, Schinkel AF, Coll B, Uthoff H, Aschwanden M, Jaeger KA, Feinstein SB: **Correlation of carotid artery atherosclerotic lesion echogenicity and severity at standard US with intraplaque neovascularization detected at contrast-enhanced US.** *Radiology* 2011, **258:**618–626.
14. Mathiesen EB, Bonaa KH, Joakimsen O: **Echolucent plaques are associated with high risk of ischemic cerebrovascular events in carotid stenosis: the tromso study.** *Circulation* 2001, **103:**2171–2175.
15. Grant EG, Benson CB, Moneta GL, Alexandrov AV, Baker JD, Bluth EI, Carroll BA, Eliasziw M, Gocke J, Hertzberg BS, Katanick S, Needleman L, Pellerito J, Polak JF, Rholl KS, Wooster DL, Zierler RE: **Carotid artery stenosis: gray-scale and Doppler US diagnosis–Society of Radiologists in Ultrasound Consensus Conference.** *Radiology* 2003, **229:**340–346.
16. Geroulakos G, Ramaswami G, Nicolaides A, James K, Labropoulos N, Belcaro G, Holloway M: **Characterization of symptomatic and asymptomatic carotid plaques using high-resolution real-time ultrasonography.** *Br J Surg* 1993, **80:**1274–1277.
17. Degnan AJ, Young VE, Gillard JH: **Advances in noninvasive imaging for evaluating clinical risk and guiding therapy in carotid atherosclerosis.** *Expert Rev Cardiovasc Ther* 2012, **10:**37–53.

18. Vancraeynest D, Pasquet A, Roelants V, Gerber BL, Vanoverschelde JL: **Imaging the vulnerable plaque.** *J Am Coll Cardiol* 2011, **57:**1961–1979.
19. Johnson JM, Kennelly MM, Decesare D, Morgan S, Sparrow A: **Natural history of asymptomatic carotid plaque.** *Arch Surg* 1985, **120:**1010–1012.
20. Reiter M, Effenberger I, Sabeti S, Mlekusch W, Schlager O, Dick P, Puchner S, Amighi J, Bucek RA, Minar E, Schillinger M: **Increasing carotid plaque echolucency is predictive of cardiovascular events in high-risk patients.** *Radiology* 2008, **248:**1050–1055.
21. Sillesen H: **Carotid artery plaque composition--relationship to clinical presentation and ultrasound B-mode imaging.** *Eur J Vasc Endovasc Surg* 1995, **10:**23–30.
22. Tegos TJ, Sohail M, Sabetai MM, Robless P, Akbar N, Pare G, Stansby G, Nicolaides AN: **Echomorphologic and histopathologic characteristics of unstable carotid plaques.** *AJNR Am J Neuroradiol* 2000, **21:**1937–1944.
23. Sztajzel R, Momjian S, Momjian-Mayor I, Murith N, Djebaili K, Boissard G, Comelli M, Pizolatto G: **Stratified gray-scale median analysis and color mapping of the carotid plaque: correlation with endarterectomy specimen histology of 28 patients.** *Stroke* 2005, **36:**741–745.
24. Nighoghossian N, Derex L, Douek P: **The vulnerable carotid artery plaque: current imaging methods and new perspectives.** *Stroke* 2005, **36:**2764–2772.
25. Nordestgaard BG, Gronholdt ML, Sillesen H: **Echolucent rupture-prone plaques.** *Curr Opin Lipidol* 2003, **14:**505–512.
26. Gronholdt ML, Nordestgaard BG, Bentzon J, Wiebe BM, Zhou J, Falk E, Sillesen H: **Macrophages are associated with lipid-rich carotid artery plaques, echolucency on B-mode imaging, and elevated plasma lipid levels.** *J Vasc Surg* 2002, **35:**137–145.
27. Moreno PR, Purushothaman KR, Sirol M, Levy AP, Fuster V: **Neovascularization in human atherosclerosis.** *Circulation* 2006, **113:**2245–2252.
28. Fleiner M, Kummer M, Mirlacher M, Sauter G, Cathomas G, Krapf R, Biedermann BC: **Arterial neovascularization and inflammation in vulnerable patients: early and late signs of symptomatic atherosclerosis.** *Circulation* 2004, **110:**2843–2850.
29. Moreno PR, Purushothaman KR, Fuster V, Echeverri D, Truszczynska H, Sharma SK, Badimon JJ, O'Connor WN: **Plaque neovascularization is increased in ruptured atherosclerotic lesions of human aorta: implications for plaque vulnerability.** *Circulation* 2004, **110:**2032–2038.
30. McCarthy MJ, Loftus IM, Thompson MM, Jones L, London NJ, Bell PR, Naylor AR, Brindle NP: **Angiogenesis and the atherosclerotic carotid plaque: an association between symptomatology and plaque morphology.** *J Vasc Surg* 1999, **30:**261–268.
31. Kumamoto M, Nakashima Y, Sueishi K: **Intimal neovascularization in human coronary atherosclerosis: its origin and pathophysiological significance.** *Hum Pathol* 1995, **26:**450–456.
32. Sluimer JC, Gasc JM, van Wanroij JL, Kisters N, Groeneweg M, Sollewijn Gelpke MD, Cleutjens JP, van den Akker LH, Corvol P, Wouters BG, Daemen MJ, Bijnens AP: **Hypoxia, hypoxia-inducible transcription factor, and macrophages in human atherosclerotic plaques are correlated with intraplaque angiogenesis.** *J Am Coll Cardiol* 2008, **51:**1258–1265.
33. Feinstein SB: **Contrast ultrasound imaging of the carotid artery vasa vasorum and atherosclerotic plaque neovascularization.** *J Am Coll Cardiol* 2006, **48:**236–243.
34. Faggioli GL, Pini R, Mauro R, Pasquinelli G, Fittipaldi S, Freyrie A, Serra C, Stella A: **Identification of carotid 'vulnerable plaque' by contrast-enhanced ultrasonography: correlation with plaque histology, symptoms and cerebral computed tomography.** *Eur J Vasc Endovasc Surg* 2011, **41:**238–248.
35. Momjian-Mayor I, Baron JC: **The pathophysiology of watershed infarction in internal carotid artery disease: review of cerebral perfusion studies.** *Stroke* 2005, **36:**567–577.
36. Siebler M, Nachtmann A, Sitzer M, Rose G, Kleinschmidt A, Rademacher J, Steinmetz H: **Cerebral microembolism and the risk of ischemia in asymptomatic high-grade internal carotid artery stenosis.** *Stroke* 1995, **26:**2184–2186.

4

Evaluation of ultrasound Tissue Velocity Imaging: a phantom study of velocity estimation in skeletal muscle low-level contractions

Frida Lindberg[1*], Mattias Mårtensson[1], Christer Grönlund[2] and Lars-Åke Brodin[1]

Abstract

Background: Tissue Velocity Imaging (TVI) is an ultrasound based technique used for quantitative analysis of the cardiac function and has earlier been evaluated according to myocardial velocities. Recent years several studies have reported applying TVI in the analysis of skeletal muscles. Skeletal tissue velocities can be very low. In particular, when performing isometric contractions or contractions of low force level the velocities may be much lower compared to the myocardial tissue velocities.

Methods: In this study TVI was evaluated for estimation of tissue velocities below the typical myocardial velocities. An in-house phantom was used to see how different PRF-settings affected the accuracy of the velocity estimations.

Results: With phantom peak velocity at 0.03 cm/s the error ranged from 31% up to 313% with the different PRF-settings in this study. For the peak velocities at 0.17 cm/s and 0.26 cm/s there was no difference in error with tested PFR settings, it is kept approximately around 20%.

Conclusions: The results from the present study showed that the PRF setting did not seem to affect the accuracy of the velocity estimation at tissue velocities above 0.17 cm/s. However at lower velocities (0.03 cm/s) the setting was crucial for the accuracy. The PRF should therefore preferable be reduced when the method is applied in low-level muscle contraction.

Keywords: Tissue Velocity Imaging, Ultrasound, Skeletal muscle, Phantom evaluation, Pulse repetition frequency

Background

Tissue Velocity Imaging (TVI) is an ultrasound based technique used for the quantitative analysis of mechanical parameters such as tissue velocity and tissue deformation [1-4]. TVI has been used clinically for many years in the field of cardiology, where the technique provides visual information on overall anatomy, regional movement- and velocity data of the myocardium together with quantitative measurements of these parameters (see [2,5,6] for an overview). All parameters are based on the velocity estimations derived from the phase shift in the ultrasound pulses that arises when they are reflected against a moving target. The method has been validated according to regional myocardial velocities and tested for inter- and intra-subject reproducibility [3,7-9]. Furthermore, TVI-based velocity and deformation parameters have been evaluated by our research group using several ultrasound scanners in a phantom study [10]. The parameters measured by TVI are considered to have a high clinical value in cardiology.

The research fields using TVI has broadened and several studies have reported using the technique on skeletal muscles [11-18]. However, there are likely important considerations to be made when applying this method, developed and evaluated for cardiac applications, in the musculoskeletal field. In cardiology the peak velocities are often of most interest. Myocardial peak velocities are normally in the range of 5–15 cm/s in resting conditions. In the studies of skeletal muscles the situation can be very different, for example in isometric contractions

* Correspondence: frida.lindberg@sth.kth.se
[1]School of Technology and Health, Royal Institute of Technology (KTH), Huddinge, Sweden
Full list of author information is available at the end of the article

or contractions with low force level. For example, Peolsson et al. reported mean velocities of 0.08 cm/s in the trapezius muscle during shoulder elevations in myalgia patients [15].

In the standard ultrasound scanner settings the pulse repetition frequency (PRF) is set to a value in order to avoid aliasing artifacts when measuring myocardial velocities. Since the velocity range is divided into a fixed number of discrete values, we hypothesize that the standard settings may have a negative impact on the accuracy of very low velocity measurements, due to too large quantification steps. This study aims to evaluate TVI for estimation of the low tissue velocities found in low force level muscle contractions. An in-house developed phantom was used to see how different PRF-settings affected the accuracy of the velocity estimations.

Methods

The phantom

A phantom set-up, used in an earlier study evaluating tissue Doppler-based velocity and deformation parameters, was redesigned for the mimicking of skeletal muscle motion [10]. In this set-up a cylindrical tissue mimicking object was made of polyvinyl alcohol (PVA) (Sigma-Aldrich, St. Louis, Missouri, USA), with a length of 125 mm and a diameter of 40 mm. In order to get it sufficiently stiff 7 thaw cycles were used. Every thaw cycle constituted of a freezing period of 12 hours at a temperature of −18°C followed by 12 hours in room-temperature, resulting in 24 hour thaw cycles. In order to get speckles similar to that of muscle tissue a small amount of graphite powder (Merck, Darmstadt, Germany) was added to the PVA when mixed with water. The concentration was by mass; water (82%), PVA (15%) and graphite (3%). The speed of sound in tissue mimicking material was measured to lie within an interval of 1530–1580 m/s. The tissue mimicking object was immersed in a mixture of glycerol (Sigma-Aldrich, St. Louis, Missouri, USA) and deionized water. The concentration was by mass; deionized water (89%) and glycerol (11%). The chosen concentration resulted in a speed of sound of 1540 m/s. A single element transducer, an oscilloscope and a micrometer were used in the measurements to estimate the speed of sound in the tissue mimicking material and the immersing fluid. The difficulty in measuring the length of the soft PVA material with a micrometer in combination with the accuracy from reading the oscilloscope lead to the inaccuracy in the measurement of the tissue mimicking material. The fluid was placed in a large plastic container, which enabled the sound to travel a much longer distance than in the phantom material, and thus the better precision.

The force generator of the dynamic phantom was an ElectroPuls E3000 (Instron, Norwood, Massachusetts, USA), normally used for dynamic testing of material properties. The ElectroPuls E3000 can be programmed to perform motions of almost any wave form, and its performed motion is measured very accurately, making it possible to compare values measured by an ultrasound system with a true value. The tissue mimicking material was connected, in the distal parts, to the ElectroPuls E3000 by two plastic rods. In order to minimize the risk of reverberation artifacts a large rubber cube was place under the midsection coinciding with the transducer position. The acoustic properties of the rubber cube effectively absorb any entering ultrasound pulse (seen in Figure 1a).

The phantom was programmed to produce three different sine wave motions, with the frequency of 0.05 Hz and amplitudes of 1mm, 5mm and 8mm, resulting in mean peak velocities of 0.03 cm/s, 0.17 cm/s and 0.26 cm/s respectively (see Table 1).

The motion performed by the electric motor of the ElectroPuls E3000 was registered by a built-in sensor on the motor shaft. The sensor measured the motor position relative to the starting position and the position was measured 1000 times per second. These position values were used to calculate the velocity of the performed motion. The repeatability of the phantom was evaluated based on the phantom data from the actual tests of the ultrasound systems, and the standard deviation was calculated to be ≤ 0.001 (mm) in all three displacement peaks, which were calculated separately in the three different sine wave motions. In Figure 2 the repeatability of the phantom for the sine waves with amplitude 1 mm and 8 mm is shown.

Ultrasound scanner and settings

The movement of the tissue mimicking material was recorded with an ultrasound scanner (Vivid7, GE Vingmed, Horten, Norway) using a 12 MHz linear transducer. The acquisition depth and width was set to 5.5 cm and 2.5 cm respectively and the different PRF settings yielded TVI frame rates from 66 to 214 frames per second. One focus point was used at a depth of 2.5 cm. An example of a TVI color-coded grayscale image is shown in Figure 1b.

Representation of velocity values

In the GE equipment the tissue velocities are estimated through autocorrelation of the phase shift of several consecutive returning ultrasound pulses. The information is translated into discrete values when the signal is converted from analog to digital and velocity is represented in a vector which is quantified by an equal number of positive and negative values, but not the value zero. The highest velocity value and the order of magnitude of each of the quantification steps depend on the

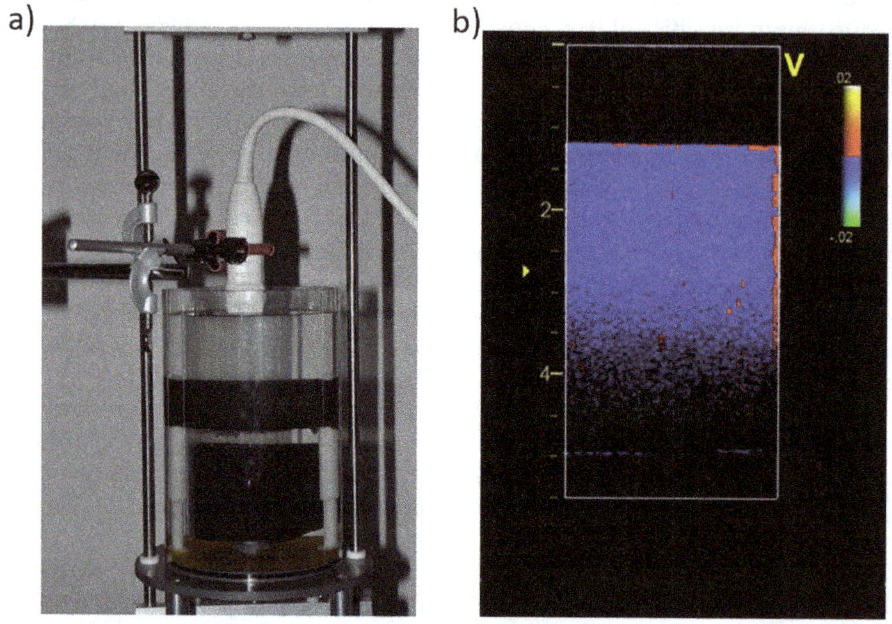

Figure 1 The phantom setup. a) shows the tissue mimicking material connected to the force generator and the linear transducer fixated above the water container. **b**) is an example of the resulting grayscale images from the ultrasound recordings. The velocity information from the TVI is color-coded and superimposed on the grayscale image. The blue color illustrates movement away from the ultrasound probe.

chosen PRF setting. A lower PRF value will result in smaller steps in the velocity vector, thus providing a more accurate representation. However, limiting the PRF will increase the risk of aliasing artifacts since the highest value in the velocity vector also will lower. According to the Nyquist theorem the distance of the phase shift should be less than half a wavelength of the sent out pulses. Since the PRF sets the time delay between the ultrasound pulses it will therefore determine the highest velocity before aliasing occurs, also known as the Nyquist limit. Three different PRF settings were included in the test protocol; 0.25 kHz, 1.0 kHz and 1.75 kHz, where 1.0 kHz is the default setting.

Table 1 Phantom motion and ultrasound settings

Phantom motion	Frequency	Amplitude	Mean peak velocities	Phantom repeatability - SD of displacement (mm)
Sine wave	0.05 Hz	1 mm	0.03 cm/s	0.001
Sine wave	0.05 Hz	5 mm	0.17 cm/s	0.001
Sine wave	0.05 Hz	8 mm	0.26 cm/s	0.001
Ultrasound settings				
PRF (kHz)	Frame rate	(/s)		
0.25	66			
1.0	168			
1.75	214			

Listed in the table are the input parameters of the phantom motion together with the frame rates corresponding to the different PRF settings tested in the study.

Test protocol and statistical analysis

The ultrasound probe was placed in the center of the tissue mimicking material at the phantom liquid surface. In the starting position the distance between the probe and tissue mimicking material was 1.2 cm. Ultrasound recordings were made while the phantom repeated one cycle of the sine motion. Ten repeated recordings were made with the three PRF settings on the three sine waves, yielding 90 recordings in total. The ultrasound probe was replaced before each recording.

The velocity information was extracted offline from the GE software EchoPac (version BT-08, GE VingMed, Horten, Norway) in a sample area of 8×16 mm centered at an image depth of 2.75 cm, in which the software calculates the mean velocity. The data was then further analyzed in MATLAB (2011b, Mathworks, Nattick, MA, USA). The phantom displacement values were used to calculate the velocity of the tissue mimicking material over time and then compared to the ultrasound velocity data. A median filter was implemented to reduce the noise in both signals.

The mean difference and standard deviation (SD) between performed and estimated velocity were calculated for the absolute peak values (three peaks) of the velocity curve. The percentage error of the true values was also calculated.

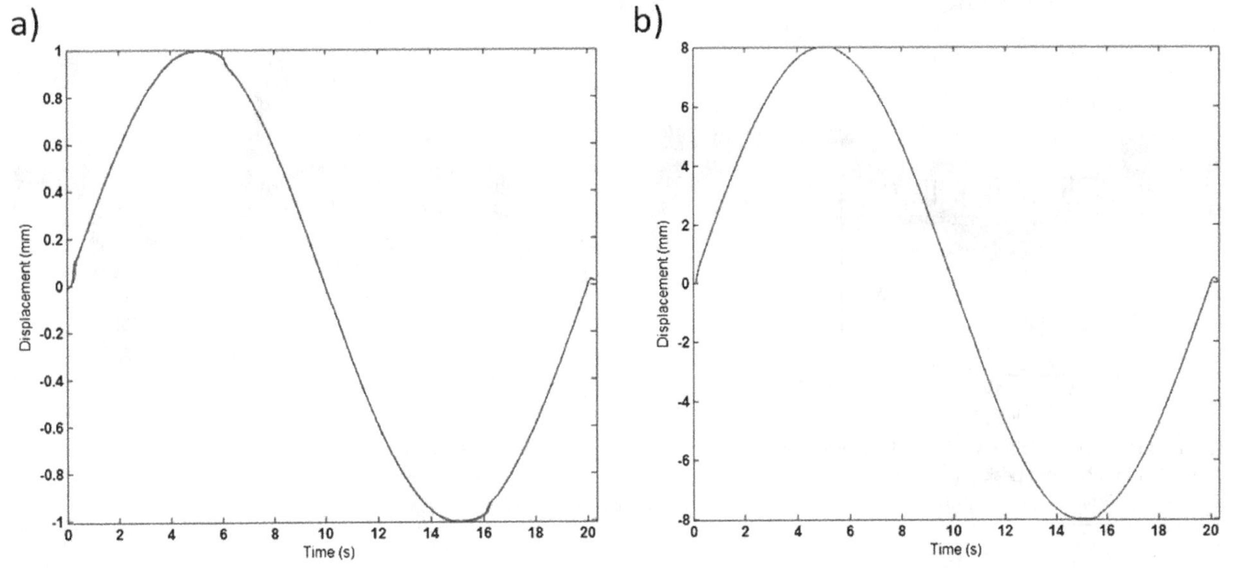

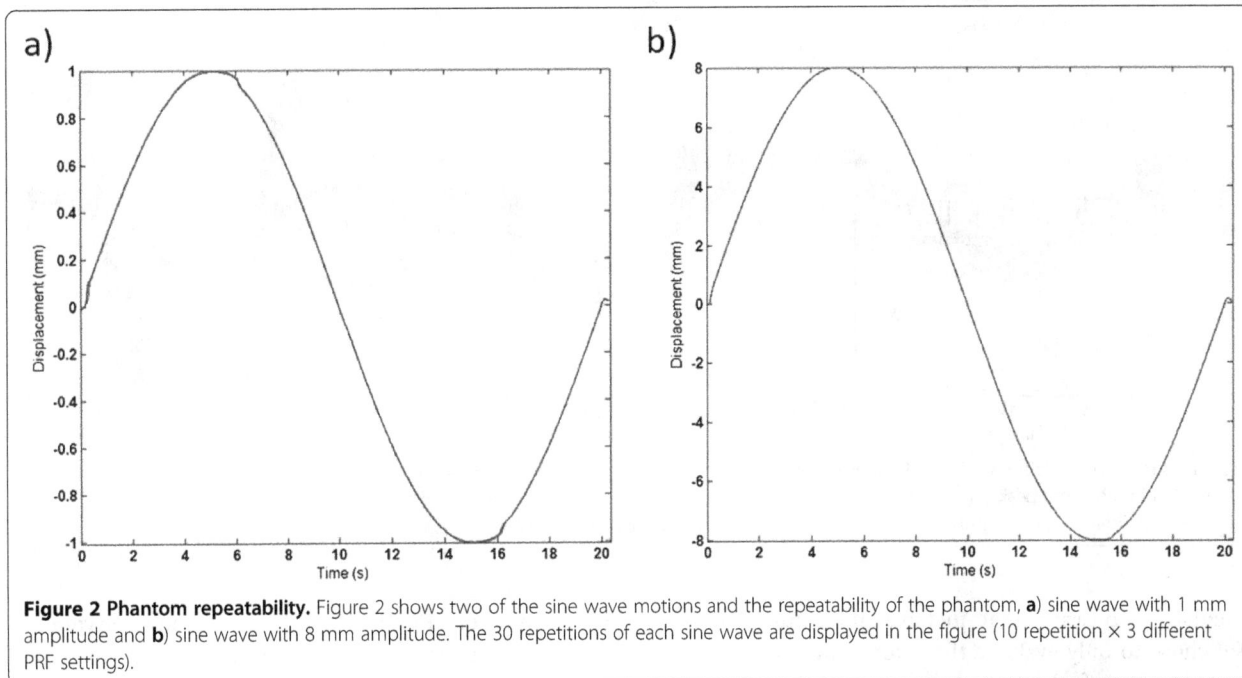

Figure 2 Phantom repeatability. Figure 2 shows two of the sine wave motions and the repeatability of the phantom, **a**) sine wave with 1 mm amplitude and **b**) sine wave with 8 mm amplitude. The 30 repetitions of each sine wave are displayed in the figure (10 repetition × 3 different PRF settings).

Results

Table 2 presents the mean difference and SD between the peak velocity values from the phantom and estimated peak velocity values from EchoPac. The error is presented as the percentage of the true value.

At very low velocities (< 0.03 cm/s) there are large differences in the TVI estimated velocities depending on the PRF-setting. With phantom peak velocity at 0.03 cm/s the error ranged from 31% up to 313% with the different PRF-settings in this study (see Figure 3). Furthermore, at the default PRF-setting (1.0 kHz) all the three peak values in all repeated measurements were estimated to 0.0724 cm/s or −0.0724 cm/s. This demonstrates the lowest possible quantification value at that setting and corresponds to an error of approx 160% of the true peak velocity. With peak velocities at 0.17 cm/s and 0.26 cm/s there is no difference in error with the three tested PFR settings, it is kept approximately around 20% (see Figure 4).

Table 2 Mean difference and estimation error

Velocity peak value (cm/s)	PRF (kHz)	Mean difference ± SD (cm/s)	Mean error (%)
0.03	0.25	0.009 ± 0.006	31
	1.0	0.045 ± 0.006	149
	1.75	0.094 ± 0.007	313
0.17	0.25	0.034 ± 0.020	20
	1.0	0.032 ± 0.016	19
	1.75	0.029 ± 0.025	17
0.26	0.25	0.057 ± 0.036	22
	1.0	0.064 ± 0.039	24
	1.75	0.057 ± 0.026	22

Table 2 show the mean differences and the standard deviation of the peak velocity values for the three sine wave motions together with the mean error (presented as the percentage of the true value).

Discussion

In this study TVI was evaluated for estimation of very low tissue velocities. An in-house developed phantom was used to see how different PRF-settings affected the accuracy of the velocity estimations. The results from the study show that for tissue velocities with peak velocities at 0.03 cm/s the PRF setting is crucial for the accuracy of the Doppler velocity estimation. However, at tissue peak velocities of order 0.3 cm/s the PRF setting has less effect on the error of the estimation.

In the analysis of the tissue mechanics, cardiac and musculoskeletal, both movement and deformation parameters are often used, such as displacement, velocity, strain, strain rate. All these parameters can be quantified and analyzed using TVI. However, it is the velocity parameter that is estimated using the autocorrelation method. The deformation parameters are calculated through the spatial gradient and temporal integration of the velocity information. This is done automatically in the off-line software. Thus, the inaccuracy of the velocity parameter will be transferred to the other parameters. If the parameter strain would have been analyzed instead it would have been more difficult to analyze how much of the error that directly could be connected to the PRF setting and how much that would be due to the

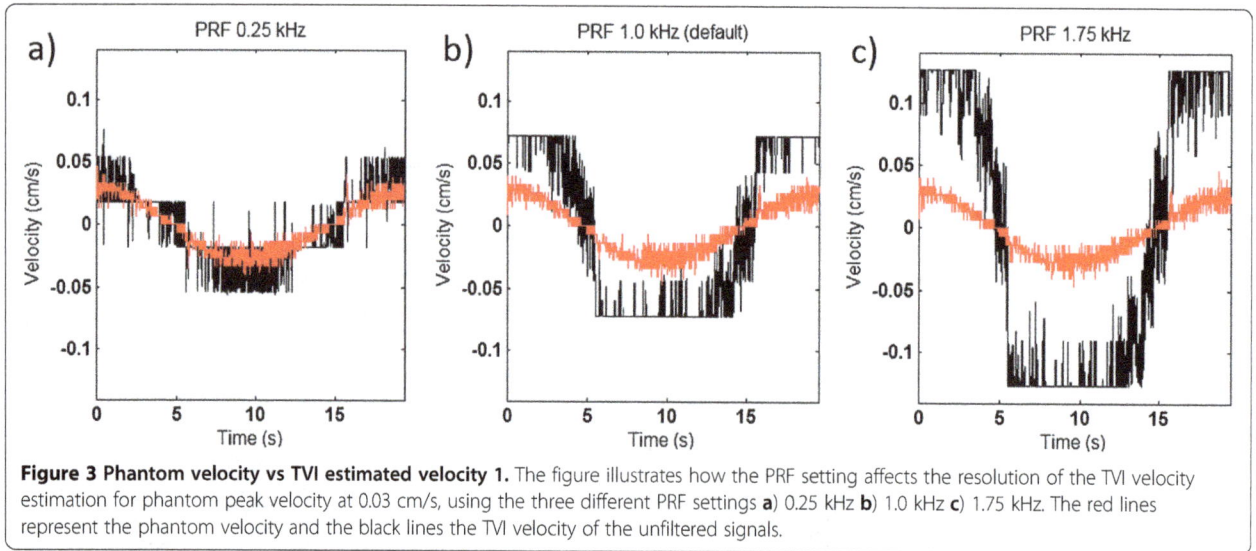

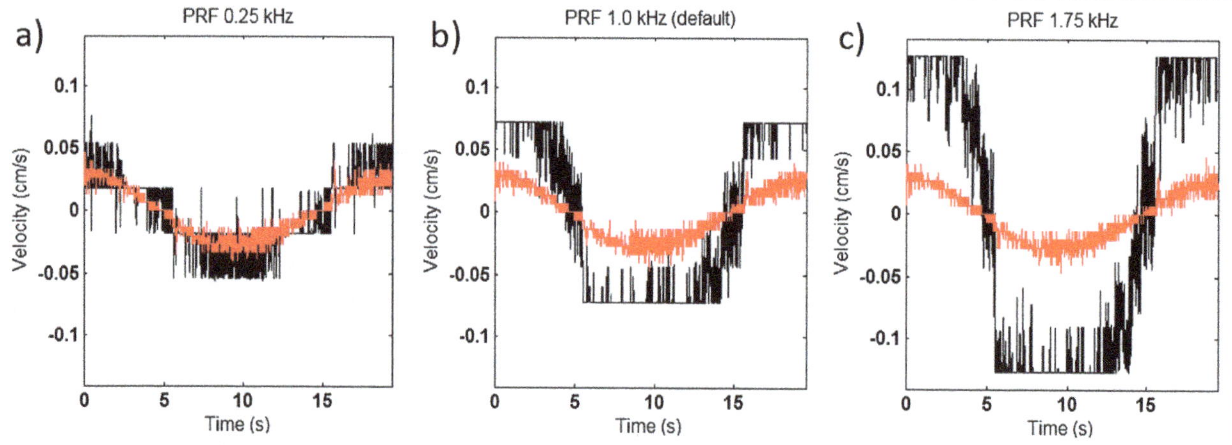

Figure 3 Phantom velocity vs TVI estimated velocity 1. The figure illustrates how the PRF setting affects the resolution of the TVI velocity estimation for phantom peak velocity at 0.03 cm/s, using the three different PRF settings **a**) 0.25 kHz **b**) 1.0 kHz **c**) 1.75 kHz. The red lines represent the phantom velocity and the black lines the TVI velocity of the unfiltered signals.

calculating software, that includes filter functions etc. We chose to only evaluate the velocity parameter in this study and therefore a non-strained phantom was used to keep the motion as homogenous as possible. The performed motion was kept in one dimension (along the ultrasound beam) eliminating errors due to out of plane motion and possible angular errors. Furthermore, the transducer was completely fixed during the acquisitions to limit any error due to transducer movements. The sine wave motion was mainly chosen for the possibility to analyze both positive and negative peak velocity values and at the same time avoid rapid acceleration of the phantom motion.

The post-processing software which calculates the deformation parameters such as strain and strain rate has earlier been evaluated for cardiac applications by Mårtensson et al. They found considerably varying results in strain and strain rate between different manufactures and also between different workstations from the same manufacture [10]. In the same study two scanners of the same type used in this study were included, however using a phased array transducer during the acquisitions. One of those scanners was equipped with exactly the same software version as the scanner used in this study. The mean error found when using that scanner for peak velocities in the range of 8–9 cm/s was in the same order as found in this study. Combined, this suggests that there is reason to believe that one can expect a mean error of this magnitude when measuring TVI velocities in skeletal muscles. It should be pointed out that the difference between individual scanners and manufactures can be significant. In addition, Doppler

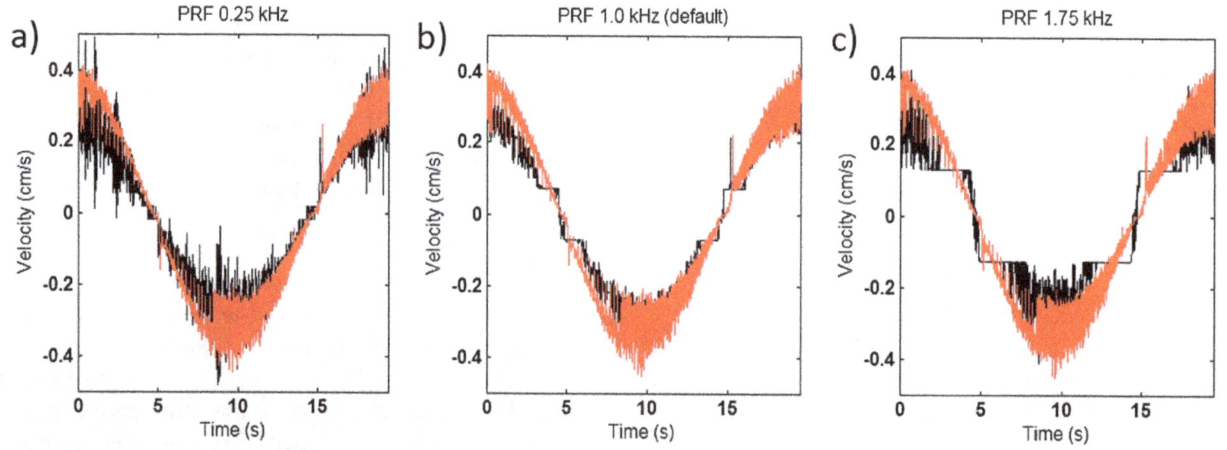

Figure 4 Phantom velocity vs TVI estimated velocity 2. The figure illustrates how the PRF setting affects the resolution of the TVI velocity estimation for phantom peak velocity at 0.26 cm/s, using the three different PRF settings **a**) 0.25 kHz **b**) 1.0 kHz **c**) 1.75 kHz. The red lines represent the phantom velocity and the black lines the TVI velocity of the unfiltered signals.

strain rate has earlier also been evaluated in slowly moving tissue (0.01-0.1 cm/s) using a phantom mimicking the gastric wall. However in this study the PRF was kept very low through all measurements and instead the sample size and sample geometry for calculating strain rate were tested [19].

To avoid aliasing it is important to keep the Nyquist limit above the peak velocities. In the GE equipment this limit is displayed as the highest/lowest velocity value of the color coding-scale. Using the lowest possible PRF setting (0.25 kHz) in this study led to a Nyquist limit at 2.0 cm/s. Is that a sufficient peak limit for measurements of skeletal muscle tissue velocities? In general, the velocities will depend on the performed motion, type of contraction, produced force and maybe also what muscle. We also believe there is a large variation between individuals. A fast dynamic contraction can surely be in the same velocity range as the myocardium [20]. However, in studies of fatigue, muscle disorders and chronic pain conditions the performed task is more likely to be of either isometric or low force type and, as reported from Peolsson et al., the velocities may be much less than 1.0 cm/s [15].

Altogether, the clinical value of the accuracy and precision will be highly dependent on the measurement to be made and the intrinsic limitations of the used equipment. We believe that TVI can be a powerful tool when it comes to analysis of intramuscular mechanics with both high spatial and temporal resolution. It also becomes a complementary method to electromyography as it provides the possibility to analyze deeper located muscles non-invasively.

Conclusions

Applying TVI on skeletal muscles one must be aware of the limitations that comes with the system. The results from the present study showed that the PRF setting did not seem to affect the accuracy of the velocity estimation at tissue velocities above 0.17 cm/s. However at lower velocities (0.03 cm/s) the setting was crucial for the accuracy. The PRF should therefore preferable be reduced when the method is applied in low-level muscle contraction. Further, the results indicate that there is an intrinsic error of the used scanner of approximately 20%. It should be carefully considered before the method is applied in a clinical setting if such an error is acceptable.

Competing interests

LÅB is co-developer and former patent holder of the analyzing software package and is having ongoing research collaboration with GE. However, no financial support for the present study has been provided from GE. The other authors declare that they have no competing interests.

Authors' contributions

FL designed and coordinated this study. FL and MM performed th data collection, data analysis and drafted the manuscript. CG and LÅB interpreted the data and critically revised the manuscript. All authors read and approved the final manuscript.

Author details

[1]School of Technology and Health, Royal Institute of Technology (KTH), Huddinge, Sweden. [2]Department of Biomedical Engineering – R&D, Radiation science, Umeå University, Umeå, Sweden.

References

1. D'Hooge J, Heimdal A, Jamal F, Kukulski T, Bijnens B, Rademakers F, Hatle L, Suetens P, Sutherland GR: **Regional strain and strain rate measurements by cardiac ultrasound: principles, implementation and limitations.** *Eur J Echocardiogr* 2000, **1**(3):154–170.
2. Sutherland GR, Di Salvo G, Claus P, D'Hooge J, Bijnens B: **Strain and strain rate imaging: a new clinical approach to quantifying regional myocardial function.** *J Am Soc Echocardiogr* 2004, **17**(7):788–802.
3. Urheim S, Edvardsen T, Torp H, Angelsen B, Smiseth OA: **Myocardial strain by Doppler echocardiography. Validation of a new method to quantify regional myocardial function.** *Circulation* 2000, **102**(10):1158–1164.
4. Stoylen A: *Strain rate imaging of the left ventricle by ultrasound. Feasibility, clinical validation and physiological aspects.* PhD Thesis: Norwegian University of Science and technology; 2001.
5. Brodin LA: **Tissue Doppler, a fundamental tool for parametric imaging.** *Clin Physiol Funct Imag* 2004, **24**(3):147–155.
6. Storaa C, Cain P, Olstad B, Lind B, Brodin LA: **Tissue motion imaging of the left ventricle–quantification of myocardial strain, velocity, acceleration and displacement in a single image.** *Eur J Echocardiogr* 2004, **5**(5):375–385.
7. Fraser AG, Payne N, Mädler CF, Janerot-Sjøberg B, Lind B, Grocott-Mason RM, Ionescu AA, Florescu N, Wilkenshoff U, Lancellotti P, *et al*: **Feasibility and reproducibility of off-line tissue doppler measurement of regional myocardial function during dobutamine stress echocardiography.** *Eur J Echocardiogr* 2003, **4**(1):43–53.
8. Gaballa M, Lind B, Storaa C, Brodin L-A: **Intra- and inter-observer reproducibility in off-line extracted cardiac tissue Doppler velocity measurements and derived variables.** *IEEE Eng Med Biol Mag* 2001, **2**:4–6.
9. Kjaergaard J, Korinek J, Belohlavek M, Oh JK, Sogaard P, Hassager C: **Accuracy, reproducibility, and comparability of Doppler tissue imaging by two high-end ultrasound systems.** *J Am Soc Echocardiogr* 2006, **19**(3):322–328.
10. Mårtensson M, Bjallmark A, Brodin LA: **Evaluation of tissue Doppler-based velocity and deformation imaging: a phantom study of ultrasound systems.** *Eur J Echocardiogr* 2011, **12**(6):467–476.
11. Grubb NR, Fleming A, Sutherland GR, Fox KA: **Skeletal muscle contraction in healthy volunteers: assessment with Doppler tissue imaging.** *Radiology* 1995, **194**(3):837–842.
12. Lindberg F, Ohberg F, Granasen G, Brodin LA, Gronlund C: **Pennation angle dependency in skeletal muscle tissue doppler strain in dynamic contractions.** *Ultrasound Med Biol* 2011, **37**(7):1151–1160.
13. Peolsson A, Brodin LA, Peolsson M: **A tissue velocity ultrasound imaging investigation of the dorsal neck muscles during resisted isometric extension.** *Man Ther* 2010, **15**(6):567–573.
14. Peolsson M, Brodin LA, Peolsson A: **Tissue motion pattern of ventral neck muscles investigated by tissue velocity ultrasonography imaging.** *Eur J Appl Physiol* 2010, **109**(5):899–908.
15. Peolsson M, Larsson B, Brodin LA, Gerdle B: **A pilot study using Tissue Velocity Ultrasound Imaging (TVI) to assess muscle activity pattern in patients with chronic trapezius myalgia.** *BMC Musculoskelet Disord* 2008, **9**:127.
16. Pulkovski N, Schenk P, Maffiuletti NA, Mannion AF: **Tissue Doppler imaging for detecting onset of muscle activity.** *Muscle Nerve* 2008, **37**(5):638–649.
17. Mannion AF, Pulkovski N, Schenk P, Hodges PW, Gerber H, Loupas T, Gorelick M, Sprott H: **A new method for the noninvasive determination of abdominal muscle feedforward activity based on tissue velocity information from tissue Doppler imaging.** *J Appl Physiol* 2008, **104**(4):1192–1201.

18. Vasseljen O, Fladmark AM, Westad C, Torp HG: **Onset in abdominal muscles recorded simultaneously by ultrasound imaging and intramuscular electromyography.** *J Electromyogr Kinesiol* 2009, **19**(2):e23–31.
19. Matre K, Ahmed AB, Gregersen H, Heimdal A, Hausken T, Odegaard S, Gilja OH: **In vitro evaluation of ultrasound Doppler strain rate imaging: modification for measurement in a slowly moving tissue phantom.** *Ultrasound Med Biol* 2003, **29**(12):1725–1734.
20. Asakawa DS, Nayak KS, Blemker SS, Delp SL, Pauly JM, Nishimura DG, Gold GE: **Real-time imaging of skeletal muscle velocity.** *J Magn Reson Imaging* 2003, **18**(6):734–739.

5

Hysterosalpingocontrast sonography (HyCoSy): evaluation of the pain perception, side effects and complications

Roberto Marci[1*], Immacolata Marcucci[2], Aurelio Aniceto Marcucci[2], Nicolina Pacini[2], Pietro Salacone[2], Annalisa Sebastianelli[2], Luisa Caponecchia[2], Giuseppe Lo Monte[1] and Rocco Rago[2]

Abstract

Background: Tubal and uterine cavity diseases commonly compromise female fertility. At the present time, hysteroscopy, laparoscopy with chromopertubation and RX-Hysterosalpingography (RX-HSG) are widely accepted screening procedures enabling the effective assessment of both tubal patency and uterine cavity. Nevertheless, consistent evidence supports the reliability of Hysterosalpingocontrast sonography (HyCoSy) in uterine cavity and tubal patency investigation, as a part of the standard infertility work-up. This prospective study was aimed at evaluating the tolerability of the technique as well as the incidence of related side effects and complications in a large series of infertile patients.

Methods: Pain perception of 632 infertile women was measured by means of an 11-point numeric rating scale. Side effects and late complications were also recorded.

Results: The mean numeric rating scale was 2.15 ± 2.0 SD. Most of the patients (374/632, 59.17%) rated HyCoSy as a non-painful procedure, whereas 24.36% (154/632) women reported mild pelvic pain and 9.96% (63/632) classified the discomfort as "moderate". Only 6.48% (41/632) of the patient population experienced severe pelvic pain. Fifteen (2.37%) patients required drug administration for pain relief. Twenty-six patients (4.11%) showed mild vaso-vagal reactions that resolved without atropine administration. No severe vaso-vagal reactions or late complications were observed.

Conclusions: HyCoSy is a well-tolerated examination and the associated vagal effects are unusual and generally mild. Consequently, we support its introduction as a first-line procedure for tubal patency and uterine cavity investigation in infertile women.

Keywords: Tubal patency, Female infertility, HyCoSy, Pain perception, Transvaginal sonography

Background

The etiology and pathophysiology of infertility are unexplained in some couples, but one-third of infertility cases are related to female factor. Tubal and uterine cavity diseases commonly compromise female fertility (14% of couples who require specialist treatment) [1]. In particular, uterine anomalies or structural abnormalities of the fallopian tubes are diagnosed in 3% and 16% infertile women, respectively [2]. For this reason, tubal and uterine examination plays a major role in the evaluation of the infertile couples and it is mandatory before assisted reproductive techniques (ART) such as intrauterine insemination or in vitro fertilization, is started [3]. At the present time, hysteroscopy [4,5], laparoscopy with chromoperturbation and Rx-Hysterosalpingography (RX-HSG) [6] are widely accepted procedures for the assessment of tubal patency and uterine cavity. However, these techniques show several limitations including: long waiting lists in some hospitals, invasiveness (or minimal invasiveness in the case of office hysteroscopy), painfulness and possible surgical and anesthesiologic risks [7]. In addition, RX-HSG is associated to exposure to

* Correspondence: roberto.marci@unife.it
[1]Department of Morphology, Surgery and Experimental medicine, University of Ferrara, Via Aldo Moro 8, Ferrara, Cona 44124, Italy
Full list of author information is available at the end of the article

ionizing radiations and involves the direct injection of a iodinated contrast agent into the uterine cavity, possibly resulting in atopic phenomena [8]. In the last 10 years, Hysterosalpingocontrast sonography (HyCoSy) has been introduced in clinical practice as an effective tool for tubal patency and uterine cavity evaluation (Figures 1, 2 and 3). This investigation is considered safe, well tolerated, rapid, easy to perform and inexpensive [9,10]. HyCoSy is a transvaginal sonography in which a galactose solution containing galactose microbubbles or an inexpensive mixture of air and saline solution is injected into the uterine cavity using a cervical catheter. Several studies [6,9-19] have shown that HyCoSy displays high specificity and sensitivity in tubal patency and uterine cavity assessment. On the contrary, only limited evidence is available on both the tolerability and the real incidence of side effects and complications related to this procedure. This prospective study was aimed at evaluating these parameters in a large series of infertile patients undergoing HyCoSy for tubal patency and the uterine cavity assessment.

Methods

Six hundred thirty-two infertile women, who referred to our clinic between January 2008 and November 2012, were consecutively enrolled. Patients underwent HyCoSy at the Andrology and Pathophysiology of Reproduction Unit of S. Maria Goretti Hospital in Latina. This work has been carried out in accordance with The Code of Ethics of the World Medical Association (Declaration of Helsinki) for experiments involving humans. Approval from the institution's ethics committee has been obtained before starting the study. The aim of the examination as well as the possible side effects and complications associated to the procedure were explained to the patients and informed consent was provided in each case before starting the procedure. The clinical data of the study group are summarized in Table 1. Exclusion criteria were a history of infertility lasting less than one year, abnormal bleeding, active pelvic infections and uterine malignancies. We performed pelvic examination, Pap smearing test and transvaginal ultrasound before HyCoSy. Vaginal and cervical swabs as well as blood samples for hormonal profile and serologic markers were also taken. Women did not receive any pain medication or antibiotic treatment before undergoing the procedure. The patients were examined in the lithotomic position, during the first phase of the menstrual cycle (day 9–11 of menstrual cycle). Patients were asked to use contraceptives or avoid sexual intercourse from the last menstrual period until the day of the exam. A preliminary transvaginal ultrasound was performed by two skilled operators with a 7 MHz probe (Logiq 5 Expert GE, GE Healthcare, United Kingdom) in order to exclude any uterine or adnexal pathology and to localize the ovaries and the interstitial part of the salpinges before the injection of the ultrasound contrast medium. The vulva and the cervix were previously disinfected with chlorhexidine. A 5 F stylet catheter (CooperSurgical, Germany) was placed into the cervical os under direct visualization and the balloon was filled with 1–1.5 ml of saline solution to fix the catheter and prevent saline backflow. Then, saline solution (0.9% sodium chloride) was slowly injected. The uterine cavity was evaluated on transverse and longitudinal images. The operator subsequently injected into the catheter a total volume of 10 to 20 mL saline solution alternated to little

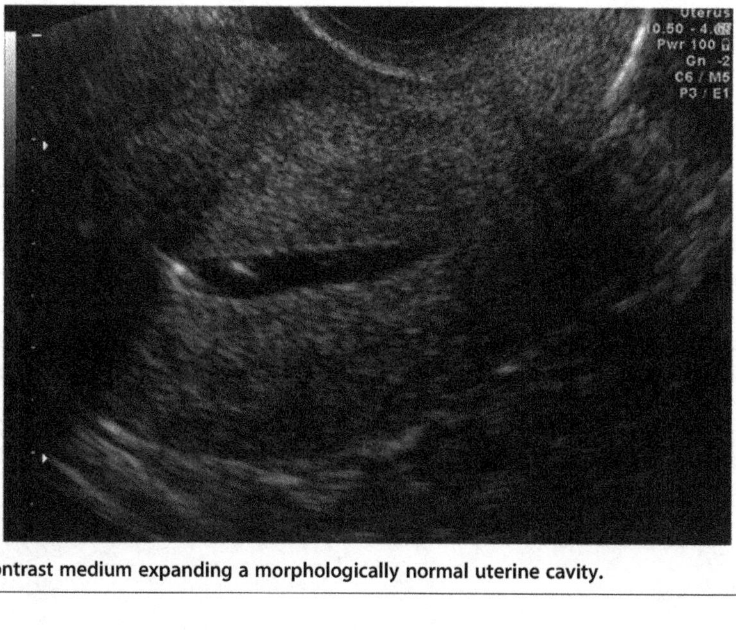

Figure 1 HyCoSy: saline contrast medium expanding a morphologically normal uterine cavity.

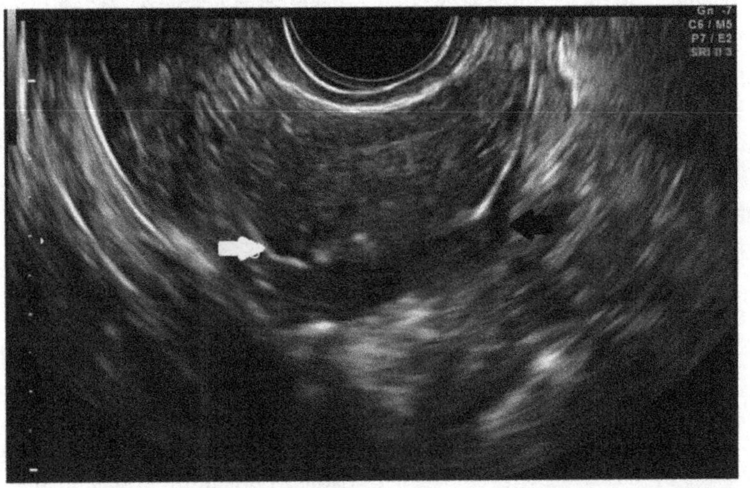

Figure 2 HyCoSy: direct visualization of bilateral tubal patency. (Black arrow: right tube; white arrow: left tube).

boluses of air. Air bubbles, that are highly echogenic, would facilitate checking the patency of the fallopian tubes. The patency of a tube was determined by the passage of air bubbles through the tube and/or the presence of liquid and air in the abdominal cavity near the ovarian fossas. At the end of the procedure, the patients were monitored for about 15 minutes in supine position in order to prevent the onset of vasovagal reactions or scapular pain, due to the irritation of the phrenic nerve. After the execution of the HyCoSy, all participants were asked about the pain (type, location, duration, irradiation) they experienced. In order to quantify pain perception during the procedure we used an 11-point (0 to 10) numerical rating scale, on which 0 corresponded to no pain at all and 10 indicated severe pain. The patients were familiarized with the scale before the procedure was performed. In accordance to Savelli et al. [20], pelvic pain was classified as "absent", "mild", "moderate" and "severe" when rated as 0, 1 to 4, 5 to 7 and 8 to 10, respectively.

Results

The mean overall numeric rating scale was 2.15 ± 2.0 SD. The duration of the procedure, from the insertion to the extraction of the catheter, ranged from 10 to 20 minutes. The majority of patients (374/632; 59.17%) considered HyCoSy a non-painful procedure, whereas 24.36% (154/632) reported mild pelvic pain and 9.96% (63/632) classified the discomfort as "moderate". Only 6.48% (41/632) of the population experienced severe

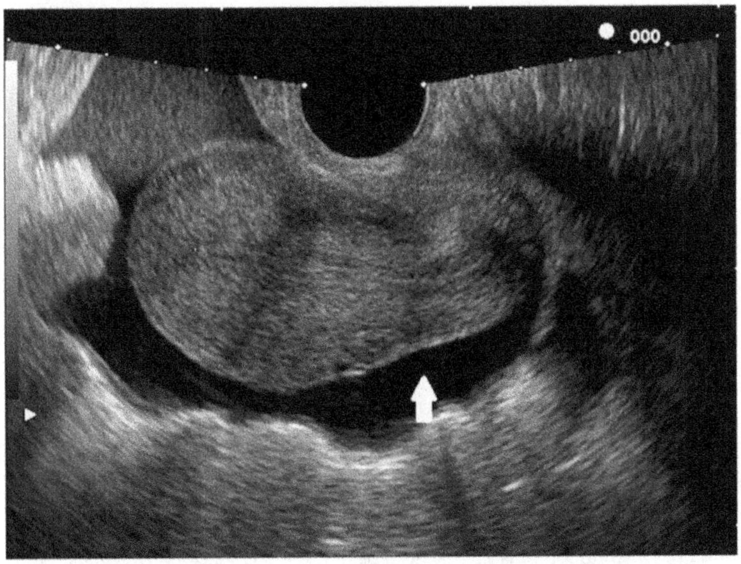

Figure 3 HyCoSy: the periuterine fluid collection (white arrow) is an indirect sign of tubal patency.

Table 1 Clinical features of the patients who underwent HyCoSy

	N (%)
N. of patients	632
Mean age (years)	33.2 ± 5.4 SD (range 22–44)
Mean infertility duration (months)	60.4 ± 31.2 SD (range 24–96)
Primary infertility	452/632 (71.5%)
Secondary infertility	180/632 (28.5%)
Associated pelvic diseases	191/632 (30.2%)
• Myomas	• 95/632 (15%)
• Pelvic endometriosis	• 54/632 (8.5%)
• Uterine congenital malformations	• 37/632 (5.8%)
• Endometrial polyps	• 5/632 (0.8%)
Tubal patency:	
• Monolateral	503/632 (79.5%)
• Bilateral	53/632 (8.3%)
• Bilateral occlusion	76/632 (12%)

pelvic pain. After HyCoSy, 15 (2.37%) patients required drug administration for pain relief. Twenty-six patients (4.11%) showed mild vaso-vagal reactions (pallor, nausea, sudation, hypotension, bradycardia) that resolved without atropine administration. No severe vaso-vagal reactions (vomiting, confusion, syncope) and late complications (haemorrhage, pelvic inflammatory disease (PID), fever) were reported. We diagnosed bilateral tubal patency in 79.5% (503/632) women, unilateral patency in 8.3% (53/632) and bilateral tubal occlusion in 12.02% (76/632). In 56/632 (8.8%) patients HyCoSy was not conclusive and the exam was repeated during the subsequent menstrual cycle. Women who underwent examination for the second time considered HyCoSy less painful than the first time (mean overall numeric rating scale 2.9 vs 6.4) (Figure 4). The second HyCoSy revealed bilateral tubal patency in 62.5% (35/56) cases and monolateral tubal patency in 21.4% (12/56), whilst diagnostic laparoscopy or RX-HSG were needed to set a definitive diagnosis in the remaining 16% (9/56) cases. In 191/632 (30%) cases we demonstrated an associated pelvic disease. The clinical features of the patient population as well as the main results of the study are summarized in Table 1 and Table 2.

Discussion

According to several studies, HyCoSy shows high overall accuracy in the evaluation of both tubal patency and uterine cavity morphology [6-19]. Furthermore, HyCoSy avoids both exposure to ionizing radiation and injection of iodinated contrast medium that could potentially result toxic. In addition, HyCoSy is inexpensive, fast and devoid of surgical and anestesthesiologic risks, as opposed to laparoscopy with chromopertubation and hysteroscopy [7,8]. As other diagnostic methods, HyCoSy does not always provide exhaustive information about

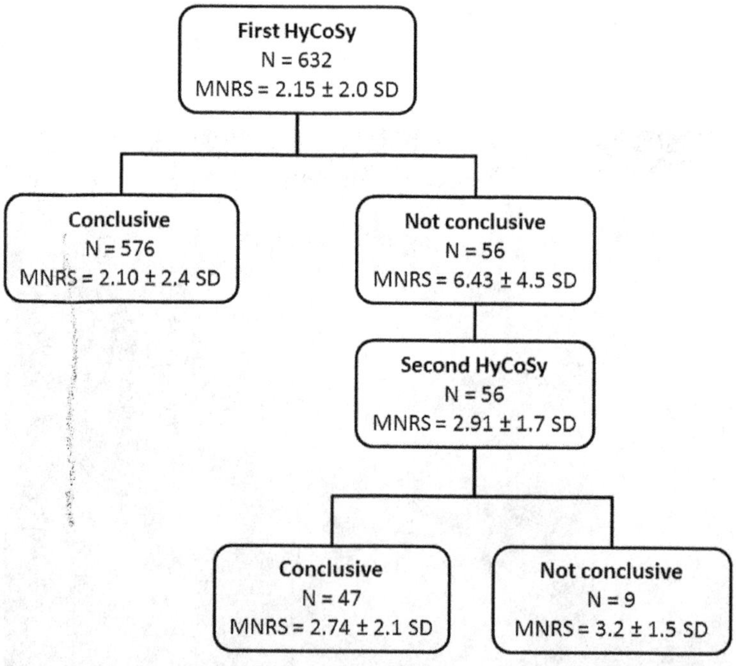

Figure 4 Flowchart representing the distribution of women who repeated HyCoSy twice (MNRS, mean numeric rating scale; SD, standard deviation).

Table 2 Pain perception, side effects and complications

	N (%)
Mean numeric rating scale	2.15 ± 2.0 SD
Pain perception:	
• Absent	374/632 (59.17%)
• Mild	154/632 (24.36%)
• Moderate	63/632 (9.96%)
• Severe	41/632 (6.49%)
Painkiller required	15/632 (2.37%)
Mild vaso-vagal reactions (pallor, nausea, sudation, hypotension, bradycardia)	26/632 (4.11%)
Severe vaso-vagal reactions (vomiting, confusion, syncope)	0/632 (0%)
Complications (haemorrhage, PID, fever)	0/632 (0%)

tubal and uterine cavity morphology [16]; in particular, it could display misleading images in case of distal tubal obstruction or complicated pelvic diseases (i.e. PID, endometriosis, previous appendicitis, abdomino-pelvic inflammation) [15]. In such doubtful clinical conditions, laparoscopy with chromoperturbation and hysteroscopy should still be considered the "gold standard" for tubal and uterine cavity assessment, respectively.

Our data prove that HyCoSy is a well-tolerated examination and it is associated to a low incidence of related complications and side-effects. The pain experienced by the patients is usually mild and comparable to the cramping pain felt during a normal menstrual cycle. Similar findings are reported by Savelli et al. in a prospective study [20]. The Authors evaluated pain perception by means of an 11-point numeric rating scale in 669 infertile women undergoing HyCoSy. The mean numeric rating scale was 2.7 ± 2.5, only 2% of patients required a painkiller for pain relief and mild or severe vasovagal reactions were observed in 4.1% and 0.8% cases, respectively. Our data concerning pain experience during HyCoSy are compared to those provided by Savelli et al. in Figure 5. In both studies only few patients reported moderate/severe pain. The only difference concerns the number of patients who felt no pain at all or mild discomfort. However, we observed that several women were frequently unable to distinguish clearly whether the sensation experienced during the examination, and in particular after the inflation of the balloon into the cervical canal, was slightly painful or just a nuisance comparable to the insertion of the vaginal speculum. As a result, we believe that the findings of the two studies are similar.

In another recent study Graziano et al. evaluated efficacy, compliance and cost effectiveness of HyCoSy, hysteroscopy, and RX-HSG for uterine cavity evaluation and tubal patency determination [21]. HyCoSy showed high sensitivity, specificity, positive predictive values (PPV) and negative predictive values (NPV) and did not display any significant difference when compared to hysteroscopy. Additionally, HyCoSy proved to be as accurate as RX-HSG in detecting a monolateral or bilateral tubal obstruction. Finally HyCoSy was associated to milder pain perception and lower costs when compared to RX-HSG and hysteroscopy. In particular, the Authors assessed pain by means of an 8-point (0 to 7) numerical rating scale on which 0 corresponded to no pain at all and 7 indicated severe pain. Pelvic pain was classified as "absent", "mild", "moderate" and "severe" when rated as 0–1, 2–3, 4–5 and 6–7, respectively. An "absent-mild" discomfort was reported in 80.84% women undergoing HyCoSy, in 52.9% women undergoing hysteroscopy and in 9.1% patients undergoing RX-HSG. Ayida et al. compared HyCoSy to conventional RX-HSG as to the tolerability of the procedure [8]. Sixty-six subfertile women underwent one of the two screening procedures, all performed by the same operator. No significant difference in reported procedure time, amount of contrast medium used, patient tolerability or adverse effects was

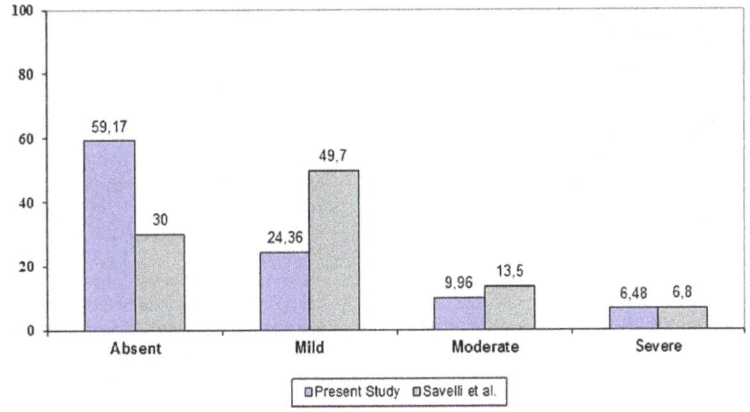

Figure 5 Evaluation of pain perception in our series and data reported by Savelli et al., 2009.

found. In a recent study by Socolov et al., the pain experience of 121 infertile women who underwent both HyCoSy and RX-HSG was analysed [10]. Pain perception was measured using a self-assessment questionnaire. On the basis of the results obtained, HyCoSy was suggested to be a well-tolerated diagnostic procedure, associated with few or mild vagal effects. During HyCoSy pain was rated as slightly higher than during RX-HSG. The correlation between pain perception and other independent variables pertaining to the HyCoSy procedure (i.e. a difficult catheter passage, amount of contrast medium injected, unilateral or bilateral tubal blockage, presence of IgG antibodies to Chlamydia, menstrual cycle phase) was also investigated **in the afore-mentioned study**. The only strong association found concerned the volume of injected contrast medium. The higher volume of contrast medium injected during HyCoSy seems to explain the significantly higher pain level reported.

Pain perception during HyCoSy could be due to uterine distension after saline solution infusion. The mechanical distension of the uterine walls could cause the release of local prostaglandins, resulting in uterine cramps [22]. Although convincing, this hypothesis has been disconfirmed by a recent study. In fact it was demonstrated that a preventive administration of antispasmodic drug such as hyoscine-N-butylbromide, a muscarinic receptor antagonist with anticholinergic effects, does not decrease pain during HyCoSy by affecting uterine contractions [23].

In addition, HyCoSy could also play a therapeutic role in subfertile women. In our infertility centre we noticed that spontaneous pregnancies often occurred in patients who underwent HyCoSy in the previous 3–6 months [24]. Lindborg et al. [25], recently suggested a valid explanation for this phenomenon: the passage of the fluid through a partially occluded tube (minor adhesions, mucus plugs) could remove minor adhesions or buildup material caused by inflammatory processes and hence restore tubal patency.

Conclusions

HyCoSy is a well-tolerated procedure and the associated vagal effects are unusual and generally mild. It is a safe, efficient and non-invasive diagnostic examination. Furthermore, it provides useful information for the management of infertile couples. Therefore we support its use as a first-line procedure for the evaluation of both the uterine cavity and the tubal patency in infertile women.

Abbreviations

(HyCoSy): Hysterosonocontrast sonography; (RX-HSG): RX-hysterosalpingography; (ART): Assisted reproductive techniques; (PID): Pelvic inflammatory disease.

Competing interests

Authors declare to have no commercial and/or financial interest with manufacturers of pharmaceuticals, laboratory supplies, and/or medical devices; they declare to have no relationship with commercial providers of medically related services.

Authors' contributions

RM has substantially contributed to design, preparation, drafting and revising the intellectual content of the final version of the manuscript. IM has substantially contributed to data collection, to the diagnostic process, to the preoperative and operative work up linked to the condition of the patient, to preparation, drafting and revising the final version of the manuscript. He also gave an extremely important intellectual support. AAM has substantially contributed to data collection, to the diagnostic process, to the preoperative and operative work up linked to the condition of the patient. NP has substantially contributed to data collection, to the diagnostic process, to the preoperative and operative work up linked to the condition of the patient. PS has substantially contributed to data collection, to the diagnostic process, to the preoperative and operative work up linked to the condition of the patient. AS has substantially contributed to data collection, to the diagnostic process, to the preoperative and operative work up linked to the condition of the patient. LC has substantially contributed to data collection, to the diagnostic process, to the preoperative and operative work up linked to the condition of the patient. GL has substantially contributed to design, preparation, drafting and revising the intellectual content of the final version of the manuscript. RR has substantially contributed to data collection, to the diagnostic process, to the preoperative and operative work up linked to the condition of the patient, to preparation, drafting and revising the final version of the manuscript. He also gave an extremely important intellectual support. All authors read and approved the final manuscript.

Author details

[1]Department of Morphology, Surgery and Experimental medicine, University of Ferrara, Via Aldo Moro 8, Ferrara, Cona 44124, Italy. [2]Department of Andrology and Pathophysiology of Reproduction, S. Maria Goretti Hospital, Latina, Italy.

References

1. Das S, Nardo LG, Seif MW: **Proximal tubal disease: the place for tubal cannulation.** *Reprod Biomed Online* 2007, **15**:383–388.
2. Spira A: **Epidemiology of human reproduction.** *Hum Reprod* 1986, **1**:111–115.
3. ESHRE Capri Workshop Group: **Diagnosis and management of the infertile couple: missing information.** *Hum Reprod Update* 2004, **10**:295–307.
4. Mencaglia L, Colafranceschi M, Gordon AG, Lindemann H, Van Herendael B, Perino A, De Placido G, Colacurci A, Van der Pas H, Tantini C, *et al*: **Is hysteroscopy of value in the investigation of female infertility?** *Acta Eur Fertil* 1988, **19**:239–241.
5. Mollo A, De Franciscis P, Colacurci N, Cobellis L, Perino A, Venlezia R, Alviggi C, De Placido G: **Hysteroscopic resection of the septum improves the pregnancy rate of women with unexplained infertility: a prospective controlled trial.** *Fertil Steril* 2009, **91**:2628–2631.
6. Saunders RD, Shwayder JM, Nakajima ST: **Current methods of tubal patency assessment.** *Fertil Steril* 2011, **95**:2171–2179.
7. Jansen FW, Kapiteyn K, Trimbos-Kemper T, Hermans J, Trimbos JB: **Complications of laparoscopy: a prospective, multicentre, observationational study.** *Br J Obstet Gynaecol* 1997, **104**:595–600.
8. Ayada G, Kennedy S, Barlow D, Chamberlain P: **A comparison of patient tolerance of hysterosalpingo-contrast sonography (HyCoSy) with Echovist ®-200 and X-ray hysterosalpingography for outpatient investigation of infertile women.** *Ultrasound Obstet Gynecol* 1996, **7**:201–204.
9. Luciano DE, Exacoustos C, Johns DA, Luciano AA: **Can hysterosalpingo-contrast sonography replace hysterosalpingography in confirming tubal blockage after hysteroscopic sterilization and in the evaluation of the uterus and tubes in infertile patients?** *Am J Obstet Gynecol* 2011, **204**(79):e1–e5.
10. Graziano A, Lo Monte G, Soave I, Caserta D, Moscarini M, Marci R: **Sonohysterosalpingography: a suitable choice in infertility workup.** *J Med Ultrasonics* 2013, **40**:225–229.

11. Lim CP, Hasafa Z, Bhattacharya S, Maheshwari A: **Should a hysterosalpingogram be a first-line investigation to diagnose female tubal subfertility in the modern subfertility workup?** *Hum Reprod* 2011, **26:**967–971.
12. Tanawattanacharoen S, Suwajanakorn S, Uerpairojkit B, Boonkasemsanti W, Virutamasen P: **Transvaginal hysterosalpingo-contrast sonography (HyCoSy) compared with chromolaparoscopy.** *J Obstet Gynaecol Res* 2000, **26:**71–75.
13. Stacey C, Bown C, Manhire A, Rose D: **HyCoSy–as good as claimed?** *Br J Radiol* 2000, **73:**133–136.
14. Hamilton JA, Larson AJ, Lower AM, Hasnain S, Grudzinskas JG: **Evaluation of the performance of hysterosalpingo contrast sonography in 500 consecutive, unselected, infertile women.** *Hum Reprod* 1998, **13:**1519–1526.
15. Volpi E, Zuccaro G, Patriarca A, Rustichelli S, Sismondi P: **Transvaginal sonographic tubal patency testing using air and saline solution as contrast mesia in a routine infertility clinic setting.** *Ultrasound Obstet Gynecol* 1996, **7:**43–48.
16. Alborzi S, Dehbashi S, Khodaee R: **Sonohysterosalpingographic screening for infertile patients.** *Int J Gynaecol Obstet* 2003, **82:**57–62.
17. Radic V, Canic T, Valetic J, Duic Z: **Advantages and disadvantages of hysterosonosalpingography in the assessment of the reproductive status of the uterine cavity and fallopian tubes.** *Eur J Radiol* 2005, **53:**268–273.
18. Exacoustos C, Zupi E, Carusotti C, Lanzi G, Marconi D, Arduini D: **Hysterosalpingo-contrast sonography compared with hysterosalpingography and laparoscopic dye perturbation to evaluate tubal patency.** *J Am assoc Gynecol Laparosc* 2003, **10:**367–372.
19. Van den Bosch T, Verguts J, Daemen A, Gevaert O, Domali E, Claerhout F, Vandenbroucke V, De Moor B, Deprest J, Timmerman D: **Pain experienced during transvaginal ultrasound, saline contrast sonohysterography, hysteroscopy and office sampling: a comparative study.** *Ultrasound Obstet Gynecol* 2008, **31:**346–351.
20. Savelli L, Pollastri P, Guerrini M, Villa G, Manuzzi L, Mabrouk M, Rossi S, Serracchioli R: **Tolerability, side effects, and complications of Hysterosalpingocontrast sonography (HyCoSy).** *Fertil Steril* 2009, **92:**1481–1486.
21. Socolov D, Boian I, Boiculese L, Tamba B, Anghelache-Lupascu I, Socolov R: **Comparison of the pain experienced by infertile women undergoing hysterosalpingo contrast sonography or radiographic hysterosalpingography.** *Int J Gynaecol Obstet* 2010, **111:**256–259.
22. Guney M, Oral B, Bayhan G, Mungan T: **Intrauterine lidocaine infusion for pain relief during saline solution infusion sonohysterography: a randomized, controlled trial.** *J Minim Invasive Gynecol* 2007, **14:**304–310.
23. Moro F, Selvaggi L, Sagnella F, Morciano A, Martinez D, Gangale MF, Ciardulli A, Palla C, Uras ML, De Feo E, Boccia S, Tropea A, Lanzone A, Apa R: **Could antispasmodic drug reduce pain during hysterosalpingo-contrast sonography (HyCoSy) in infertile patients? A randomized double-blind clinical trial.** *Ultrasound Obstet Gynecol* 2012, **39:**260–265.
24. Giugliano E, Cagnazzo E, Bazzan E, Patella A, Marci R: **HyCoSy: is possible to quantify the therapeutic effect of a diagnostic test?** *Clin Exp Reprod Med* 2012, **39:**161–165.
25. Lindborg L, Thorburn J, Bergh C, Strandell A: **Influence of HyCoSy on spontaneous pregnancy: a randomized controlled trial.** *Hum Reprod* 2009, **24:**1075–1079.

6

Dynamic ultrasound imaging — A multivariate approach for the analysis and comparison of time-dependent musculoskeletal movements

Tommy Löfstedt, Olof Ahnlund, Michael Peolsson and Johan Trygg*

Abstract

Background: Muscle functions are generally assumed to affect a wide variety of conditions and activities, including pain, ischemic and neurological disorders, exercise and injury. It is therefore very desirable to obtain more information on musculoskeletal contributions to and activity during clinical processes such as the treatment of muscle injuries, post-surgery evaluations, and the monitoring of progressive degeneration in neuromuscular disorders.

The spatial image resolution achievable with ultrasound systems has improved tremendously in the last few years and it is nowadays possible to study skeletal muscles in real-time during activity. However, ultrasound imaging has an inherent problem that makes it difficult to compare different measurement series or image sequences from two or more subjects. Due to physiological differences between different subjects, the ultrasound sequences will be visually different – partly because of variation in probe placement and partly because of the difficulty of perfectly reproducing any given movement.

Methods: Ultrasound images of the biceps and calf of a single subject were transformed to achieve congruence and then efficiently compressed and stacked to facilitate analysis using a multivariate method known as O2PLS. O2PLS identifies related and unrelated variation in and between two sets of data such that different phases of the studied movements can be analysed. The methodology was used to study the dynamics of the Achilles tendon and the calf and also the Biceps brachii and upper arm. The movements of these parts of the body are both of interest in clinical orthopaedic research.

Results: This study extends the novel method of multivariate analysis of congruent images (MACI) to facilitate comparisons between two series of ultrasound images. This increases its potential range of medical applications and its utility for detecting, visualising and quantifying the dynamics and functions of skeletal muscle.

Conclusions: The most important results of this study are that MACI with O2PLS is able to consistently extract meaningful variability from pairs of ultrasound sequences. The MACI method with O2PLS is a powerful tool with great potential for visualising and comparing dynamics between movements. It has many potential clinical applications in the study of muscle injuries, post-surgery evaluations and evaluations of rehabilitation, and the assessment of athletic training interventions.

Keywords: Ultrasound, Medical imaging, Wavelet transform, Musculoskeletal movements, Multivariate data analysis, O2PLS, Speckle tracking

* Correspondence: johan.trygg@chem.umu.se
Computational Life Science Cluster (CLiC), Department of Chemistry, Umeå University, Umeå, Sweden

Background

Medical imaging is a rich source of information in the diagnostic process. Variation in characteristics of interest can be identified, compared, and correlated to specific symptoms and clinical findings by analysing patterns observed within the imaged tissues. These patterns can be used to determine whether tissues are benign or malign, and intact or repaired. Imaging can thus be used to test the effectiveness of remedies and evaluate the effects of treatments for specific diseases.

The aim of our studies is to develop tools to detect, visualise and quantify skeletal muscle dynamics and functionality using ultrasound imaging and multivariate image analysis. The strategic significance of such tools is very high since they could be applied in muscle rehabilitation programmes (including sports medicine) and the treatment of neurological disorders (e.g. whiplash and fibromyalgia) and pain-related conditions (e.g. back pain).

The quality of ultrasound imaging has evolved rapidly, and modern equipment is capable of recording images with good spatial resolution at high frame rates. This makes ultrasound imaging suitable for the analysis of both structural and functional aspects of muscles. For example, it has been used to study tendon injuries in sports medicine [1] and inflammation processes [2,3].

Ultrasound imaging has been used to study tissue movements for a couple of decades. A period of training is required before good registrations can be captured, but studies focusing on ultrasound validation of the tendon tracking have accurately quantified tendon displacements without reference to anatomical landmarks [4], and exhibit high repeatability within and between both subjects and examiners [5,6].

There are important differences between structural imaging studies and dynamic studies of functional movements. In the first case, the patient remains still while the clinician moves the ultrasound probe. Conversely, in dynamic studies, the patient is asked to perform a movement and the clinician holds the ultrasound probe still relative to an anatomical landmark [7,8]. The latter approach was adopted in this work. Furthermore, structural assessments are based on single images while dynamic analyses are based on series of images recorded while the patient performs specific movements. Dynamic and structural studies thus have different and complementary emphases.

Ultrasound images of tissue consist of a set of intensity values that form a mosaic image in shades of grey. This mosaic consists of speckles that create patterns, which can be regarded as "fingerprints" of specific tissue components. If the probe remains in the same position during a movement, the changes in the speckle patterns represent movements in the tissue. These movements can be directly and actively followed using speckle-tracking software. A Region of Interest (ROI) is an area that is identified in the first frame of an ultrasound sequence and then followed frame by frame. Movements of the tissue over the course of an image sequence can be "observed" and quantified by monitoring changes in the position of the ROI. If the discrete wavelet transform is used, these changes in intensity, which represent actual muscle tissue movements, are indirectly and passively observed as they pass by the "observer" (the variable, the wavelet coefficient). When images of this kind are analyzed using techniques such as O2PLS, movements of specific muscle tissues are represented by multiple variables that together describe individual phenomena within the sequence. The data analysis aspect is therefore to identify the systematic structures in the pixel variations present in the subsequent images that best describe the movement being performed.

Ultrasound imaging has an inherent problem when comparing two different measurement series or comparing image sequences from two or more subjects. Since different subjects will invariably have various physiological differences, there will be visual differences between their ultrasound sequences. This is partly due to differences in probe placement and partly to the difficulty of exactly duplicating any given movement.

This paper describes a method that facilitates the comparison of two ultrasound sequences based on combining the O2PLS method and Multivariate Analysis of Congruent Images (MACI). MACI [9,10] is a powerful tool for analysing and visualising the dynamics of muscle tissues in ultrasonic B-mode grey scan image sequences [10]. It is based on the discrete wavelet transform that effectively compresses image sequences while preserving information relating to time and shape.

This article explains the flexibility of MACI and demonstrates that it can be readily used to compare ultrasound image sequences. The method has two components: the discrete wavelet transform and multivariate data analysis using O2PLS. The wavelet transform is used to extract position, size and shape information that is present in greyscale B-scan ultrasound image sequences captured while performing muscular movements. This approach has two key advantages over conventional image analysis [9]. First, while conventional methods deal only with the intensities of individual pixels, MACI also analyses pixel intensities across larger regions as a whole. This eliminates problems with non-congruency. Second, the application of O2PLS to the wavelet-transformed images makes it possible to compare sequences and identify similarities and differences. In previous studies, we have performed MACI using PCA [10] rather than O2PLS. O2PLS is advantageous in this context because it can be used to compare two full length registrations, e.g. one from a healthy individual and another from an injured person, or registrations from a person before and after an intervention. Third, the results of multivariate O2PLS analyses can be further manipulated using a range of statistical tools to perform comparisons, cluster analyses, discrimination analyses, and so on. All of these increase the scope for describing the functional and dynamic aspects of skeletal muscle movements.

Methods

Modelling Tissue Dynamics

The basis of image analysis is that an $M \times N$ two-dimensional digital intensity image can be regarded as a function, $I(x, y)$, with an intensity value for every point (x, y) of the image [11].

When several such 2D images are stacked upon one-another, a multivariate image space is created. In this work, stacks of ultrasound images were created in which each layer of the stack represented a specific time point. In such a multivariate image space, when looking from the top of the stack, each location (i.e. pixel) is represented by a series of greyscale values (with one value for each image in the sequence) and so the stack contains a very large amount of highly correlated data. Various unfolding procedures can be used to analyse these 3D data structures [12-14].

The feature extraction procedure used in this work is based on the discrete 2D wavelet transform (2D-DWT). In this method, images are compressed by choosing the wavelet coefficients that hold the most information about the ultrasound sequence. These coefficients are found by ordering them according to their variance (importance) and choosing the n variables with the highest variance, i.e. the coefficients with the highest information content. The selected wavelet coefficients are then stored in a regular two-way data table where each row represents an image and each column contains the wavelet coefficients for the images. Multivariate analysis is then performed on the two-way data tables of wavelet coefficients.

O2PLS

O2PLS is an extension of Partial least squares regression (PLS-R) and Orthogonal projections to latent structures (OPLS) [15] invented by Johan Trygg in 2002 [16,17]. O2PLS creates a model linking two matrices X and Y. In this article, X and Y are two ultrasound sequences that could represent two movements performed by the same subject or the same movements performed by two subjects. In O2PLS, the variation in X and Y is divided into four parts. The first two describe the joint $X \leftrightarrow Y$ covariation, i.e. what in X is linearly related to Y, and what in Y is linearly related to X. The remaining parts describe what in X is unrelated to Y and what in Y is unrelated to$X$. All of these parts can be analysed separately. O2PLS is very similar to PLS regression [18-20] and OPLS, and has properties in common with both methods, but O2PLS increases the *interpretability* of the resulting model.

The O2PLS model comprises the four model matrices and two residual matrices. The relationships between these matrices are as follows:

$$X = T_k P_k^T + T_{o,l} P_{o,l}^T + E$$

and

$$Y = U_k C_k^T + U_{o,m} Q_{o,m}^T + F$$

where the o subscript refers to the unrelated variation in X and Y, k, l and m are the number of latent variables in each matrix, T contains the X-scores, P contains the X-loadings, U contains the Y-scores, and Q contains the Y-loadings. E and F are the residual matrices.

O2PLS was performed using SIMCA-P+ 12.0 (MKS Umetrics AB, Umeå, Sweden). The cross validation procedure in SIMCA-P+ 12.0 was used to determine how many related and unrelated components should be used. Note that the number of components needed for any given analysis depends on the purpose of the study. The number of components suggested by cross validation is equal to the number of dimensions in the space that are significantly different from noise. Conversely, it is usually sufficient to consider only the two "largest" dimensions (components) to identify the movement phases (as discussed below). When analysing other important forms of variation, however, it may be necessary to consider greater numbers of components in order to extract the most important information.

Multivariate analysis of congruent images

Multivariate analysis of congruent images (MACI) is used to find and express patterns over multivariate image spaces in order to classify or study relationships between images [9]. The main goals of multivariate image analysis are first to compress the highly correlated data in terms of a few linear combinations of the intensity values, and second to preserve the spatial information in the images.

A set of images is said to be congruent if they have been properly pre-processed (i.e. transformed) such that each element in any given image corresponds to the same element in all of the other images. If the image series is not fully congruent to begin with (as is generally true), it must be made so [4,12-14,21]. In this work, the discrete 2D wavelet transform (2D-DWT) using the Symlet 8 wavelet basis was applied to each image in the series to make them congruent. The 2D-DWT was used to extract spatial (position) and frequency (shape and size) data from the images.

Once obtained, the wavelet coefficients for each image (i.e. observation) are recorded in the rows of an ordinary two-way data table that can be analysed using conventional multivariate methods such as PCA or O2PLS to extract information. In this work, these data sets were analysed using MACI in conjunction with O2PLS.

The development of wavelet-based texture analysis methods has greatly expanded the scope of multivariate data analysis techniques of this kind in recent years [22].

The principles of MACI are illustrated in Figure 1, which shows the transformation of a series of B-scan ultrasound images into a score plot using the 2D-DWT.

Speckle tracking

The acoustic patterns in an ultrasound signal change in response to the activation of the muscle being scanned when the probe is held in a fixed position relative to an anatomical landmark. These acoustic markers, or speckle patterns, remain relatively stable over time and can therefore be followed frame-by-frame in a sequence of images [23].

In the examples discussed below, speckle tracking was performed using an in-house post-processing software package in order to obtain a reference analysis of some of the different phases of the movements and to show how much movement there is in different anatomical regions at different times.

The first step in speckle tracking is to specify a rectangular region of interest (ROI) in a particular frame. The objective is then to find the region in the next frame that is most similar to the selected region according to some criterion. The objective is thus to find the values of Δx and Δy that minimise

$$\epsilon = \sum_{y} \sum_{x} [I(x,y,t) - I(x+\Delta x, y+\Delta y, t+1)]^2 w(x,y),$$

Where I is the image intensity, x and y are the pixel coordinates at time (or for frame) t, and w is a weighting function that takes a value of 1 in the simplest case.

In the examples presented below, the ROIs were defined in the first frame of each series and the movements were captured in the following frames using a frame-by-frame approach. There are two directional components to the movements of the ankle: towards and away from the knee (dorsal and plantar flexion, respectively). Vector flow fields were created from the speckle tracks in order to illustrate changes in direction and to highlight the movement patterns of the different anatomical regions in each phase.

The algorithm does not always follow speckles correctly when the analysed tissue changes rapidly or is significantly deformed. This can also happen if out-of-plane motions occur. However, current research indicates that despite these limitations, speckle tracking is well suited for studying skeletal muscle movements [24,25].

The speckle tracking algorithm used in the in-house speckle tracking software is the recent optical flow method developed by Farnebäck [26], as implemented in the open source computer vision library (OpenCV) version 2.0 (http://opencv.willowgarage.com/wiki/).

The accuracy and reproducibility of results obtained using our in-house speckle tracking software has been tested, yielding good to excellent intra-class correlation coefficients (unpublished data).

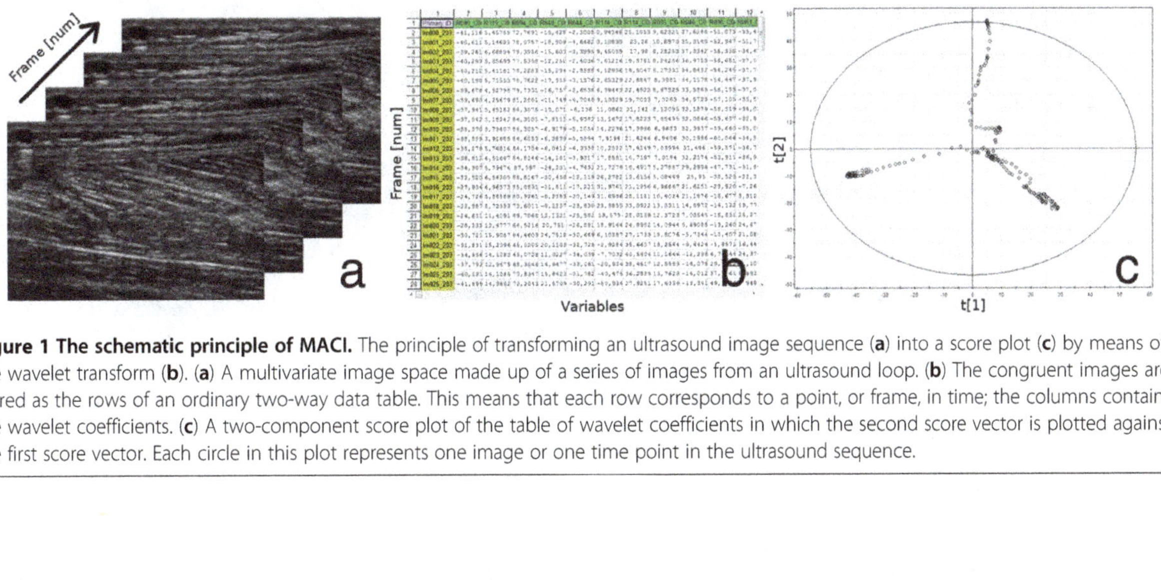

Figure 1 The schematic principle of MACI. The principle of transforming an ultrasound image sequence (**a**) into a score plot (**c**) by means of the wavelet transform (**b**). (**a**) A multivariate image space made up of a series of images from an ultrasound loop. (**b**) The congruent images are stored as the rows of an ordinary two-way data table. This means that each row corresponds to a point, or frame, in time; the columns contain the wavelet coefficients. (**c**) A two-component score plot of the table of wavelet coefficients in which the second score vector is plotted against the first score vector. Each circle in this plot represents one image or one time point in the ultrasound sequence.

Experimental setup

Two examples are presented to illustrate the usefulness of O2PLS MACI. The first example illustrates its reliability and deals with captures of the Achilles tendon in a single subject performing a specific ankle movement. The second example concerns two very disjunctive captures (one longitudinal and one transversal) of the biceps brachii of the same subject, performing a maximal voluntary contraction.

When capturing the ultrasound loops, the ultrasound system (Vivid 7, GE Healthcare, Horten, Norway) was used in conjunction with a linear 12 MHz ultrasound probe. Movements were captured at 78.6 frames per second (FPS) with a resulting time resolution of approximately 13 ms between frames; the lateral resolution was 0.5 mm.

Since only the captures of the first example were controlled, the captures of the second example had to be synced during post-processing. This was done by specifying a beginning and an end frame for the movement, and linearly removing frames located between these two points within the longer sequence.

Example 1: Capturing the movement of the Achilles tendon

The first example deals with an unloaded passive dorsal flexion ankle movement and illustrates the reliability of the O2PLS-MACI method, demonstrating that O2PLS extracts the same information from two separate sequences showing the same healthy subject performing a single movement. The movement was performed over a period of ~7.3 s with the ankle being moved from 20 degrees plantar to 15 degrees dorsal flexion. This movement was repeated twice in each sequence. The hand-held probe was positioned longitudinally over the posterior portion of the Achilles tendon, 3 cm proximal to the lateral malleolus. The anatomical regions that were captured are shown in Figure 2b.

Example 2: Longitudinal and transversal captures

The second example demonstrates that the method facilitates comparisons between two orthogonal ultrasound registrations, in this case a longitudinal and transversal projection of the same muscle (the biceps brachii). Two ultrasound sequences of the biceps brachii were captured during a 20% maximal voluntary contraction (MVC) calculated from an MVC (isometric contraction). The ultrasound probe was placed in two perpendicular orientations on the first and second runs. For the first run, it was held in a longitudinal direction such that the ultrasound sequence captured the muscles along the muscle fibres. For the second, the probe was rotated along its own axis such that it was oriented in a transverse direction and the resulting ultrasound sequence captured the intersection of the muscle fibres. The two registrations thus have only a small area in common corresponding to the thickness of the probe. The arm was fixed at an angle of 120 degrees angle (where 180 degrees corresponds to full flexion of the arm) in a KinCom dynamometer. The maximal voluntary contraction (MVC) was determined and the movement was performed at 20% of the MVC for ~3.6 s.

As one might expect, these two ultrasound sequences are visually very different, as seen in Figure 2c and Figure 2d. However, despite their visual differences, the registrations are assumed to contain enough common

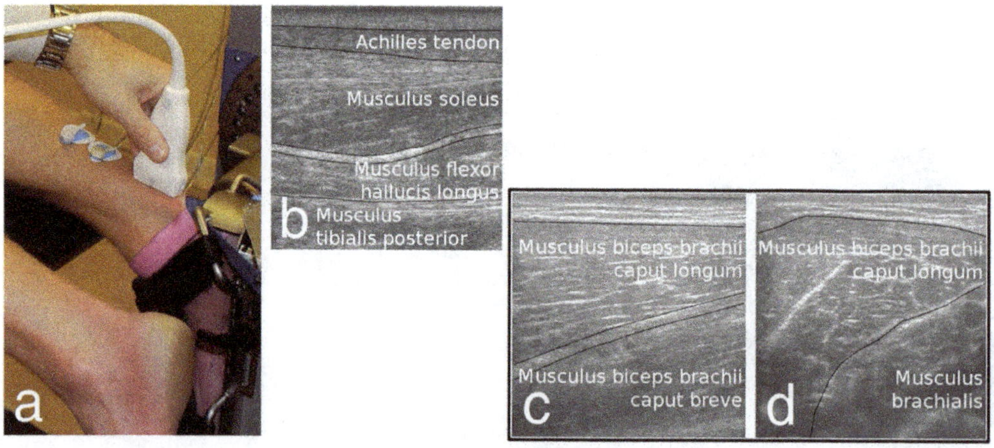

Figure 2 Experimental setup and the resulting ultrasound sequences. (**a**) The passive movement (Example 1) was performed lying face down with the foot strapped to an isokinetic dynamometer. The ultrasound probe was then held in the researcher's hand, just above the subject's malleolus. (**b**) The anatomy of the calf viewed from the probe surface towards the interior of the calf. The marked anatomic areas are the areas discussed in Example 1. Figures (**c**) and (**d**) show the anatomical regions in the biceps considered in Example 2. (**c**) is the longitudinal capture and (**d**) is the transversal capture.

information about the actual underlying movement to enable the extraction and analysis of the similarities and differences in the movements.

Ethical consideration

The research was conducted with informed consent, and has been exempted from formal ethical approval by the Regional Ethical Review Board.

Results

The results show that the O2PLS models for these experiments do very well at describing the relationships between sequences of registrations. O2PLS can thus be used not only for similar sequences of the same muscles, but also for sequences captured in different ways. In all cases, it was possible to identify and correlate the different phases of the movements in both sequences.

Example 1: Captures of the Achilles tendon

When MACI was first applied to ultrasound sequences, it was used in conjunction with PCA [10]. While PCA can be used to construct models for each sequence, it cannot readily be used to study the relationships between the resulting models. When O2PLS is used instead to model the relationship between the sequences instead, one obtains a clear picture of the correlations between the sequences that can be studied in detail.

The O2PLS model that was obtained had 24 predictive (i.e. shared) components that described 73% of the variance in the first capture and 64% of the variance in the second, with no orthogonal components. This means that a significant amount of shared variation was found, and neither sequence contained any information that was distinguishable from noise and not present in the other.

See Figure 3 for a visual correlation of the frames during the ankle movement. The first and second O2PLS components are shown in Figures 3a and b, respectively,

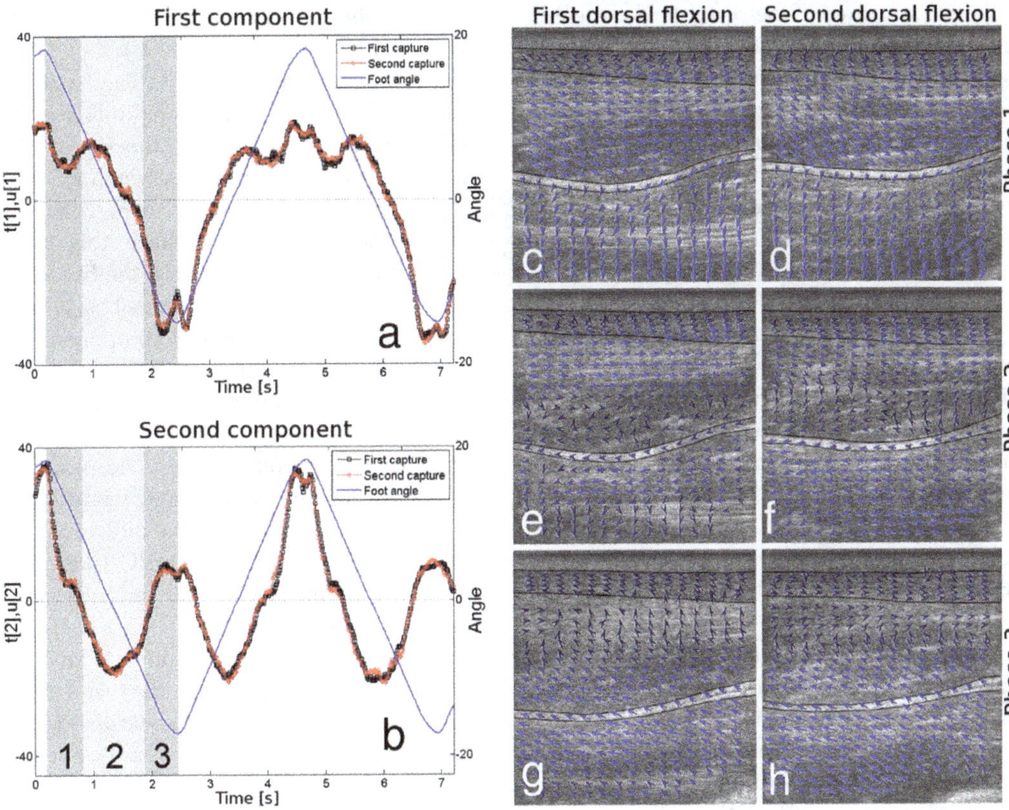

Figure 3 Example 1: Reliability study focusing on the Achilles tendon. The first (**a**) and second (**b**) score vectors are plotted together with the average angle measured by the isokinetic dynamometer for the two movements. Both the plantar and the dorsal flexions are clearly captured by both score vectors. The dorsal flexion is divided into three phases: Phase 1 is the end of the plantar flexion, Phase 2 is the transition from plantar to dorsal flexion and Phase 3 is the beginning of the dorsal flexion. The phases are marked in both Figure (**a**) and (**b**); in the case of Figure (**b**), the different phases are indicated by the numbers 1, 2 and 3. The corresponding speckle tracking vector field plots are shown in (**c**) and (**d**) for Phase 1, (**e**) and (**f**) for Phase 2 and (**g**) and (**h**) for Phase 3. The directions of the vectors indicate the direction of motion of the corresponding tissues.

together with the goniometric data for the ankle as it moves between the directions of flexion. The turning phases of the movement were thus easily identified.

Four movement phases are clearly visible when looking at the ultrasound sequences. These are the plantar flexion turning point, the dorsal flexion, the dorsal flexion turning point, and the plantar flexion. The first three of these phases are highlighted in Figures 3a and b as Phase 1, 2 and 3. Speckle tracking vector flow fields [27,28] were created for each of these phases in order to illustrate how the phases differ. These vector fields are shown in Figures 3c-h for the first and the second captures. Figures 3c and d correspond to Phase 1 (the plantar flexion turning point), Figures 3e and f to Phase 2 (the dorsal flexion), and Figures 3g and h to Phase 3 (the dorsal flexion turning point). Four calf regions were analysed when these vector fields were created (see Figure 2), namely the Achilles tendon, Musculus soleus, Musculus flexor hallucis longus, and Musculus tibialis posterior, along with the fascia between the Soleus and Hallucis muscles. The outlines of these regions are indicated in Figures 3c-h (the Musculus flexor hallucis longus and Musculus tibialis posterior were analysed together). The arrows of the vector field represent the movement within each area, with the length of each arrow corresponding to the speed and length of the movement in its vicinity. Note that the arrow lengths are comparable within each image but cannot be used to make comparisons between the different images in Figure 3c-h.

Note in Figures 3a-b how well the components correlate with respect to both the first and second components. Actually, all 24 of the predictive components in T and U have correlation coefficients exceeding 0.94. This means that the ultrasound sequences are very similar and can be modelled together very well.

Overall, this example demonstrates that when two controlled repetitive movements were analysed using O2PLS, identical dynamic behaviour was observed in both sequences.

Example 2: Longitudinal and transversal captures

The two sequences examined in this example are very different, but the purpose of the O2PLS method is to extract common information present in both sequences. In this case the relevant information concerns dynamic aspects of the movement being studied.

The O2PLS analyses of these sequences did indeed capture a common underlying dynamic behaviour. As can be seen in Figures 4a and c, there is a similar and congruous pattern in both sequences. The O2PLS model that was found had 18 predictive components (describing 87% of the variance in the longitudinal and 80% of the variance in the transversal capture) and one component in the longitudinal capture that was orthogonal to the transversal capture. This means that a significant amount of shared variation was found, and that something of significance happened in the longitudinal capture that did not exist in the transversal capture.

The movement as performed had three phases: a contraction phase (during muscle activation), a static contraction phase (when the muscle was constantly tensed) and a relaxation phase (when the arm returned to its start position). These three phases are very well described by this O2PLS model, and especially in the first component. The contraction phase is actually composed of two sub-phases, which are indicated in Figures 4a-c and are referred to as Phase 1 and Phase 2. Phase 1 lasts from ~0.3 s to ~0.6 s and Phase 2 lasts from ~0.6 s to ~1.0s. The former mainly involves the short head of the Biceps brachii while the latter mainly involves the long head. This can also be seen in the speckle tracking vector field plots shown in Figures 4d and f, which correspond to Phase 1 and Phase 2, respectively.

The static contraction phase lasts from ~1.0 s to ~2.7 s and the dynamic eccentric phase lasts from ~2.7 s to the end of the sequence at ~3.6 s. The relaxation phase is shown as Phase 4 in Figures 4a-c.

The orthogonal component in Figure 4b suggests that something happened in the longitudinal capture during the static contraction phase, in the area marked as Phase 3 in Figures 4a-c. Specifically, a twitch in Phase 3 in both heads of the Biceps brachii is apparent in the longitudinal ultrasound sequence. Since this twitch did not occur in the transversal capture, the behaviour was captured in the orthogonal component, $t_{o,1}$, of the longitudinal capture. This orthogonal component also had high values during the contraction phase and at the end of the relaxation phase, indicating that differences occurred there as well.

The second component, Figure 4c, suggests that there is dynamic activity in the static contraction phase as well; this is probably due to the difficulty of maintaining a constant force during the MVC (this was also mentioned in reference [10] as well and thus once again confirms previous findings [29]).

One interesting thing to notice is that even though the muscle is relaxed at the start and the end of the movement, the score plots shown in Figures 4a and c do not begin and end at the same position with the same score value. This is probably because of a slight difference in tension in the muscles before and after the movement.

A drawback of this experiment is the lack of EMG data. However, the force curve obtained from the KinCom gave information regarding the length of the activation phase capturing the submaximal phase of the MVC (20%) movement.

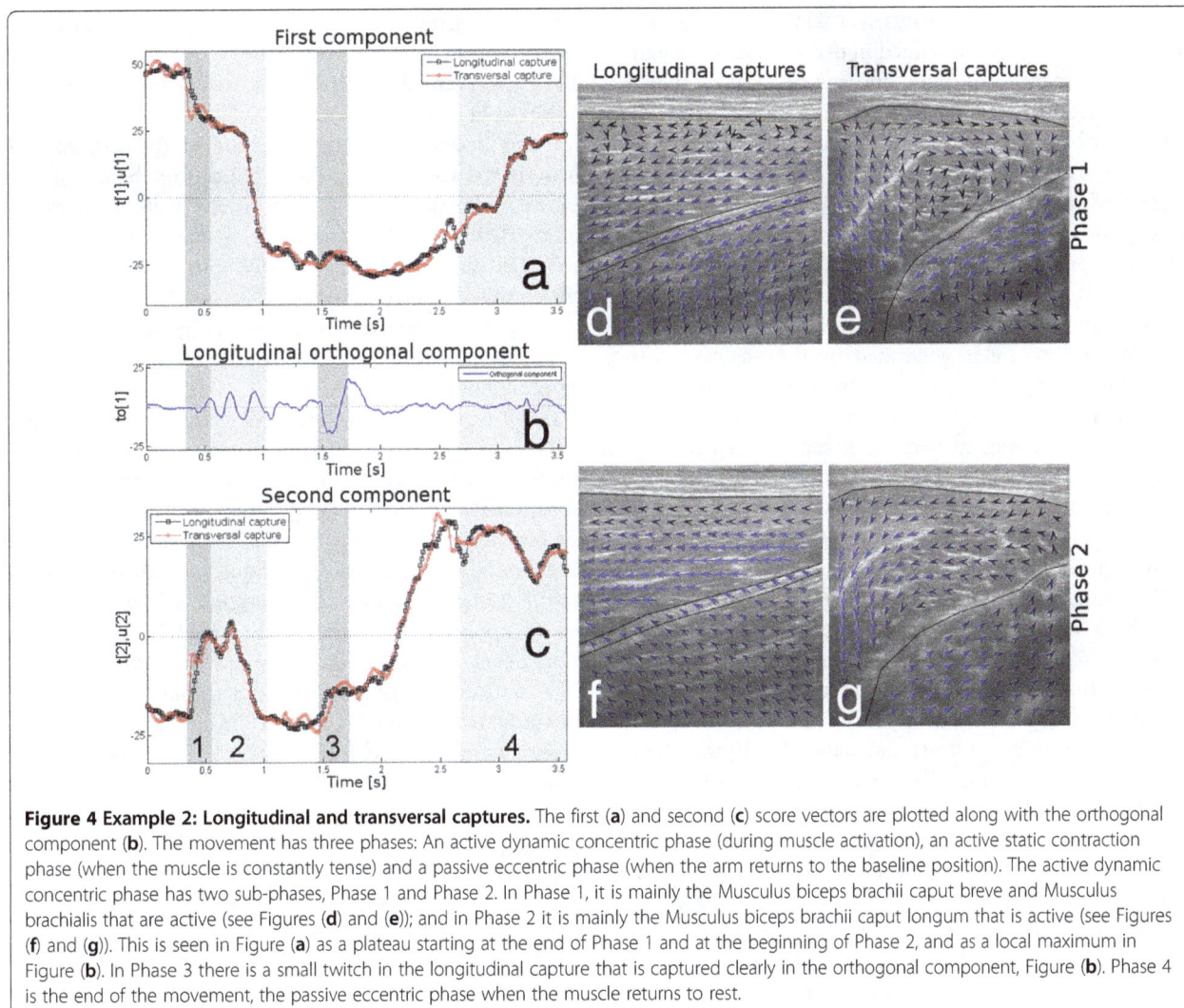

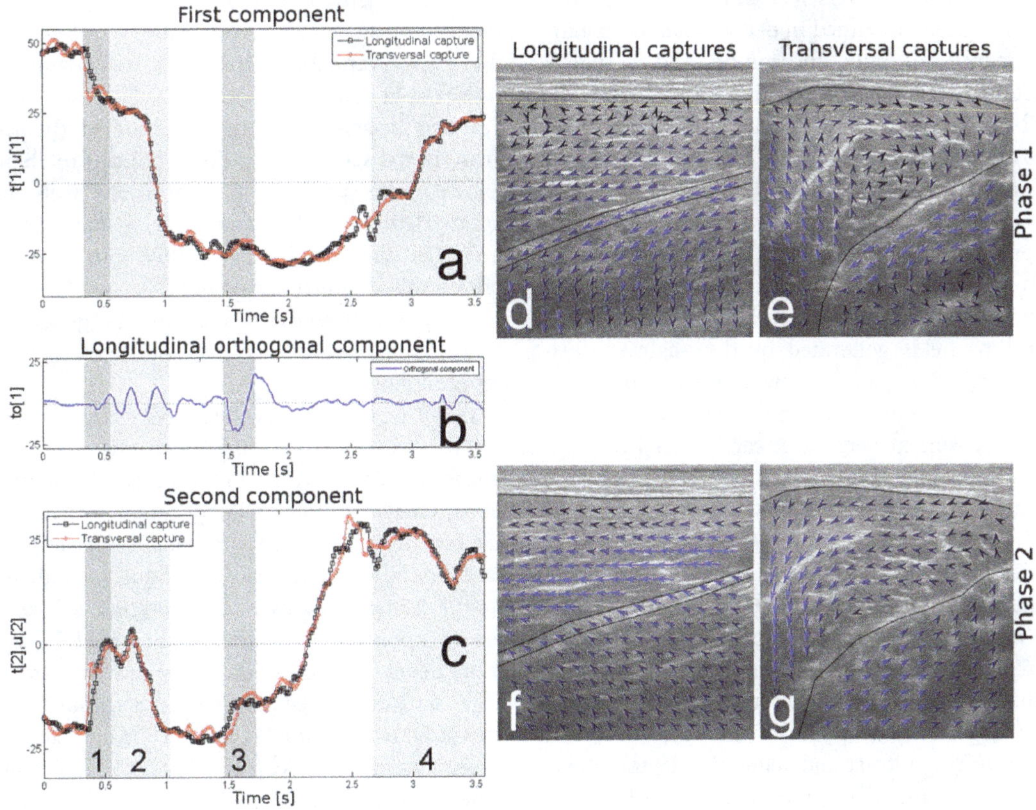

Figure 4 Example 2: Longitudinal and transversal captures. The first (**a**) and second (**c**) score vectors are plotted along with the orthogonal component (**b**). The movement has three phases: An active dynamic concentric phase (during muscle activation), an active static contraction phase (when the muscle is constantly tense) and a passive eccentric phase (when the arm returns to the baseline position). The active dynamic concentric phase has two sub-phases, Phase 1 and Phase 2. In Phase 1, it is mainly the Musculus biceps brachii caput breve and Musculus brachialis that are active (see Figures (**d**) and (**e**)); and in Phase 2 it is mainly the Musculus biceps brachii caput longum that is active (see Figures (**f**) and (**g**)). This is seen in Figure (**a**) as a plateau starting at the end of Phase 1 and at the beginning of Phase 2, and as a local maximum in Figure (**b**). In Phase 3 there is a small twitch in the longitudinal capture that is captured clearly in the orthogonal component, Figure (**b**). Phase 4 is the end of the movement, the passive eccentric phase when the muscle returns to rest.

Discussion

The main conclusion from these studies is that the combination of O2PLS with MACI represents a very useful and important extension to the MACI method. When used in conjunction with O2PLS, MACI can accurately identify and explain the common variation found in two ultrasound sequences. MACI modelling with PCA, as described in [10], provides a method for effectively compressing and extracting dynamic behaviour in a single video sequence. The O2PLS version of this method described herein facilitates comparisons between two blocks of data (two video sequences). O2PLS extracts common variation and allows for the analysis of discrepancies and non-related variation between the two blocks.

It is very useful to be able to compare different functional movements when using ultrasound image analysis to study musculoskeletal processes. When using the MACI method with PCA, only one ultrasound sequence could be described at a time. Conversely, when using O2PLS it is possible to analyse two full-length registrations simultaneously. This greatly increases the scope of the method, making it possible to compare registrations from a healthy and an injured person, different phases of a specific movement, or registrations from a person before and after an intervention. As such, the method clearly has considerable potential for use in medical applications.

The O2PLS method is an inductive, data-driven approach that extracts the information that is the most important for describing a particular sequence. It is thus the method rather than the analyst that decides which parts of the image should be examined. This unbiased data exploration technique therefore has great potential in clinical situations.

The O2PLS MACI method will thus add value to medical image analysis in different ways. Traditional image analysis methods focus on extracting specific features from single sequences. Conversely, O2PLS MACI extracts all of the information contained in every image pertaining to the movement in question and can be used to analyse them simultaneously in a comparative fashion. It could potentially be used to analyse the dynamics within individual muscles and tendons. Alternatively, image fields showing several muscles could be analysed in order to describe activity patterns.

It was possible to separate the studied functional movements into distinct phases that correspond to actual directions of motion as verified by visual inspection. The vector flow fields generated by the analyses illustrate the movements occurring within each phase in more detail, providing information that is extremely useful in a medical context because it can be used to compare the effects of different movements and determine how a specific intervention improves a given situation or to identify correlations between interventions and subjective symptoms or clinical findings.

The second case study examined in this work suggests that the angle of the ultrasound probe does not greatly affect the results obtained. This is encouraging, because it means that it would not be necessary to ensure that the probe was positioned in exactly the same way each time when capturing ultrasound sequences in the clinic. That is to say, the underlying movements can be compared even when sequences are captured from different angles or in slightly different ways.

Some variation is inevitable in all ultrasound registrations. Functional movements are also in and of themselves hard to repeat exactly, even among athletes who strive for years to achieve high levels of consistency when performing specific movements. It is therefore interesting to consider the variation between two repetitions of individual movements, both in terms of the common factors and the differences between them. As such, it is important to use standardized protocols that facilitate such comparisons whenever possible.

This study was methodological rather than clinical. The results presented suggest that the new method has considerable potential in the clinic but more testing and development will be required before it can be used in clinical applications, and the limitations of the case studies presented should be considered in this context.

Conclusions

MACI with O2PLS is able to consistently extract meaningful variability from ultrasound sequences. The O2PLS MACI method is thus applicable to studies of intra-individual relationships in ultrasound sequences of musculoskeletal tissues.

All of the studied sequences were modelled well, i.e. there were strong correlations between the O2PLS score vectors and the overlap between the sequences was substantial. Any variation present in both analysed sequences can thus be extracted efficiently, indicating that the shared variation corresponds to dynamic behaviours that exist in both movements.

When the shared variation was studied, the patterns that arose in the score vectors corresponded to changes in the nature of the movement (i.e. transitions from one phase to another) that could be verified by visual inspection. This indicates that MACI with O2PLS can identify different phases of functional movements.

Analyses of repeated movements generated similar score patterns, implying that the method exhibits good repeatability.

MACI with O2PLS is thus a powerful tool for studying variations and relationships between images in ultrasound image sequences with a broad range of potential applications. One such potential application concerns studies on the functionality healthy and injured muscles or the effects of training. It could also be useful for studying neuromotor related diseases such as multiple sclerosis. The potential applications of the method will be explored in more detail in future studies from our laboratories.

To our knowledge, there were previously no methods for inductively studying whole image sequences. The development of MACI with O2PLS has now made it possible to do this.

Competing interests

TL received financial support from MKS Umetrics AB, Umeå, Sweden.

Authors' contributions

TL performed the data analysis and wrote the manuscript together with OA and MP. MP generated the data. JT and MP designed and coordinated the study. All of the authors read and approved the final manuscript.

Acknowledgements

The authors would like to thank Dr. Anthony Arndt for the collaboration when using his lab equipment. This research was supported by the Swedish Research Council (JT) grant no. 2011-6044, MKS Umetrics AB (TL), and Young Investigator award, Umeå University, Sweden (JT).

References

1. Nørregaard J, Larsen CC, Bieler T, Langberg H: **Eccentric exercise in treatment of Achilles tendinopathy.** *Scand J Med Sci Sports* 2007, **17**:133–138.
2. Grassi W, Filippucci E, Busilacchi P: **Musculoskeletal ultrasound.** *Best Practice & Research Clinical Rheumatology* 2004, **18**:813–826.
3. Kane D, Balint PV, Sturrock R, Grassi W: **Musculoskeletal ultrasound - a state of the art review in rheumatology. Part 1: Current controversies and issues in the development of musculoskeletal ultrasound in rheumatology.** *Rheumatology* 2004, **43**:823–828.
4. Korstanje JW, Selles R, Stam H, Hovius S, Bosch J: **Development and validation of ultrasound speckle tracking to quantify tendon displacement.** *J Biomech* 2010, **43**:1373–1379.
5. Arndt A, Bengtsson A-S, Peolsson M, Thorstensson A, Movin T: **Non-uniform displacement within the Achilles tendon during passive ankle joint motion.** *Knee Surgery Sports Traumatology, Arthroscopy* 2011.
6. Oxborough D, George K, Birch KM: **Intraobserver Reliability of Two-Dimensional Ultrasound Derived Strain Imaging in the Assessment of the Left Ventricle, Right Ventricle, and Left Atrium of Healthy Human Hearts.** *Echocardiography* 2012, **29**:793–802.

7. Cameron A, Rome K, Hing W: **Ultrasound evaluation of the abductor hallucis muscle: Reliability study.** *Journal of Foot and Ankle Research* 2008, **1**:12.
8. Koppenhaver SL, Hebert JJ, Fritz JM, Parent EC, Teyhen DS, Magel JS: **Reliability of Rehabilitative Ultrasound Imaging of the Transversus Abdominis and Lumbar Multifidus Muscles.** *Archives of Physical Medicine and Rehabilitation* 2009, **90**:87–94.
9. Eriksson L, Wold S, Trygg J: **Multivariate analysis of congruent images (MACI).** *J Chemometr* 2005, **19**:393–403.
10. Peolsson M, Löfstedt T, Vogt S, Stenlund H, Arndt A, Trygg J: **Modelling human musculoskeletal functional movements using ultrasound imaging.** *BMC Medical Imaging* 2010, **10**.
11. Gonzalez RC, Woods RE: *Digital Image Processing.* 2nd edition. New Jersey: Prentice Hall; 2002.
12. Esbensen K, Geladi P: **Strategy of multivariate image analysis (MIA).** *Chemometrics Intell Lab Syst* 1989, **7**:67–86.
13. Geladi P: **Some special topics in multivariate image analysis.** *Chemometrics Intell Lab Syst* 1992, **14**:375–390.
14. Geladi P, Isaksson H, Lindqvist L, Wold S, Esbensen K: **Principal component analysis of multivariate images.** *Chemometrics Intell Lab Syst* 1989, **5**:209–220.
15. Trygg J, Wold S: **Orthogonal projections to latent structures (O-PLS).** *J Chemometr* 2002, **16**:119–128.
16. Trygg J: **O2-PLS for quantitative and qualitative analysis in multivariate calibration.** *J Chemometr* 2002, **16**:283–293.
17. Trygg J, Wold S: **O2-PLS a two-block (X-Y) latent variable regression (LVR) method with an integral OSC filter.** *J Chemometr* 2003, **17**:53–64.
18. Höskuldsson A: **PLS Regression Methods.** *J Chemometr* 1988, **2**:211–228.
19. Wold H: **Nonlinear Estimation by Iterative Least Square Procedures.** In *Research Papers in Statistics: Festschrift for J Neyman.* Edited by David FN. London: Volume Wiley; 1966:411–444.
20. Wold S, Martens H, Wold H: **The multivariate calibration problem in chemistry solved by the PLS method.** In *Matrix Pencils.* 973rd edition. Edited by Kågström B, Ruhe A. Heidelberg: Springer Berlin; 1983:286–293. Lecture Notes in Mathematics.
21. Stenlund H, Gorzsás A, Persson P, Sundberg B, Trygg J: **Orthogonal Projections to Latent Structures Discriminant Analysis Modeling on in Situ FT-IR Spectral Imaging of Liver Tissue for Identifying Sources of Variability.** *Anal Chem* 2008, **80**:6898–6906.
22. Bharati MH, Liu JJ, MacGregor JF: **Image texture analysis: methods and comparisons.** *Chemometrics Intell Lab Syst* 2004, **72**:57–71.
23. Korinek J, Wang JW, Sengupta PP, Miyazaki C, Kjaergaard J, McMahon E, Abraham TP, Belohlavek M: **Two-dimensional strain - a Doppler-independent ultrasound method for quantitation of regional deformation: Validation in vitro and in vivo.** *J Am Soc Echocardiogr* 2005, **18**:1247–1253.
24. Amundsen BH, Helle-Valle T, Torp H, Crosby J, Støylen A, Ihlen H, Smiseth O, Slørdahl SA: **Ultrasound speckle tracking reduces angle dependency of myocardial strain estimates - Validation by sonomicrometry.** In *Euroecho 8. European Association of Echocardiography.*; 2004.
25. Helle-Valle T, Crosby J, Edvardsen T, Lyseggen E, Amundsen BH, Smith HJ, Rosen BD, Lima JAC, Torp H, Ihlen H, Smiseth OA: **New noninvasive method for assessment of left ventricular rotation - Speckle tracking echocardiography.** *Circulation* 2005, **112**:3149–3156.
26. Farnebäck G: **Two-Frame Motion Estimation Based on Polynomial Expansion.** In *Proceedings of the 13th Scandinavian Conference on Image Analysis.* Sweden: June-July; Gothenburg; 2003:363–370.
27. Revell JD, Mirmehdi M, McNally DS: **Musculoskeletal motion flow fields using hierarchical variable-sized block matching in ultrasonographic video sequences.** *J Biomech* 2004, **37**:511–522.
28. Lin C-H, Lin MC-J, Sun Y-N: **Ultrasound motion estimation using a hierarchical feature weighting algorithm.** *Computerized Medical Imaging and Graphics* 2007, **31**:178–190.
29. Ito L, Kawakami Y, Ichinose Y, Fukashiro S, Fukunaga T: **Nonisometric behavior of fascicles during isometric contractions of a human muscle.** *J Appl Physiol* 1998, **85**:1230–1235.

7

The use of high-frequency ultrasound imaging and biofluorescence for *in vivo* evaluation of gene therapy vectors

Nicola Ingram[1*], Stuart A Macnab[2], Gemma Marston[1], Nigel Scott[3], Ian M Carr[1], Alexander F Markham[1], Adrian Whitehouse[2] and P Louise Coletta[1]

Abstract

Background: Non-invasive imaging of the biodistribution of novel therapeutics including gene therapy vectors in animal models is essential.

Methods: This study assessed the utility of high-frequency ultrasound (HF-US) combined with biofluoresence imaging (BFI) to determine the longitudinal impact of a Herpesvirus saimiri amplicon on human colorectal cancer xenograft growth.

Results: HF-US imaging of xenografts resulted in an accurate and informative xenograft volume in a longitudinal study. The volumes correlated better with final *ex vivo* volume than mechanical callipers ($R^2 = 0.7993$, $p = 0.0002$ vs. $R^2 = 0.7867$, $p = 0.0014$). HF-US showed that the amplicon caused lobe formation. BFI demonstrated retention and expression of the amplicon in the xenografts and quantitation of the fluorescence levels also correlated with tumour volumes.

Conclusions: The use of multi-modal imaging provided useful and enhanced insights into the behaviour of gene therapy vectors *in vivo* in real-time. These relatively inexpensive technologies are easy to incorporate into pre-clinical studies.

Keywords: Biofluorescence, Ultrasound, Gene therapy, Imaging, Multi-modal, Colorectal cancer

Background

The use of non-invasive and accurate methods to determine tumour volume, as well as biodistribution and transduction imaging of novel therapeutics, is essential in experimental models *in vivo*. In particular, for gene therapy studies, knowledge of maintenance, expression and efficacy of the vector is a fundamental part of the testing process [1]. However, this is rarely achieved during the *in vivo* study of a novel gene therapy strategy, as often only longitudinal calliper measurements of xenograft growth or final histology after treatment are carried out. The spread or loss of a vector is rarely detected during the course of the experiment and for cancer treatment, not all therapies will result in a reduction in tumour volume. Therefore it is important to be able to examine the impact of a gene therapy vector during the *in vivo* testing phase using different assessment criteria, whilst being mindful of adhering to the principles of reduction, refinement and replacement in animal experiments.

Ultrasound is a non-invasive method that has been utilised recently for tumour growth studies *in vivo* and is used in the clinic for staging colorectal cancer among others [2,3]. High-frequency ultrasound (HF-US) machines are available for small animal imaging. They are relatively easy to use and give high resolution greyscale images of mouse anatomy [4]. They also give functional information on the vascular structure of xenografts through the use of contrast agents and are relatively inexpensive and portable compared to MRI machines [5]. Mechanical callipers, however, are still utilised extensively for therapeutic agent testing, especially in gene therapy applications on xenografts [6]. These are very cheap, non-invasive and allow multiple

* Correspondence: n.ingram@leeds.ac.uk
[1]School of Medicine, University of Leeds Brenner Building, St James's University Hospital, Leeds LS9 7TF, UK
Full list of author information is available at the end of the article

repeated measurements with no anaesthetic required. However, mechanical callipers assume that the growth of xenografts is always ellipsoid and can only measure growth above the skin surface of the animal. In addition, calliper measurements are also affected by skin thickness, subcutaneous fat layer thickness and compressibility of the tumour [7]. From our experience of xenograft growth in gene therapy and other therapeutic studies, we know that this ellipsoid growth pattern is rarely observed, especially as the tumour volume becomes large (above approximately $300mm^3$).

A gene encoding a fluorescent or luminescent protein is often incorporated into gene therapy vectors in order to enumerate transduction efficiencies *in vitro* [8,9]. Moreover, these markers are also very useful for *in vivo* studies. Optical imaging chambers can be used to image the biodistribution of a vector when administered and can give an indication of the transduction efficiency in the target cells [10]. Optical imaging systems also allow the maintenance of a vector to be determined throughout the course of treatment, as well as examining the genetic stability of the vector over time. The first paper to prove that optical imaging could be used to measure tumour growth used bioluminescence of tumour cells in rat brain and was compared to MRI scans for tumour volume [11]. Imaging of stably-transfected cell lines containing red or green fluorescent protein (RFP or GFP) has been used to measure tumour and metastatic growth [12,13]. Recent work has also shown that fluorescent intensity correlates better with tumour volume than fluorescent area [14].

In the study described herein, we aimed to determine whether the use of HF-US measurements were more accurate than mechanical callipers in assessing xenograft volumes of tumour cells which were infected before injection with an experimental gene therapy vector. The use of HF-US to provide anatomical information on tumour growth and BFI to monitor expression of a gene therapy vector in longitudinal studies, were also analysed. The vector we used was a Herpesvirus saimiri (HVS) amplicon which contains the minimal elements for episomal maintenance without infectious capabilities [9,15]. This gamma-2 Herpesvirus amplicon can incorporate large amounts of heterologous DNA using a HVS-BAC (bacterial artificial chromosome) system and infects a broad range of human cells. The amplicon was previously stably transfected into the SW480 colorectal cancer cell line and contains a constitutively active GFP gene [16]. The presence of the GFP gene enabled monitoring of its persistence during xenograft growth in this study.

Methods

Tumour model

The colorectal cancer cell line, HCT116 was stably-transfected with an episomally-maintained Herpesvirus saimiri amplicon incorporating the GFP gene under the control of the Cytomegalovirus (CMV) promoter. These cells were grown in Dulbecco's Modified Eagle Medium (DMEM, Invitrogen) supplemented with 10% (v/v) foetal calf serum, and 4ul/ml Hygromycin B (Sigma, Poole U.K.) in 5% CO_2 at 37°C until there were enough cells for xenograft set up (approximately 3-4 weeks from infection). Parental cell lines were grown in DMEM and serum but no Hygromycin B. Two days before injection the amplicon-transfected cells were transferred to medium without any Hygromycin B.

1×10^6 each of the parental and amplicon-containing cells were collected in 100ul of serum-free DMEM and injected subcutaneously into the right flank of 8-10 week old female CD1 nude mice to form xenografts. 6 mice per group were used. All experiments were performed following local ethical approval and in accordance with the Home Office Animal Scientific Procedures Act 1986.

Tumour volume measurement with mechanical callipers

Tumours were measured with mechanical callipers three times per week once the tumour became palpable (approximately 7-10 days following injection). Tumour volume was calculated as follows, unless otherwise stated: [17]

$$\text{Tumor volume} = 1/2(\text{greatest longitudinal diameter} \times \text{greatest transverse diameter}^2)$$

After 40 days a final calliper measurement was taken, the xenografts were excised and weighed. If tumours exceeded the maximum permitted size of 17mm diameter, the mice were sacrificed earlier. Mechanical calliper measurements were then taken in three dimensions *ex vivo* and the following tumour volume was calculated, unless otherwise stated:

$$\text{Tumor volume} = \text{length} \times \text{height} \times (\pi/6)$$

Anatomical imaging and tumour volume measurement using HF-US

Once per week, mice were anaesthetised using 3% (v/v) isofluorane and xenografts were imaged using a Vevo 770 high-frequency ultrasound machine (FUJIFILM VisualSonics, Inc, Toronto, Canada) equipped with a 40 MHz transducer. The focal depth of the transducer was placed at the mid-point of the centre of the tumour whilst scanning. A 3D scan of the tumour was then performed using the minimum step size possible for the length of tumour and regions of interest were drawn around the xenograft at approximately every 5 frames by an operator with extensive experience of HF-US and analysis [4]. A tumour volume was then calculated using the Vevo 770 version 3 software by creating a 3D reconstruction of these xenografts.

Measurement of biofluorescence

Before sacrifice at day 40, xenografts were imaged in an IVIS Spectrum (PerkinElmer, Inc, Massachusetts, USA). Standard settings for GFP were used (excitation 500nm and emission detected at 540nm) in epi-illumination at high intensity. Binning was set at 8, field of view was 13.1cm and f stop was 2. Regions of interest of the same size were drawn around each xenograft and the total radiant efficiency ([photons/s]/[$\mu W/cm^2$]) was calculated within this using Living Image version 4.2 software (PerkinElmer, Inc, Massachusetts, USA).

Histology and morphology of xenografts

Once the xenographs were excised, photographs were taken of the intact tumours. The tumours were then cut in half and fixed in 4% (w/v) paraformaldehyde in PBS overnight. After processing and embedding in wax, sections were dewaxed, rehydrated and stained with haematoxylin and eosin. Sections were assessed by an experienced histopathologist.

Statistical analysis

Analysis of the tumour volumes and vector expression obtained by these methods used Pearson correlations. Positive correlations produced a positive R^2 value and were considered significant if $p < 0.05$. Agreement between the methods was then further analysed by Bland-Altman plots where the central line (mean of differences or bias) and 2 standard deviation (SD) limits of agreement were generated. The bias was considered significant if 0 was not included within these standard deviation lines. These calculations were carried out using GraphPad Prism version 5 (GraphPad Software, Inc, La Jolla, California, USA).

Results

Comparison of tumour growth curves generated using mechanical callipers or HF-US

HF-US was used to determine the tumour volume during the growth course of the xenografts derived from the parental cell line and amplicon-infected cell line and compared to the volume calculated from mechanical calliper measurements. The tumour volumes generated from the two methods are shown in Figure 1. The amplicon-infected xenograft tumours grew more slowly than the parental cells and this was detected by both measurement methods. Tumour volumes by HF-US generated smaller calculated tumour volumes than those using mechanical callipers. At day 28 for example, calliper assessed xenograft tumour volumes were calculated to be more than twice the volumes generated using HF-US imaging. This difference was even greater for the amplicon-infected xenografts as these were 3.3 times larger when measured using mechanical callipers compared to HF-US.

Comparison of tumour volume measurement methods to the volume calculated using *ex vivo* calliper measurements

HF-US measurements correlated more closely than mechanical callipers (denoted as *in vivo* callipers on the graphs) to the final *ex vivo* calliper measurement at the end of the period of xenograft growth which is our most accurate measurement (Figure 2 a and b). Thus the tumour growth curves in Figure 1 are an over-estimation if mechanical callipers are used compared to HF-US measurements. Alternative formulae for tumour volume calculation for both *in vivo* and *ex vivo* calliper measurements were examined and compared to HF-US (Table 1) [17]. As before, HF-US measurements correlated more closely to either *ex vivo* volume formula than any *in vivo* volume formula and no difference in correlation was

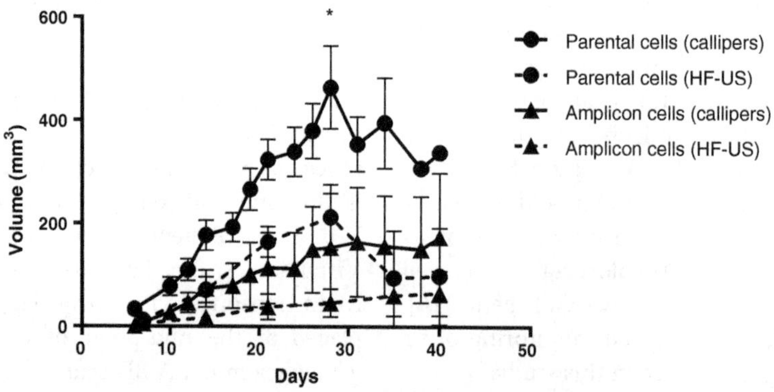

Figure 1 Longitudinal growth of xenograft tumours using mechanical callipers and HF-US. Growth of xenografts generated from each line using mechanical Vernier callipers on the external surface of the animal (*in vivo* calliper volume – solid lines) and using 3D high-frequency ultrasound scans and calculating volumes by drawing regions of interest on each frame (dotted lines). Mean volume +/- standard deviation of each group is shown (n = 5 for calliper measurements and 6 for HF-US) * denotes that mice were culled in this group after this point due to large tumour volumes (n = 2 from day 28).

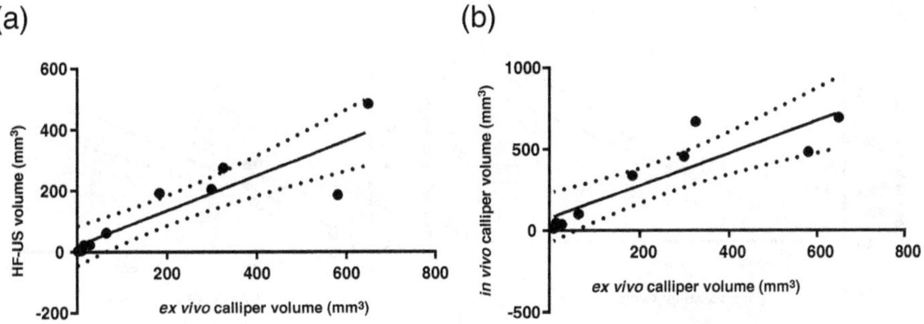

Figure 2 HF-US correlates more closely to the *ex vivo* tumour volume than using mechanical callipers *in vivo*. The tumour volume generated by HF-US correlates more closely with the final *ex vivo* calliper volume than the *in vivo* calliper volume. **(a)** The Pearson correlation plot of HF-US volumes versus *ex vivo* volumes has a higher R^2 value ($R^2 = 0.7993$, 95% CI = 0.6342-0.9724,p = 0.0002, two-tailed) than *in vivo* calliper volumes versus *ex vivo* volumes **(b)** ($R^2 = 0.7867$, 95% CI = 0.5421-0.9761, p = 0.0014, two-tailed). The solid line denotes line of best fit and dotted lines indicate the 95% confidence band, n = 10.

found between the two *ex vivo* volume formulae and HF-US volumes. Using the formula $\pi/6 \times (L \times W)^{3/2}$ for *in vivo* calliper volumes gave a higher correlation to both HF-US volumes and to mass of tumour than the other two equations.

Comparison of tumour volume measurement methods to final tumour mass

After sacrifice, the resulting xenograft tumours were excised and weighed. Using Pearson correlation coefficients and linear regression analysis, final *in vivo* calliper measurements had a lower correlation coefficient to tumour mass than HF-US. The tumour volumes calculated from *ex vivo* calliper measurements of the excised xenograft had the highest correlation coefficient to tumour mass (Figure 3 a, b and c and Table 1). Bland-Altman graphs show a smaller 95% confidence interval between HF-US volumes and the *ex vivo* calliper measurement compared to the confidence interval between final *in vivo* calliper and the *ex vivo* calliper measurements (Figure 4a and b). This demonstrates a smaller difference between HF-US and the *ex vivo* calliper measurement methods than between *in vivo* and *ex vivo* callipers.

HF-US imaging and BFI of tumour anatomy and gene therapy vector expression

In addition to HF-US, the use of BFI allowed the persistence and expression of the amplicon to be tracked *in vivo*. The HF-US images and photographs show that the amplicon-containing xenografts grew in distinct lobes

Table 1 Pearson correlation coefficients of xenograft tumour volumes using different ellipsoid formulae and measured using mechanical callipers, HF-US or mass

		$\pi/6 \times L \times W \times H$	$0.5 \times L \times W \times H$	HF-US	Mass (g)
$0.5 \times L \times W^2$	R^2	0.7867	0.7867	0.8576	0.7843
	95% CI	0.5421-0.9761	0.5421-0.9761	0.7110-0.9827	0.4811-0.9792
	p	0.0014	0.0014	0.0001	0.0034
$\pi/6 \times L \times W^2$	R^2	0.7867	0.7867	0.8576	0.7843
	95% CI	0.5421-0.9761	0.5421-0.9761	0.7110-0.9827	0.4811-0.9792
	p	0.0014	0.0014	0.0001	0.0034
$\pi/6 \times (L \times W)^{3/2}$	R^2	0.8325	0.8325	0.8636	0.8492
	95% CI	0.6300-0.9817	0.6300-0.9817	0.7223-0.9835	0.6184-0.9860
	p	0.0006	0.0006	0.0001	0.0011
HF-US	R^2	0.7993	0.7993		0.8470
	95% CI	0.6342-0.9724	0.6342-0.9724		0.6135-0.9857
	p	0.0002	0.0002		0.0012
Mass (g)	R^2	0.9254	0.9254		
	95% CI	0.7580-0.9946	0.7580-0.9946		
	p	0.0005	0.0005		

Three different formulae for generating *in vivo* tumour volumes using callipers are shown to the left and two different formulae for *ex vivo* tumour volumes using callipers on top. Each have been subject to pairwise comparison to determine the different correlation coefficients.

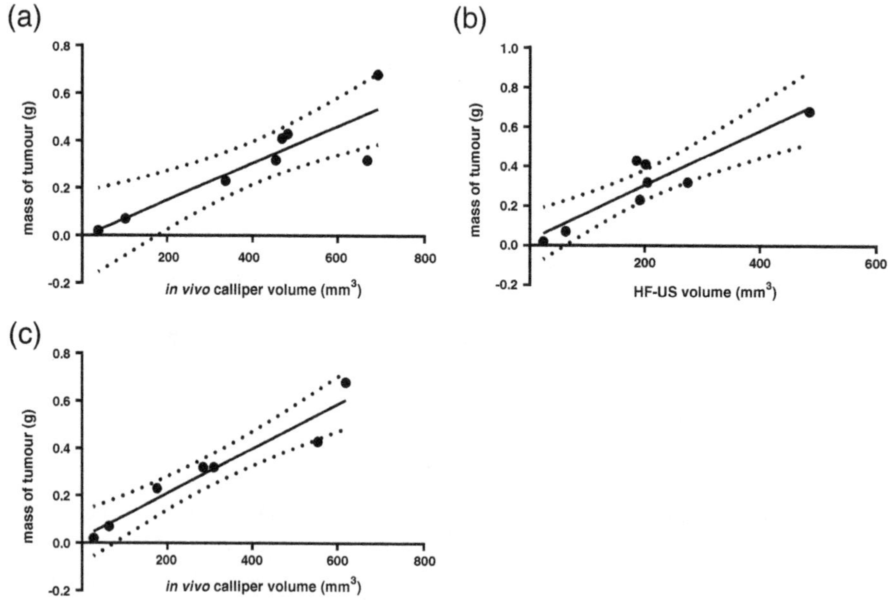

Figure 3 ***Ex vivo*** **callipers and HF-US correlated well to tumour mass.** Final tumour mass correlated most strongly with *ex vivo* calliper volume. Pearson correlations showed that *in vivo* calliper volumes correlated the least with tumour mass (Figure 3**a**, $R^2 = 0.7843$, 95% CI = 0.4811-0.9792, $p = 0.0034$), followed by HF-US volume (Figure 3**b**, $R^2 = 0.8470$, 95% CI = 0.6135-0.9857, $p = 0.0012$) whereas *ex vivo* calliper volume showed the best correlation (Figure 3**c**, $R^2 = 0.9254$, 95% CI = 0.7580-0.9946, $p = 0.0005$). Smaller tumours were not accurately weighed by the balance therefore n = 8.

unlike the parental cell xenografts. These distinct lobes were visible even from day 8 on the HF-US images in comparison to the parental cell xenografts, thus allowing very early detection of anatomic differences between the two groups *in vivo* which was not possible to elucidate from calliper measurements alone. The detailed greyscale anatomical images using HF-US showed both lighter and darker areas (derived from areas that are more or less echogenic to ultrasound) (Figure 5). The relatively lighter areas within the xenograft were not adipose tissue and corresponded to denser tumour tissue and from histology we observed that the darker areas are necrotic tissue and when the tumours were excised open, a liquid interior core was found (Figure 6a). Amplicon infection of the cells caused formation of syncitia (fused cells) during xenograft growth, which was not evident in the parental

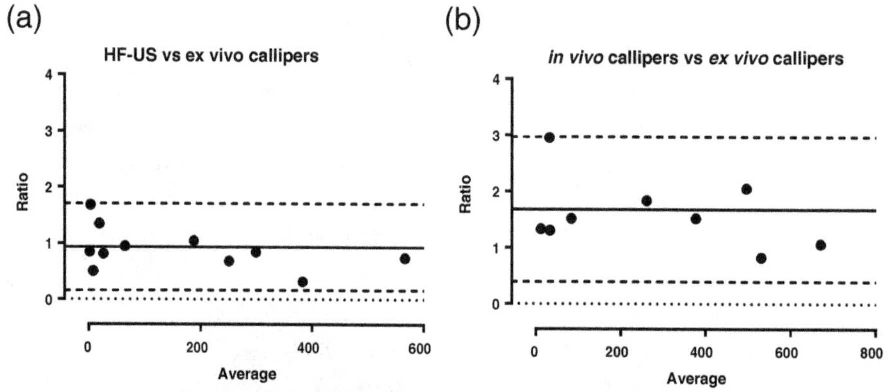

Figure 4 Bias assessment of each method for tumour volume calculation. HF-US volumes show less bias than *in vivo* calliper volumes when compared to *ex vivo* calliper volumes. The ratios of HF-US to *ex vivo* calliper volumes (y-axis) were compared to the average value of the measurements (x-axis). Bland-Altman plots were generated comparing the bias between HF-US and *ex vivo* calliper volumes **(a)** and *in vivo* calliper volumes compared to *ex vivo* calliper volumes **(b)**. The solid line denotes the bias (the average of the differences between the two measurement methods) and the dashed lines define the 95% confidence limits. The dotted line defines zero. HF-US could detect much smaller tumour volumes than callipers therefore n = 11 in **(a)** and n = 10 in **(b)**.

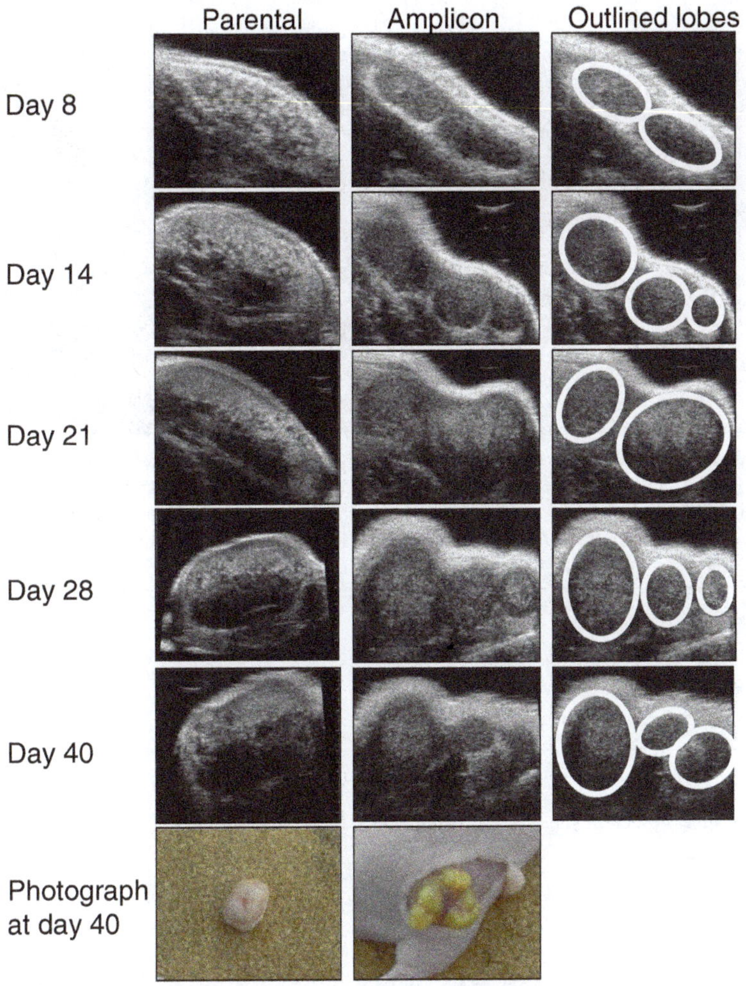

Figure 5 High-frequency ultrasound imaging showing anatomical detail of xenograft growth that corresponds with *ex vivo* examination. HF-US images of representative xenografts at the indicated day of growth. The first column shows images from an uninfected xenograft (parental cell line). Note that by day 28 the imaging plane was changed to be able to fit the xenograft into the field of view and scan over the whole tumour to generate the 3D image. The second column shows the amplicon infected xenograft. The third column outlines the lobes visible in the amplicon xenograft. The photographs in the column are of each xenograft at day 40 showing the distinct lobes of the amplicon infected xenograft compared to the uninfected xenograft.

cell xenografts, as shown in Figure 6b. The presence of lobes seen by HF-US can also be discerned in the fluorescent image taken by the IVIS Spectrum instrument (Figure 6c).

Correlation of total radiant efficiency (fluorescence) and tumour volume measurements

The measurement of levels of fluorescence was determined for the amplicon-infected xenografts using an IVIS Spectrum and the Living Image software and plotted alongside the *ex vivo* calliper volume (Figure 7a). These measurements show a similar pattern for the amplicon cell line in terms of fluorescence emission and calliper-derived tumour volume. *In vivo* calliper measurements on the final day of growth were less significantly correlated to fluorescence measurements than calliper measurements of the *ex vivo* xenografts (*in vivo* callipers, $R^2 = 0.8882$, 95% CI = 0.3568-0.9963, p = 0.0164 compared with *ex vivo* callipers, $R^2 = 0.9417$ 95% CI = 0.5518-0.9938, p = 0.0050) (Figure 7b and c). HF-US volume measurements had a better correlation coefficient to fluorescence measurements than the *ex vivo* calliper measurements ($R^2 = 0.8895$, 95% CI = 0.5606-0.9939, p = 0.0048) (Figure 7d). However, it must be noted these are based on small numbers in each group, as only the amplicon-infected cells contained GFP and not the parental cells.

Discussion

Multimodal imaging in gene therapy applications is a useful tool to shed light on the behaviour of vectors during *in vivo* testing. In this study, the use of HF-US imaging identified anatomical differences during growth

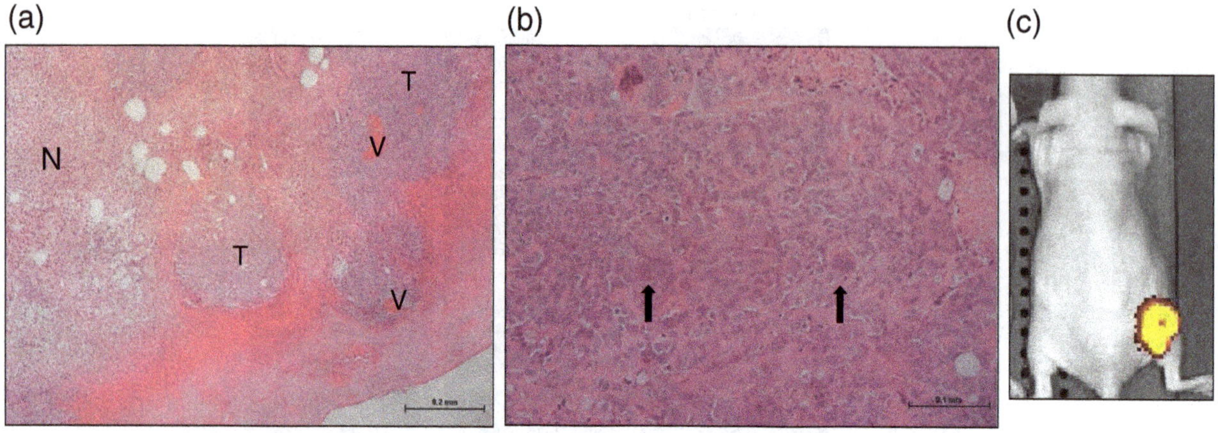

Figure 6 Histological examination of the tumours. Haematoxylin and Eosin stained sections of xenografts. **(a)** Parental cell xenografts typically showed islands of viable tumour (T) containing blood vessels (V) with large areas of necrosis (N). **(b)** amplicon infected xenografts show syncitia (arrowed) present amongst the tumour cells, which were not observed in any of the parental cell line xenografts. **(c)** The IVIS Spectrum image clearly shows the fluorescence emission from the xenograft lobes in an amplicon-infected xenograft, pseudo-coloured with the software default settings of red to yellow for increasing intensity of signal (parental cell line xenografts contained no GFP and showed no signal by BFI).

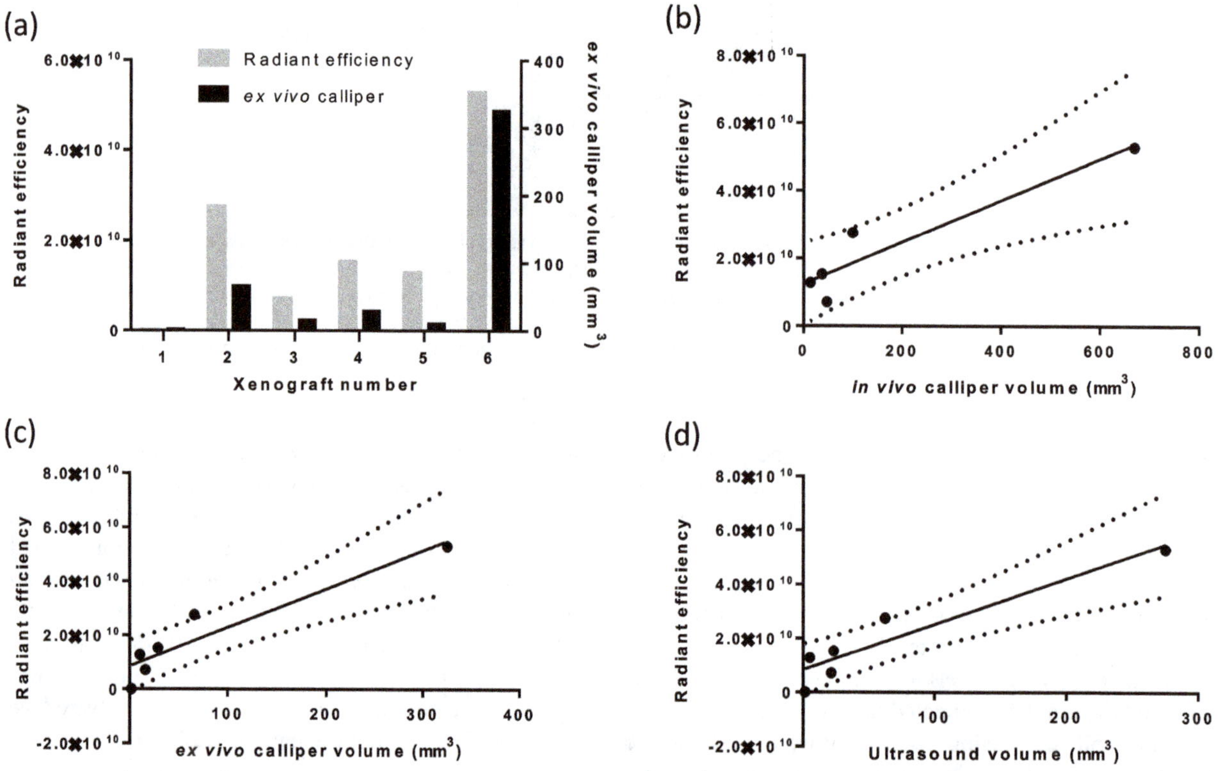

Figure 7 Total radiant efficiency correlates with xenograft tumour volume. (a) The total radiant efficiency of each amplicon-infected xenografts is plotted on the left y-axis of the graph alongside the *ex vivo* calliper tumour volume which is plotted on the right y-axis of the graph. Total radiant efficiency compared to *in vivo* calliper volume is shown **(b)**, $R^2 = 0.8882$, 95% CI = 0.3568-0.9963, $p = 0.0164$ ($n = 5$ as one xenograft was too small to be measured by callipers *in vivo*). Total radiant efficiency compared to *ex vivo* calliper volumes is shown in **(c)**, $R^2 = 0.9417$ 95% CI = 0.5518-0.9938, $p = 0.0050$, $n = 6$. Total radiant efficiency compared to HF-US volumes is shown in **(d)**, $R^2 = 0.8895$, 95% CI = 0.5606-0.9939, $p = 0.0048$, $n = 6$.

between the parental cell line and the vector-transfected cell line in a xenograft model, even from day 8 after implantation. It has been shown that HF-US can more accurately measure tumour volume compared to the traditional mechanical callipers, as demonstrated in this paper and by others [2,18]. The use of different ellipsoid volume formulae to generate the tumour volumes from calliper measurements made small differences in accuracy where the highest correlation to mass was found using $\pi/6 \times (L \times W)^{3/2}$ rather than the more commonly used $0.5 \times L \times W^2$ as described previously (although based on only one paper [17]). Correlation to determining volume by water displacement would be the gold standard and would be a useful addition to this study. HF-US volume generation and mechanical calliper measurements by multiple operators would also be valuable for determining variability as these measurements are subject to bias from operators. Jensen and colleagues compared volumes determined by microCT, ^{18}F-FDG-microPET and external callipers, to an *ex vivo* reference volume calculated by weight and density [19]. They demonstrated that micro-CT was more accurate and reproducible between observers than either external callipers or ^{18}F-FDG-microPET. They also showed that ^{18}F-FDG-microPET was not so useful for determining tumour size, although there was some correlation ($R^2 = 0.75$). This was similar to our findings with biofluorescence imaging. As with our study, this functional tumour imaging modality is useful for metabolic imaging and should give an indication of the effect of a gene therapy vector on tumour viability. In the current study, HF-US accurately showed the slower tumour growth of the vector-transfected cell line compared to the parental cell line, as predicted from *in vitro* cell growth curves [16]. However, lobe formation was unexpected. We are currently investigating whether this is due to the GFP gene or other components of the vector backbone. We also demonstrated the utility of the different greyscale textures in monitoring different patterns of growth. The discrimination of areas of necrosis and high vascularity (using contrast agents) was also possible. This should allow real-time monitoring of agents that currently have little apparent effect on tumour volume but may have useful effects of anti-angiogenesis or inducing cell senescence. HF-US would be of particular use for very small xenografts, orthotopic models to in transgenic mice such as the *Apc*$^{Min/+}$ mouse, where callipers cannot access the tumour. Indeed, gene therapy vectors are also used in non-cancer applications such as diabetes or organ regeneration, where callipers may not be used to measure disease progress or regression. In these cases, HF-US would be invaluable in monitoring progress longitudinally without sacrifice of mice.

In addition to HF-US images, the use of biofluorescence allowed monitoring of tumour growth patterns and correlated well with final tumour volumes (although it must be noted this was based on small numbers with a wide variation). This technique is a simple and very quick method of visualising the tumour and much less expensive than ^{18}F-FDG-microPET, for example. Bio-fluorescence is also applicable to patients. It is currently being trialled in surgery on human tumours to define tumour margins for resection [20]. The monitoring of these two cell lines grown as xenografts showed that the presence and expression of the vector was maintained within the tumour over the duration of the experiment. This information is of great value for gene therapy applications as silencing of the vector can occur, which may not be evident from growth curves or even from immunohistochemistry on *ex vivo* tumour sections for vector proteins. Linkage of the therapeutic gene of interest to a fluorescent marker gene via an IRES (internal ribosomal entry site) sequence or as a fusion protein would yield valuable information on the efficacy of expression during the time course of an *in vivo* experiment. It may also be used to reduce costs by eliminating animals in which the introduction of a vector by injection has not been successful.

Conclusions

In conclusion we believe that multi-modal imaging provides useful and enhanced insights into the behaviour of gene therapy vectors *in vivo*. Addition of imaging to gene therapy protocols would be straightforward especially in the case of relatively inexpensive ultrasound and biofluorescence imaging. The use of multi-modal imaging can give important information on the behaviour of gene therapy vectors in real-time, rather than traditional calliper measurements and final histological examination.

Abbreviations

HF-US: High-frequency ultrasound; BFI: Biofluorescent imaging; HVS: Herpesvirus saimiri; GFP: Green fluorescent protein.

Competing interests

The authors declare no competing interests financial or otherwise.

Authors' contributions

NI carried out the experiments, analysed the data and wrote the manuscript. SAM generated the stably-infected cell line. GM imaged xenografts by HF-US and generated tumour volumes. IMC generated the amplicon. NS provided histological information on the resulting xenografts. AFM provided discussion of the results. AW was involved in study design, discussion of results and generation of the amplicon. PLC was involved in study design, discussion of results and manuscript editing. All authors read and approved the final manuscript.

Acknowledgements

This study was funded by EPSRC grant number EP/I000623/1 and YCR grant number L332.

Author details

[1]School of Medicine, University of Leeds Brenner Building, St James's University Hospital, Leeds LS9 7TF, UK. [2]School of Molecular and Cellular Biology, Faculty of Biological Sciences and Astbury Centre for Structural

Molecular Biology, University of Leeds, Leeds LS2 9JT, UK. [3]Department of Histopathology, Bexley Wing, St James's University Hospital, Leeds LS9 7TF, UK.

References

1. Waerzeggers Y, *et al*: **Methods to monitor gene therapy with molecular imaging.** *Methods* 2009, **48**(2):146–160.
2. Cheung AM, *et al*: **Three-dimensional ultrasound biomicroscopy for xenograft growth analysis.** *Ultrasound Med Biol* 2005, **31**(6):865–870.
3. Samee A, Selvasekar CR: **Current trends in staging rectal cancer.** *World J Gastroenterol* 2011, **17**(7):828–834.
4. Abdelrahman MA, *et al*: **High-Frequency Ultrasound for In Vivo Measurement of Colon Wall Thickness in Mice.** *Ultrasound Med Biol* 2012, **38**(3):432–442.
5. Lee DJ, *et al*: **Relationship between retention of a vascular endothelial growth factor receptor 2 (VEGFR2)-targeted ultrasonographic contrast agent and the level of VEGFR2 expression in an in vivo breast cancer model.** *J Ultrasound Med* 2008, **27**(6):855–866.
6. Zhao Y, *et al*: **Increased antitumor capability of fiber-modified adenoviral vector armed with TRAIL against bladder cancers.** *Mol Cell Biochem* 2011, **353**(1–2):93–99.
7. Euhus DM, *et al*: **Tumor measurement in the nude mouse.** *J Surg Oncol* 1986, **31**(4):229–234.
8. Sims K, *et al*: **In vitro evaluation of a 'stealth' adenoviral vector for targeted gene delivery to adult mammalian neurones.** *J Gene Med* 2009, **11**(4):335–344.
9. Smith PG, *et al*: **Herpesvirus saimiri-based vector biodistribution using noninvasive optical imaging.** *Gene Ther* 2005, **12**(19):1465–1476.
10. Prasad KM, *et al*: **Robust cardiomyocyte-specific gene expression f ollowing systemic injection of AAV: in vivo gene delivery follows a Poisson distribution.** *Gene Ther* 2011, **18**(1):43–52.
11. Rehemtulla A, *et al*: **Rapid and quantitative assessment of cancer treatment response using in vivo bioluminescence imaging.** *Neoplasia* 2000, **2**(6):491–495.
12. Yang M, *et al*: **Whole-body optical imaging of green fluorescent protein-expressing tumors and metastases.** *Proc Natl Acad Sci U S A* 2000, **97**(3):1206–1211.
13. Snyder C, *et al*: **Complementarity of ultrasound and fluorescence imaging in an orthotopic mouse model of pancreatic cancer.** *BMC Cancer* 2009, **9**(1):106.
14. Abou-Elkacem L, *et al*: **Comparison of muCT, MRI and optical reflectance imaging for assessing the growth of GFP/RFP-expressing tumors.** *Anticancer Res* 2011, **31**(9):2907–2913.
15. Smith PG, *et al*: **Efficient infection and persistence of a herpesvirus saimiri-based gene delivery vector into human tumor xenografts and multicellular spheroid cultures.** *Cancer Gene Ther* 2005, **12**(3):248–256.
16. Macnab SA, *et al*: **Herpesvirus saimiri-mediated delivery of the adenomatous polyposis coli tumour suppressor gene reduces proliferation of colorectal cancer cells.** *Int J Oncol* 2011, **39**(5):1173–1181.
17. Tomayko MM, Reynolds CP: **Determination of subcutaneous tumor size in athymic (nude) mice.** *Cancer Chemother Pharmacol* 1989, **24**(3):148–154.
18. Ayers GD, *et al*: **Volume of preclinical xenograft tumors is more accurately assessed by ultrasound imaging than manual caliper measurements.** *J Ultrasound Med* 2010, **29**(6):891–901.
19. Jensen MM, *et al*: **Tumor volume in subcutaneous mouse xenografts measured by microCT is more accurate and reproducible than determined by 18F-FDG-microPET or external caliper.** *BMC Med Imaging* 2008, **8**:16.
20. Keller MD, *et al*: **Autofluorescence and diffuse reflectance spectroscopy and spectral imaging for breast surgical margin analysis.** *Lasers Surg Med* 2010, **42**(1):15–23.

8

The diagnostic validity of musculoskeletal ultrasound in lateral epicondylalgia

Valentin C Dones III[1*], Karen Grimmer[1], Kerry Thoirs[2], Consuelo G Suarez[3] and Julie Luker[1]

Abstract

Background: Ultrasound is considered a reliable, widely available, non-invasive and inexpensive imaging technique for assessing soft tissue involvement in Lateral epicondylalgia. Despite the number of diagnostic studies for Lateral Epicondylalgia, there is no consensus in the current literature on the best abnormal ultrasound findings that confirm lateral epicondylalgia.

Methods: Eligible studies identified by searching electronic databases, scanning reference lists of articles and chapters on ultrasound in reference books, and consultation of experts in sonography. Three reviewers (VCDIII, KP, KW) independently searched the databases using the agreed search strategy, and independently conducted all stages of article selection. Two reviewers (VCDIII, KP) then screened titles and abstracts to remove obvious irrelevance. Potentially relevant full text publications which met the inclusion criteria were reviewed by the primary investigator (VCDIII) and another reviewer (CGS).

Results: Among the 15 included diagnostic studies in this review, seven were Level II diagnostic accuracy studies for chronic lateral epicondylalgia based on the National Health and Medical Research Council Hierarchy of Evidence. Based from the pooled sensitivity of abnormal ultrasound findings with homogenous results ($p > 0.05$), the hypoechogenicity of the common extensor origin has the best combination of diagnostic sensitivity and specificity. It is moderately sensitive [Sensitivity: 0.64 (0.56-0.72)] and highly specific [Specificity: 0.82 (0.72-0.90)] in determining elbows with lateral epicondylalgia. Additionally, bone changes on the lateral epicondyle [Sensitivity: 0.56 (0.50-0.62)] were moderately sensitive to chronic LE. Conversely, neovascularity [Specificity: 1.00 (0.97-1.00)], calcifications [Specificity: 0.97 (0.94-0.99)] and cortical irregularities [Specificity: 0.96 (0.88-0.99)] have strong specificity for chronic lateral epicondylalgia. There is insufficient evidence supporting the use of Power Doppler Ultrasonogrophy, Real-time Sonoelastography and sonographic probe-induced tenderness in diagnosing LE.

Conclusions: The use of Gray-scale Ultrasonography is recommended in objectively diagnosing lateral epicondylalgia. The presence of hypoechogenicity and bone changes indicates presence of a stressed common extensor origin-lateral epicondyle complex in elbows with lateral epicondylalgia. In addition to diagnosis, detection of these abnormal ultrasound findings allows localization of pathologies to tendon or bone that would assist in designing an appropriate treatment suited to patient's condition.

Keywords: Systematic review, Diagnosis, Musculoskeletal ultrasound, Lateral epicondylalgia, Lateral epicondylitis, Tennis elbow

* Correspondence: DONVC001@mymail.unisa.edu.au
[1]International Centre for Allied Health Evidence, University of South Australia, Adelaide, South Australia
Full list of author information is available at the end of the article

Background

Lateral Epicondylalgia is the most common cause of lateral elbow pain [1]. It is generally attributed to osteotendinous irritation of the common extensor origin in which pathological changes in the tendinous origins of Extensor Carpi Radialis Brevis (ECRB) and Extensor Digitorum Communis (EDC) muscles [2-8] are commonly implicated.

In this review, the term 'Lateral epicondylalgia' represents pain in the lateral elbow area involving the lateral epicondyle and the common extensor origin regardless of the nature (inflammatory or non-inflammatory), acuity of elbow symptoms (acute or chronic) and other sources of pathology. Considering the term 'Lateral epicondylalgia' is irrelevant to the nature, acuity and sources of pathology of lateral elbow symptoms [9], the name 'Lateral epicondylalgia' encompasses lateral epicondylitis [10], lateral elbow tendinosis [11], lateral elbow enthesopathy [12,13], or lateral elbow epicondylopathy [14].

There is currently no gold standard in diagnosing Lateral epicondylalgia [15]. However in both clinical practice and research, the Cozen, Mill, and Maudsley tests are commonly used provocation tests which are considered positive if they replicate lateral elbow pain [15]. The Cozen test is the only one recommended by the United Kingdom Health Safety Executive Workshop to diagnose Lateral epicondylalgia [16]. However, the diagnostic capacity of these three clinical provocation tests to confirm Lateral epicondylalgia is under-investigated [15].

Consequently, health care professionals are increasingly using musculoskeletal ultrasound to identify tendon pathologies which may be associated with Lateral Epicondylalgia [17]. Musculoskeletal Ultrasound is reported to be reliable, widely available, non-invasive and inexpensive [17].

Gray-scale Ultrasonography is the most commonly used musculoskeletal ultrasound in detecting pathological changes in tendons [17]. It was suggested by Grassi et al. to be the reference standard for diagnostic imaging in rheumatologic conditions [17]. However, there is currently no consensus on the best musculoskeletal ultrasound finding to confirm Lateral epicondylalgia.

In Gray-scale Ultrasonography, a high resolution and high frequency transducer is essential to clearly demonstrate the special resolution of superficial soft tissue structures [18]. The echotexture of muscles, tendon and bones have been observed differently in real-time, using transducer heads with varying frequency bands, for instance:

- Gibbon: 7.5 or 10 MHz [18]
- Bianchi and Martinoli: 5–15 MHz [19] and
- Robinson: 9–17 MHz [20]

Another musculoskeletal ultrasound technology has recently emerged to objectively assess Lateral epicondylalgia, namely Power Doppler Ultrasonography and Real-time Sonoelastography. The poor scanning ability of the Colour Doppler Ultrasonography in detecting slow blood flow and separating blood flow from background noise is addressed by the Power Doppler Ultrasonography. Power Doppler Ultrasonography is useful when optimal Doppler angles (of 60 degrees or less) cannot be obtained. It scans longer segments of vessels and more individual vessels [21]. With its improved ability to detect increased blood flow, it appears to have the highest diagnostic validity for chronic Lateral epicondylalgia [22,23]. Real-Time Sonoelastography assesses tissue elasticity through compression [22]. With the common extensor origin suspected of weakening due to intratendinous focal changes, its compressibility is increased compared to healthy tendons indicating tendon degeneration [22]. De Zordo et al. [22] and Khoury and Cardinal [23] suggested Real-time Sonoelastography can be a powerful adjunct to the diagnosis of Lateral epicondylalgia.

A manual technique which evolved from the use of musculoskeletal ultrasound is sonographic probe-induced tenderness. During musculoskeletal ultrasound scan, the operator uses a small part of one end of the musculoskeletal ultrasound probe which is equivalent to the tip of the index finger on a painful elbow specifically where a musculoskeletal ultrasound pathologic lesion (i.e. hypoechogenicity) is reported. The musculoskeletal ultrasound lesion is found relevant only if tenderness is elicited [24]. This intervention was suggested to increase the accuracy of identifying the exact zone of abnormality and useful in confirming the location of the pathology in elbows with Lateral epicondylalgia [24].

Aims

This review was primarily undertaken with the aims of establishing the diagnostic validity of Gray-scale Ultrasonography (the index test) for Lateral epicondylalgia, using a clinical (provocation test) diagnosis of Lateral epicondylalgia as the reference standard. A secondary aim was to establish any improvements in diagnostic sensitivity of musculoskeletal ultrasound in determining Lateral epicondylalgia when using Colour Doppler Ultrasonography, Power Doppler Ultrasonography, Real-time Sonoelastography, sonographic probe-induced tenderness or high frequency transducer head.

Methods

Eligibility

Studies were included if they reported on humans with Lateral epicondylalgia, reported at least one clinical provocation testing as a reference standard, and reported any statistic relating to the diagnostic validity of musculoskeletal ultrasound for Lateral epicondylalgia. Diagnostic validity could be available using any estimate (e.g. sensitivity, specificity, likelihood ratio or predictive values) or if these could be calculated from available data. There were no age restrictions on participants.

Literature was searched between January 1990 and May 2013, this time period reflecting the evolution of musculoskeletal ultrasound equipment and techniques. Studies that included participants diagnosed with other types of lateral elbow pain such as fibromyalgia or osteoarthritis were excluded.

Information sources

Eligible studies were identified by primary and secondary searching. Primary searching involved a comprehensive search of EMBASE, OVID, ICONDA, International Pharmaceutical Abstracts, Cochrane and DARE (Database of Abstracts of Reviews of Effectiveness), PUBMED, Google Scholar, Web of Science, Web of Knowledge, EBSCO (CINAHL, SPORTDiscus, Academic Search Premier, Health Source: Nursing/Academic Edition, ERIC, PsycInfo), Science Direct databases, HighWire Press, PubMed Central, Scopus, PsycARTICLES, Informit e-library collections, Biomed Central Gateway, and TRIP Database were searched. No language limitations were applied. Secondary searching involved pearling reference lists of published articles, or chapters on ultrasound in reference books, and by consulting experts in the field of sonography.

Search strategy

Boolean terms and three sets of keywords were used in search strategies which included:

Keywords 1: sensitivity OR specificity OR diagnostic accuracy OR diagnosis OR accuracy, AND

Keywords 2: lateral epicondylitis OR tennis elbow OR radial epicondyalgia OR lateral epicondylalagia OR extensor tendinopathy OR epicondylitis lateralis humeris OR lateral elbow tendinopathy OR lateral epicondylosis OR tennis elbow OR lateral tennis elbow, AND

Keywords 3: sonography OR ultrasound OR musculoskeletal ultrasound

Study selection

Three reviewers (VCDIII, KP, KW) independently searched the databases using the agreed search strategy, and independently conducted all stages of article selection. Two reviewers (VCDIII, KP) then screened titles and abstracts and agreed on 19 articles possibly relevant to this review. Full texts were retrieved. Studies were then reviewed by VCDIII and another reviewer (CGS).

The PRISMA flow diagram illustrated the process of identifying relevant studies used in this systematic review (Figure 1). At all stages of the review process, the reviewers reached consensus by discussion. A third independent reviewer was available for arbitration, but was not used.

Hierarchy and methodological quality

The National Health and Medical Research Council (NHMRC) hierarchy for evidence for diagnostic studies was applied [25]. As recommended by Fontela et al. [26], the Quality Assessment for Diagnostic Accuracy Studies (QUADAS) [27] (Additional file 1: Appendix 1. QUADAS checklist) and the Standards for Reporting of Diagnostic Accuracy (STARD) [28] (Additional file 1: Appendix 2. STARD checklist) and tools were applied to appraise the methodological quality. The STARD identified the quality of reporting study procedures and results, and QUADAS graded the methodological quality. To improve the rigor in grading STARD, relevant data were extracted prior to grading an item (Additional file 1: Appendix 2. STARD checklist). Each item was graded as well covered, adequately addressed, poorly addressed, and not addressed. Items which were assigned scores of well covered and adequately addressed were given a score of 1, otherwise 0.

The full text included articles were independently appraised by two reviewers; QUADAS [27] (VCDIII, JL) and STARD [28] (VCDIII, CGS). All disagreements were resolved during discussion without intervention from a third party.

Data extraction process

Data extraction was performed independently by VCDIII and CGS using a specifically-designed data extraction tool, which integrated STARD (Additional file 1: Appendix 2. STARD checklist). Data were extracted on authors, year, country where study was performed, characteristics of the study population, sample size, inclusion and exclusion criteria, details of index texts used and results. Missing data were requested through e-mail from corresponding authors, by the primary author. Only authors of one paper provided missing data.

Data analysis

Where statistical estimates of diagnostic validity were missing, raw data were extracted from frequency tables by the primary author, or were derived from published sensitivity and specificity results Calculations were verified by an epidemiologist (KG).

Pooling of musculoskeletal ultrasound findings

Data were pooled where possible, to determine the standardised sensitivity and specificity of musculoskeletal ultrasound administrations (Gray-scale Ultrasonography, Colour Doppler Ultrasonography, Power Doppler Ultrasonography and Real-time Sonoelastography). To

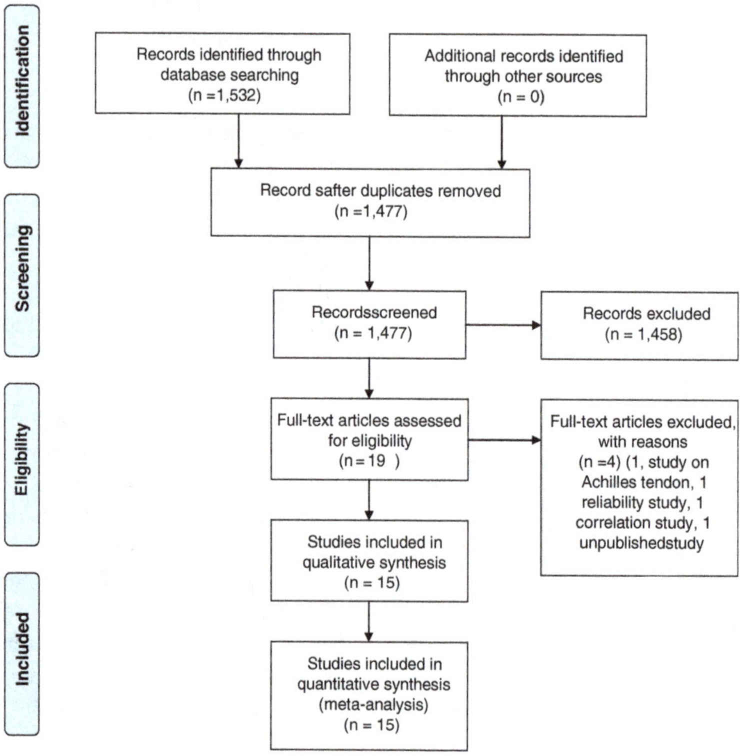

Figure 1 The PRISMA flow diagram. *Key:* PRISMA, Preferred Reporting Items for Systematic Reviews and Meta-Analyses.

appropriately pool the musculoskeletal ultrasound results, two steps were taken to identify similar studies. The first step identified the studies which used the same criteria in determining a musculoskeletal ultrasound abnormality. From this subset of studies, the second step identified those which used similar descriptions of: a. inclusion criteria, b. type and frequency of transducer head used, c. qualification of the reader of the image, d. duration of elbow symptoms, e. age of the participant, and f. the reference standard used.

MetaDisc 1.4 was used to compute for the pooled sensitivity and specificity and heterogeneity of musculoskeletal ultrasound findings from the subset of similar studies, described above [29]. P-values <0.05 indicated presence of significant heterogeneity in pooled results on sensitivity and specificity. Inconsistency square test for homogeneity (I^2) (in percentage) was computed to determine the degree of variability in study results. It describes the percentage of variation across studies that are due to heterogeneity rather than chance [30]. $I^2 = 100\% \times (Q\text{-}df)/Q$ where Q is distributed as a chi-square statistic with K (number of studies) minus 1 degree of freedom and df is degrees of freedom [30].

High frequency versus low frequency range

With the frequency range recommended by Bianchi and Martinoli [19] and Robinson [20], this review categorised the musculoskeletal ultrasound frequency into high frequency range of 9–17 MHz [20] and low frequency range of 5–15 MHz [19] and tested its ability to detect abnormal musculoskeletal ultrasound findings. Musculoskeletal ultrasound results of diagnostic studies were excluded if:

- The frequency of the transducer head used to scan the elbows was not mentioned in the study.
- The study used sonographic probe-induced tenderness to confirm the presence of musculoskeletal ultrasound findings in elbows with Lateral epicondylalgia. This maneuver replicates the elbow pain which could potentially influence the testers' objectivity in localizing the pathology within the elbow and interpreting the obtained images.

The transducer head (high frequency or low frequency) that effectively detected presence of abnormal musculoskeletal ultrasound findings in elbows with Lateral epicondylalgia was recommended as the frequency range for diagnosing Lateral epicondylalgia.

Results

Study selection

The number of database 'hits' was comparable between the three independent researchers, indicating that it was unlikely that important studies had been missed. Titles and abstracts of potentially relevant articles from these 'hits' were similarly identified between the three independent searches. From a total of 1,532 potentially relevant citations from the database searches, 15 full-text studies were eligible for inclusion. The study consort diagram is outlined in Figure 1 and hits identified per database are provided in Additional file 1: Appendix 3. Search results.

Levels of evidence

No systematic reviews on diagnostic validity of musculoskeletal ultrasound findings on Lateral epicondylalgia elbows were found. Seven studies were classified as level II, five studies as level III-1, and three studies as level III-2. Each level corresponded with the description of included studies and the articles identified were reported in Additional file 1: Appendix 4. NHMRC Hierarchy of Evidence.

Agreement between assessors

The agreement in STARD scores between the two reviewers (VCDIII, CGS) was good (weighted $k = 0.671$ (95% confidence interval 0.590-0.752). Disagreements were principally due to either reading errors, or differences in interpretation.

However when using QUADAS, the agreement between reviewers (VCDIII, JL) was only fair [weighted $k = 0.381$ (95% confidence interval 0.242-0.520). Disagreements were most common in criteria 1, 2, 9, and 12. Before reconsidering the scores, the reviewers agreed on the following: a. criterion 1: studies which recruited a group of healthy controls to compare against the participants with Lateral epicondylalgia were graded as "no"; b. criterion 2: studies which itemised the inclusion and exclusion criteria were graded as "yes"; c. criterion 9: studies which gave minimum details on clinical examination procedure were graded as "yes"; d. criterion 12: knowledge of the tester of the symptomatic side were graded as "no."

Standards for Reporting of Diagnostic Accuracy (STARD) grades are reported for each included paper in Additional file 1: Appendix 5. STARD Grades. Ten STARD items were reported in fewer than 50% studies: identification as diagnostic study (27%), report on reference standard and its rationale (47%), recruitment period (47%), use of reliability tests (13%), time interval between the clinical examination and musculoskeletal ultrasound (20%), severity of symptoms (20%), adverse events (7%), diagnostic accuracy and 95% confidence interval (27%), subgroup analysis (20%) and estimates of reliability (13%).

Quality Assessment for Diagnostic Accuracy Studies (QUADAS) scores are presented in Additional file 1: Appendix 6. Quality Assessment for Diagnostic Accuracy Studies (QUADAS) scores. Forms of bias found in the studies include: spectrum bias (n = 15/15, or 100% of the studies, criterion 1), disease progression bias (n = 9/15, or 60%, criterion 4), incorporation bias (n = 1/15, or 7% of the studies, criterion 7), test review bias (n = 3/15, 20% of the studies, criterion 10), reference review bias (n = 1/15, 7% of the studies, criterion 11), and clinical review bias (n = 14/15, 93% of the studies, criterion 12). Details were insufficient on the following:

- how uninterpretable test results were handled (n = 14/15, 93% of the studies, criterion 13).
- information on selection criteria (n = 5/15, 33% of the studies, criterion 2)
- classification of target condition (2/15, 13 % of the studies, and criterion 3),
- procedure used for clinical examination (n = 15/15, or 100% of the studies, criterion 9) and
- procedure used in musculoskeletal ultrasound (n = 1/15, 7% of the studies, criterion 8).

Descriptions of included studies

The characteristics of the 15 included studies and the reference sample population are reported in Additional file 1: Appendix 7. Description of diagnostic studies. Considering these included studies, fourteen [14] were published since 2000, potentially reflecting advances in musculoskeletal ultrasound technology, and an increasing focus on diagnostic validity studies.

In this review, the elbow with Lateral epicondylalgia was described as the symptomatic elbow. For individuals with one Lateral epicondylalgia elbow, the non-Lateral epicondylalgia elbow was the asymptomatic elbow. The elbows of participants who did not have Lateral epicondylalgia on either elbow were described as non-symptomatic.

Twelve (12) of the 15 studies compared the musculoskeletal ultrasound results of:

- symptomatic vs asymptomatic elbows [23,31];
- symptomatic vs non-symptomatic elbows [24,32-36] and
- symptomatic vs combined asymptomatic and non-symptomatic elbows [22,37-39].

Different brands of musculoskeletal ultrasound machines with frequencies of transducer heads ranging from 5 to 19 MHz were used in the included studies. Four studies used Colour Doppler Ultrasonography [23,32,35,40] and three studies [33,36,37] used Power Doppler Ultrasonography to detect neovascularity in the common extensor origin. One study used Real-Time

Sonoelastrographic scanner to assess for the compressibility of the common extensor origin [22].

During the scanning procedure, elbows were either extended [33] or flexed [22-24,32,34-41] with the forearm either pronated [32,34,35,37,40], supinated [23] or in neutral position [22,23,33,34,38]. Two studies did not report on the position of the elbows during scan [31,42]. The images were scanned by radiologists in 10 studies [22,23,32-35,38,40-42], sonographers in two studies [31,37], radiologist and sonographer in one study [36], radiologist and body imager in one study [39] and orthopaedic surgeon in one study [24].

There were 666 patients included in the 15 studies; of who 297 were males (45.6%) and 369 were females (55.4%) Ages ranged from 16 to 70 years. Maffulli et al. (1990) [42] tested the youngest age group who were composed of tennis players (16–36 years old). The reported mean duration of elbow symptoms in 12 studies was more than 6 weeks [22,24,31,32,34-37,39-42] making Lateral epicondylalgia presentation of a chronic nature. One study [33] did not specifically identify the duration of symptoms but attributed most of their musculoskeletal ultrasound findings to chronicity of Lateral epicondylalgia. Two studies did not indicate their participants' duration of elbow symptoms [23,38].

Twelve of the 15 studies [31-42] indicated the reference population from which their participants were drawn. In these studies, the patients were recruited from hospitals [32,33,35], local community [34], clinics [37,40], outpatients [31,41], self-referred [37], or referred by health care practitioners [33-40] or were tennis players [42]. The comorbidities and treatment of included patients were variably reported across all included studies.

In nine studies which reported the number of case and control participants [22,24,32-36,38,39], there was a total of 270 patients with Lateral epicondylalgia (128 males, 142 females) compared to 259 healthy participants (91 males, 168 females). The age range of patients with Lateral epicondylalgia (min-max: 13–70 years) was comparable to the healthy group (min-max: 17–71 years).

Diagnostic value of the tests

For six studies, 2×2 contingency tables could not be constructed because of the following issues:

- A control group was lacking [40-42].
- Musculoskeletal Ultrasound findings for the control were not reported [23,36].
- Only over-all diagnostic sensitivity and specificity and diagnostic odds ratio were reported [38].

Additional file 1: Appendix 8. Sensitivity and Specificity of MSUS findings in elbows LE lists the diagnostic sensitivity and specificity for each musculoskeletal ultrasound technique and musculoskeletal ultrasound finding in each study from which statistics could be extracted. Studies which reported scanning of asymptomatic and non-symptomatic elbows but did not report findings on diagnostic specificity were labeled as not reported. Studies which did not investigate on the diagnostic specificity of asymptomatic and non-symptomatic elbows were labeled as not applicable.

Studies utilizing the same criteria in determining an abnormal musculoskeletal ultrasound finding are grouped as Criteria (e.g. A or B) and are reported in Additional file 1: Appendix 9. Criteria used to determine abnormal MSUS findings. Other variables that were common between the 15 diagnostic studies are reported in Additional file 1: Appendix 10. Similarities of collected MSUS data in 15 diagnostic studies. Common across all 15 studies were: a. the use of provocation tests as basis for recruitment; b. the use of transducer heads whose frequencies ranged between 5–15 MHz; c. participants with mean age between 30–55 years; and d. qualified interpreters of images.

Table 1 reports the pooled sensitivity and specificity of the musculoskeletal ultrasound findings from the comparable subset of papers, including 95% CI, p-value and I-squared for heterogeneity and the number of investigations from which results were combined. Separate analysis on studies which added sonographic probe-induced tenderness [24,32], increased blood flow on common extensor origin [40] and those studies which only used provocation tests as part of the reference standard were performed. Studies whose diagnostic sensitivity and specificity cannot be pooled were labeled as not applicable. Table 1 reports that:

- Hypoechogenicity of the common extensor origin has the best combination of diagnostic sensitivity [Sensitivity: 0.64 (0.56-0.72)] and specificity [Specificity: 0.82 (0.72-0.90)].
- Bone changes on the lateral epicondyle [Sensitivity: 0.56 (0.50-0.62)] were moderately sensitive in confirming elbows with chronic Lateral epicondylalgia.
- Neovascularity [Specificity: 1.00 (0.97-1.00)], calcifications [Specificity: 0.97 (0.94-0.99)] and cortical irregularities [Specificity: 0.96 (0.88-0.99)] have strong specificity for chronic Lateral epicondylalgia.
- No sufficient evidence supported the use of Colour Doppler Ultrasonography, Power Doppler Ultrasonography, Real-time Sonoelastography and sonographic probe-induced tenderness in confirming the presence of chronic Lateral epicondylalgia.

Forest plots were constructed from the groups of studies which reported the same diagnostic criteria in determining

Table 1 Pooled diagnostic validity of musculoskeletal ultrasound abnormalities in elbows with LE

MSUS findings	N = investigations	Sensitivity	p-value, I^2	N = investigations	Specificity	p-value, I^2
Over-all GS changes	3 [25,28,31]	0.77 (0.69-0.84)	0.81,0	3 [25,28,31]	0.73 (0.66-0.80)$	0.08,61
PDU + GS changes	4 [26,27,31]	0.69 (0.64-0.73)	<0.0001,97	4 [26,27,31]	0.82 (0.76-0.86)$	<0.001,85
Hypoechogenicity (criterion A)	2 [25,30]	0.65 (0.56-0.73)	0.74, 0	0	NA	NA
Hypoechogenicity (criterion B using RTSE)	3 [16]	0.64 (0.55-0.73)	<0.0001,89	3 [16]	0.96 (0.91-0.99)$	<0.01,82
Hypoechogenicity (criterion A with probe)	3 [18,25,30]	0.64 (0.56-0.72)	0.80,0	2 [18,25]	0.82 (0.72-0.90)$	0.61,0
Calcifications	3 [26-28]	0.33 (0.28-0.38)	<0.0001,96	3 [26-28]	0.97 (0.94-0.99)#	0.16,45
Neovascularity (PDU)	2 [27,31]	0.26 (0.21-0.32)	<0.0001,98	2 [27,31]	1.00 (0.97-1.00)$	0.10,63
Thickness (criterion A)	2 [30,31]	0.42 (0.32-0.53)	<0.01,88	0	NA	NA
Thickness (criterion B)	4 [27,28]	0.51 (0.47-0.55)	<0.0001, 95	4 [27,28]	0.80 (0.75-0.84)#	<0.0001, 94
Enthesopathy	2 [25]	0.38 (0.29-0.47)	<0.0001, 98	0	NA	NA
Cortical irregularities (criterion A)	2 [28,30]	0.20 (0.14-0.29)	0.53,0	0	NA	NA
Cortical spurs (criterion A)	2 [30,34]	0.13 (0.07-0.21)	0.03, 78	0	NA	NA
Bone changes (cortical irregularities or spurs) (criterion A)	2 [27,31]	0.56 (0.50-0.62)	0.41,0	2 [27,31]	0.84 (0.78-0.88)$	<0.0001, 96
Cortical irregularities (criterion A with sonographic probe-induced tenderness)	3 [26,28,30]	0.20 (0.14-0.27)	0.79,0	2 [26,28]	0.96 (0.88-0.99)#	0.34,0
Partial tear	2 [30,35]	0.29 (0.12-0.27)	0.02,80	0	NA	NA
Full tear	2 [30,35]	0.02 (0.00-0.06)	0.14,55	0	NA	NA

Key: GS, Gray-scale, I^2, Iconsistency-square test for homogeneity; LE, Lateral Epicondylalgia; MSUS, musculoskeletal ultrasound; N, number; NA, not applicable; PDU, Power Doppler Ultrasonography; RTSE, Real-time Sonoelastography; #, healthy elbows; $, combined asymptomatic and healthy elbows.

abnormal musculoskeletal ultrasound findings. An example of one Forest plot for over-all Gray-scale changes is presented in Figure 2. The remaining Forest plots are presented in Additional file 1: Appendix 11. Forest Plots of on Diagnostic Validity of Abnormal MSUS findings, Figures S3–S16.

High frequency (9–17 MHz) versus low frequency range (5–15 MHz)

The following studies were excluded from the analysis in determining the ability of the two frequency ranges in detecting abnormal musculoskeletal ultrasound findings in elbows with Lateral epicondylalgia. The reasons were as follows:

- Obradov and Anderson [32] utilised sonographic probe-induced tenderness to confirm an musculoskeletal ultrasound finding which could have influenced the final diagnosis given.
- Noh et al. [24] did not report the frequency of the transducer head used.
- De Zordo et al. [22] used Real-Time Sonoelastography to scan elbows with Lateral epicondylalgia.

Comparing the nearness of the pooled diagnostic sensitivity and specificity of the abnormal musculoskeletal ultrasound findings in Table 1 with the pooled diagnostic sensitivity and specificity of the abnormal musculoskeletal ultrasound findings based on the frequency of the transducer head used in Table 2, the following trends were observed:

- Low frequency transducer heads appear to detect hypoechogenicity and enthesopathy of the common extensor origin more frequently than high frequency transducer heads.
- High frequency transducer heads appear to detect calcifications and neovascularity of the common extensor origin more frequently than low frequency transducer heads.
- Based on the frequency of the transducer head used, there was not enough pool-able data determining the diagnostic specificity of abnormal musculoskeletal ultrasound findings.

Table 2 reports the pooling of diagnostic sensitivity and specificity (when applicable) of musculoskeletal ultrasound findings using high and low frequency ranges of transducer head.

The reference standard

There were a number of ways in which a clinical diagnosis of Lateral epicondylalgia was used as reference standard. The Cozen test [22,24,31,33-35,37-42] was the most commonly used provocation test, and in five studies [31,33,35,38,40], this was the only test used to Lateral epicondylalgia. Other tests used (alone or in conjunction

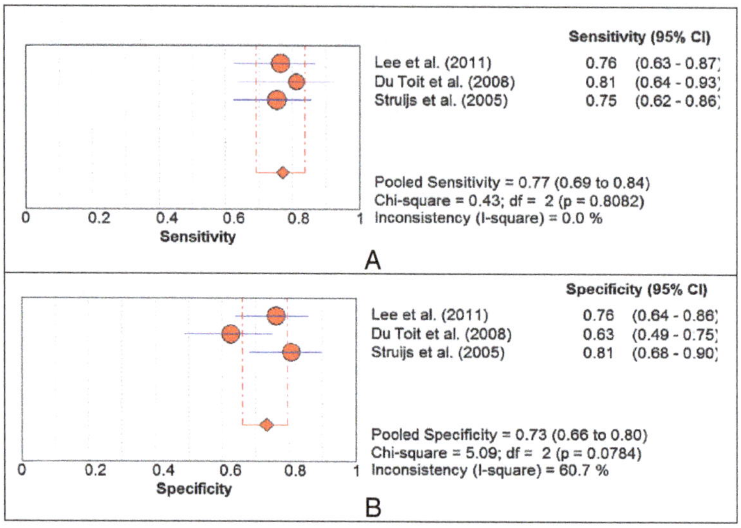

Figure 2 Forest plots for over-all gray-scale changes. A. Sensitivity, **B**. Specificity.

with others) were Maudsley [37,41,42], handgrip [39], sonographic probe-induced tenderness [32], resisted wrist supination [32], chair-lift test [34], and coffee-cup test [34]. Studies which used more than one provocation test did not report the sequence in which these tests were applied on the patients. In all included studies, the positions of the elbow and shoulder joints during provocation tests were not reported.

Other criteria used to clinically diagnose Lateral epicondylaliga were the following: a. surgical and histopathologic

Table 2 Diagnostic sensitivity and specificity based on frequency of the transducer head

MSUS findings	High frequency		Low frequency	
	N	Sns,p-value,I^2 SpC, p-value,I^2	N	SnS, p-value,I^2 SpC, p-value,I^2
Hypoechogenicity	2 [17,28]	0.35(0.22-0.50), 0.0001,93 NA	5 [25,29,30,33]	0.71(0.63-0.77),0.0009,79 NA
Calcifications	3 [17,27,28]	0.26(0.22-0.32),0.0001,89 NA	4 [25,29,30,35]	0.11(0.07-0.16),0.0081,75 NA
Neovascularity	3 [17,27,31]	0.28(0.23-0.24),<0.00001,97 100(98–100),0.25,28	3 [29,30,34]	0.40(0.31-0.49),<0.0001,99 NA
Thickness	4 [17,27,28,31]	0.53(0.49-0.57),<0.0001,93 NA	3 [30,33,36]	0.27(0.21-0.33),0.0003,81 NA
Enthesopathy	1 [17]	0.64(0.24-0.91) NA	3 [25,35,36]	0.31(0.23-0.39),<0.0001,96 NA
Bone changes (cortical irregularities or bone spurs)	2 [27,31]	0.56(0.50-0.62),0.41,0 NA	0	NA NA
Cortical irregularities	1 [28]	0.18(0.08-0.31) NA	1 [30]	0.22(0.13-0.34) NA
Cortical spurs	0	NA NA	2 [30,33]	0.13(0.07-0.21),0.03,78 NA
Partial tear	1 [17]	0.38(0.09-0.76) NA	2 [30,35]	0.06(0.02-0.11),0.10, 62 NA
Full tear	0	NA NA	2 [30,35]	0.02(0.00-0.06),0.14,55 NA

Key: I^2, Inconsistency-square test for homogeneity; MSUS, musculoskeletal ultrasound; N, number; NA, not applicable; SnS, sensitivity; SpC, specificity.

results [39], reduced grip strength [22,34,37], duration of lateral elbow pain [24,31,32,37,41] and previous sonographic findings [40].

Discussion

This is the first known systematic review supporting the use of Gray-scale Ultrasonography as operated by qualified practitioners in detecting abnormal musculoskeletal ultrasound findings to confirm presence of Lateral epicondylalgia in individuals whose lateral elbow pain can be replicated by provocation test. There was insufficient evidence in the use of Colour Doppler Ultrasonography, Power Doppler Ultrasonography, Real-time Sonoelastography, sonographic probe-induced tenderness and high frequency transducer head to increase the diagnostic validity of musculoskeletal ultrasound in confirming Lateral epicondylalgia.

Hypoechogenicity of the common extensor origin has the best combination of diagnostic sensitivity and specificity being moderately sensitive and highly specific in determining elbows with Lateral epicondylalgia. Sonographically, hypoechogenicity can be detected on a normal background or in areas of degeneration and partial rupture. Hypoechogenicity of the common extensor origin, however, varies depending on the scanned area (anterior, middle, posterior sections) [22].

Bone changes on the lateral epicondyle were moderately sensitive to chronic Lateral epicondylalgia. Although cortical irregularities are suggested features of chronic stage of musculoskeletal disease [43-45], it is less frequently detected in Lateral epicondylalgia elbows compared to focal hypoechogenicity. This suggests a greater involvement of the common extensor origin in Lateral epicondylalgia.

Neovascularity, calcifications and cortical irregularities were strongly specific but poorly sensitive for chronic Lateral epicondylalgia. There is little clarity on the role of these findings in the diagnosis of Lateral epicondylalgia. Neovascularity is a vascular hyperplasia found in elbows with Lateral epicondylalgia [45]. It may be an infrequent indicator of the failed attempt of the common extensor origin to heal. However, the neovascularity in elbows with Lateral epicondylalgia does not contain patent lumens and does not correlate with improved healing [45,46]. Additionally, calcifications were inconsistently detected in elbows with Lateral epicondylalgia despite being considered a main feature of degenerative tendon changes [1,43]. This may indicate traumatic more than degenerative cause for the pathological changes in elbows with Lateral epicondylalgia.

There is no statistical evidence to recommend the use of Colour Doppler Ultrasonography, Power Doppler Ultrasonography, Real-time Sonoelastography, sonographic probe-induced tenderness and high frequency transducer heads in improving the diagnosis for Lateral epicondylalgia being that:

- Neovascularity is an inconsistent musculoskeletal ultrasound abnormality in elbows with Lateral epicondylalgia. Despite that neovascularity is commonly absent in healthy elbows (as indicated by its high specificity when using Power Doppler Ultrasonography), its diagnostic ability in confirming presence of Lateral epicondylalgia in elbows with pain has inconsistent results [34,36,37]. The diagnostic sensitivity and specificity of Real-time Sonoelastography is high yet comparable to the diagnostic sensitivity of Gray-scale Ultrasonography and diagnostic specificity of Colour Doppler Ultrasonography. Gray-scale Ultrasonography and Colour Doppler Ultrasonography are often practical to use in the clinical setting [17].
- The diagnostic utility of sonographic probe-induced tenderness may just be limited to replication of elbow pain without sufficient evidence of increasing the accuracy of locally identifying the site of abnormality in elbows of individuals with Lateral epicondylalgia.

Based on the mean age of participants, and duration of Lateral epicondylalgia symptoms reported in the papers included in this systematic review, we recommend the use of the pooled results for sensitivity and specificity of musculoskeletal ultrasound abnormalities as guide in objectively determining Lateral epicondylalgia in individuals aged between 16–70 years, with chronic Lateral epicondylalgia.

Conclusion

The use of Gray-scale Ultrasonography (with 5-17 MHz transducer head) without sonographic probe-induced tenderness in detecting hypoechogenicity of the common extensor origin in elbows with pain was moderately sensitive [Sensitivity: 64 (56-72)] and highly specific [Specificity: 82 (72-90)] in determining elbows with Lateral epicondylalgia. The use of Power Doppler Ultasonography and Real-time Sonoelastography is expensive, and the evidence found in the review suggested that this technology did not significantly add to the sensitivity and specificity of Gray-scale Ultrasonography in detecting abnormal musculoskeletal findings in elbows with pain.

Additional file

Additional file 1: Appendix 1. QUADAS checklist. **Appendix 2.** STARD checklist. **Appendix 3.** Search results. **Appendix 4.** NHMRC Hierarchy of Evidence. **Appendix 5.** STARD Grades. **Appendix 6.** Quality Assessment for Diagnostic Accuracy Studies (QUADAS) scores. **Appendix 7.**

Description of diagnostic studies. **Appendix 8**. Sensitivity and Specificity of MSUS findings in elbows LE. **Appendix 9**. Criteria used to determine abnormal MSUS findings. **Appendix 10**. Similarities of collected MSUS data in 15 diagnostic studies. **Appendix 11**. Forest Plots of on Diagnostic Validity of Abnormal MSUS findings.

Abbreviations

Asx: Asymptomatic; CSA: Cross sectional area; Df: Degrees of freedom; ECRB: Extensor carpi radialis brevis; EDC: Extensor digitorum communis; I^2: Inconsistency square test for homogeneity; LE: Lateral epicondylalgia; MHz: Megahertz; MSUS: Musculoskeletal ultrasound; NA: Not applicable; NR: Not reported; NSx: Non-symptomatic; PDU: Power Doppler ultrasonography; PRISMA: Preferred reporting items for systematic reviews and meta-analyses; Q: Chi-square statistics with number of studies; QUADAS: Quality assessment for diagnostic accuracy studies; RTSE: Real-time sonoelastography; SnS: Sensitivity; SpC: Specificity; STARD: Standards for reporting of diagnostic accuracy.

Competing interests

We certify that no party having a direct interest in the results of the research supporting this article has or will confer a benefit on us or on any organization with which we are associated AND, if applicable, we certify that all financial and material support for this research and work are clearly identified in the title page of the manuscript. The authors declare that they have no competing interests.

Authors' contribution

The following authors are listed based on their contributions. Conception and design of study: VCDIII, KG. Analysis and interpretation of data: VCDII, KG, KT, CGS, JL. Writing of the manuscript: VCDIII, KG, KT, CGS, JL. All authors read and approved the final manuscript.

Acknowledgment

We would like to acknowledge the staff of the International Centre for Allied Health Evidence specifically Khushnum Pastakia for assisting us in critically appraising the papers involved in this review. We also wish to thank Kylie Wall and Olivia Thorpe for searching the databases and referencing this manuscript, respectively.

Author details

[1]International Centre for Allied Health Evidence, University of South Australia, Adelaide, South Australia. [2]Division of Health Sciences, University of South Australia, C8-26, Centenary Building, GPO Box 2471, Adelaide, SA 5001, Australia. [3]Department of Rehabilitation Medicine, Faculty of Medicine and Surgery, University of Santo Tomas, Manila, Philippines.

References

1. Regan W, Wold LE, Coonrad R, Morrey BF: **Microscopic histopathology of chronic refractory lateral epicondylitis.** *Am J Sports Med* 1992, 20:746–749.
2. Bunata RE, Brown DS, Capelo R: **Anatomic factors related to the cause of tennis elbow.** *J Bone Joint Surg Am* 2007, **89**:1955–1963.
3. Faro F, Wolf JM: **Lateral epicondylitis: review and current concepts.** *J Hand Surg Am* 2007, **32**:1271–1279.
4. Oskarsson E, Gustafsson BE, Pettersson K, Aulin KP: **Decreased intramuscular blood flow in patients with lateral epicondylitis.** *Scand J Med Sci Sports* 2007, **17**:211–215.
5. Erak S, Day R, Wang A: **The role of supinator in the pathogenesis of chronic lateral elbow pain: a biomechanical study.** *J Hand Surg Am* 2004, **29**:461–464.
6. Fairbank SM, Corlett RJ: **The role of the extensor digitorum communis muscle in lateral epicondylitis.** *J Hand Surg Am* 2002, **27**:405–409.
7. Albrecht S, Cordis R, Kleihues H, Noack W: **Pathoanatomic findings in radiohumeral epicondylopathy. A combined anatomic and electromyographic study.** *Arch Orthop Trauma Surg* 1997, **116**:157–163.
8. Briggs CA, Elliott BG: **Lateral epicondylitis. A review of structures associated with tennis elbow.** *Anat Clin* 1985, **7**:149–153.
9. Waugh E: **Lateral epicondylalgia or epicondylitis: what's in a name?** *Orthop Sports Phys Ther* 2005, **35**:200–202.
10. Boyer MI, Hastings H 2ND: **Lateral tennis elbow: "is there any science out there?".** *J Shoulder Elb Surg* 1999, **8**:481–491.
11. Stasinopoulos D, Johnson MI: **'Lateral elbow tendinopathy' is the most appropriate diagnostic term for the condition commonly referred-to as lateral epicondylitis.** *Med Hypotheses* 2006, **67**:1400–1402.
12. Jaen-Diaz JI, Cerezo-Lopez E, Lopez-De Castro F, Mata-Castrillo M, Barcelo-Galindez JP, De La Fuente J, Balius-Mata R: **Sonographic findings for the common extensor tendon of the elbow in the general population.** *J Ultrasound Med* 2010, **29**:1717–1724.
13. Kamien M: **A rational management of tennis elbow.** *Sports Med* 1990, **9**:173–191.
14. Muehlberger T, Buschmann A, Ottomann C, Toman N: **Aetiology and treatment of a previously denervated "tennis" elbow.** *Scand J Plast Reconstr Surg Hand Surg* 2009, **43**:50–53.
15. Lebrun C: **What are the best diagnostic criteria for lateral epicondylitis?** In *Evidence-based Orthopaedics: the Best Answers to Clinical Questions.* Edited by Wright JG. London: Elsevier Health Sciences; 2008:148–157.
16. Palmer K, Walker-Bone K, Linaker C, Reading I, Kellingray S, Coggon D, Cooper C: **The Southampton examination schedule for the diagnosis of musculoskeletal disorders of the upper limb.** *Ann Rheum Dis* 2000, **59**:5–11.
17. Grassi W, Filippucci E, Farina A, Cervini C: **Sonographic imaging of tendons.** *Arthritis Rheum* 2000, **43**:969–976.
18. Gibbon WW: **Musculoskeletal ultrasound.** *Baillieres Clin Rheumatol* 1996, **10**:561–588.
19. Bianchi S, Martinoli C: *Ultrasound of the Musculoskeletal System.* Germany: Springer-Verlag Berlin Heidelberg; 2007:605–614.
20. Robinson P: **Sonography of common tendon injuries.** *AJR Am J Roentgenol* 2009, **193**:607–618.
21. Hamper UM, Dejong MR, Caskey CI, Sheth S: **Power doppler imaging: clinical experience and correlation with color doppler US and other imaging modalities.** *Radiographics* 1997, **17**:499–513.
22. De Zordo T, Lill SR, Fink C, Feuchtner GM, Jaschke W, Bellmann-Weiler R, Klauser AS: **Real-time sonoelastography of lateral epicondylitis: comparison of findings between patients and healthy volunteers.** *Am J Roentgenol* 2009, **193**:180–185.
23. Khoury V, Cardinal E: **"Tenomalacia": a new sonographic sign of tendinopathy?** *Eur Radiol* 2009, **19**:144–146.
24. Noh KH, Moon YL, Jacir AM, Kim KH, Gorthi V: **Sonographic probe- induced tenderness for lateral epicondylitis: an accurate technique to confirm the location of the lesion.** *Knee Surg Sports Traumatol Arthrosc* 2010, **18**:836–839.
25. Coleman K, Norris S, Weston A, Grimmer-Somers K, Hillier S, Merlin T, Middleton P, Tooher R, Salisbury J: NHMRC additional levels of evidence and grades for recommendations for developers of guidelines STAGE 2 CONSULTATION Early 2008-end June 2009, viewed 26 March 2011, http://www.nhmrc.gov.au/guidelines/publications/cp65.
26. Fontela PS, Pant Pai N, Schiller I, Dendukuri N, Ramsay A, Pai M: **Quality and reporting of diagnostic accuracy studies in TB, HIV and malaria: evaluation using QUADAS and STARD standards.** *PloS One* 2009, **4**:e7753.
27. Whiting P, Rutjes AW, Reitsma JB, Bossuyt PM, Kleijnen J: **The development of QUADAS: a tool for the quality assessment of studies of diagnostic accuracy included in systematic reviews.** *BMC Med Res Methodol* 2003, **3**:25.
28. Bossuyt PM, Reitsma JB, Bruns DE, Gatsonis CA, Glasziou PP, Irwig LM, Lijmer JG, Moher D, Rennie D, de Vet HC: **Towards complete and accurate reporting of studies of diagnostic accuracy: the STARD initiative. The standards for reporting of diagnostic accuracy group.** *Croat Med J* 2003, **44**:635–638.
29. Zamora J, Abraira V, Muriel A, Khan K, Coomarasamy A: **Meta-DiSc: a software for meta-analysis of test accuracy data.** *BMC Med Res Methodol* 2006, **6**:31.
30. Higgins JP, Thompson SG: **Quantifying heterogeneity in a meta-analysis.** *Stat Med* 2002, **21**:1539–1558.
31. Struijs PA, Spruyt M, Assendelft WJ, van Dijk CN: **The predictive value of diagnostic sonography for the effectiveness of conservative treatment of tennis elbow.** *AJR Am J Roentgenol* 2005, **185**:1113–1118.
32. Obradov M, Anderson PG: **Ultrasonographic findings for chronic lateral epicondylitis.** *JBR-BTR* 2012, **95**:66–70.

33. Toprak U, Baskan B, Ustuner E, Oten E, Altin L, Karademir MA, Bodur H: **Common extensor tendon thickness measurements at the radiocapitellar region in diagnosis of lateral elbow tendinopathy.** *Diagn Interv Radiol* 2012, **18:**566–570.
34. Lee MH, Cha JG, Jin W, Kim BS, Park JS, Lee HK, Hong HS: **Utility of sonographic measurement of the common tensor tendon in patients with lateral epicondylitis.** *AJR Am J Roentgenol* 2011, **196:**1363–1367.
35. Zeisig E, Ohberg L, Alfredson H: **Extensor origin vascularity related to pain in patients with tennis elbow.** *Knee Surg Sports Traumatol Arthrosc* 2006, **14:**659–663.
36. Connell D, Burke F, Coombes P, Mcnealy S, Freeman D, Pryde D, Hoy G: **Sonographic examination of lateral epicondylitis.** *AJR Am J Roentgenol* 2001, **176:**777–782.
37. du Toit C, Stieler M, Saunders R, Bisset L, Vicenzino B: **Diagnostic accuracy of power Doppler ultrasound in patients with chronic tennis elbow.** *Br J Sports Med* 2008, **42:**872–876.
38. Levin D, Nazarian LN, Miller TT, O'kane PL, Feld RI, Parker L, Mcshane JM: **Lateral epicondylitis of the elbow: US findings.** *Radiology* 2005, **237:**230–234.
39. Lin J, Fessell D, Jacobson J, Weadock W, Hayes C: **An illustrated tutorial of musculoskeletal ultrasonography: part 1, introduction and general principles.** *AJR Am J Roentgenol* 2000, **175:**637–645.
40. Miller TT, Shapiro MA, Schultz E, Kalish PE: **Comparison of sonography and MRI for diagnosing epicondylitis.** *J Clin Ultrasound* 2002, **30:**193–202.
41. Zeisig E, Fahlstrom M, Ohberg L, Alfredson H: **A two-year sonographic follow-up after intratendinous injection therapy in patients with tennis elbow.** *Br J Sports Med* 2010, **44:**584–587.
42. Tarhan S, Unlu S, Ovali Z, Pabuscu Y: **Value of ultrasonography on diagnosis and assessment of pain and grip strength in patients with lateral epicondylitis.** *Turk J Rheumatol* 2009, **24:**123–130.
43. Maffulli N, Khan KM, Puddu G: **Overuse tendon conditions: time to change a confusing terminology.** *Arthroscopy* 1998, **14:**840–843.
44. Chard MD, Cawston TE, Riley GP, Gresham GA, Hazleman BL: **Rotator cuff degeneration and lateral epicondylitis: a comparative histological study.** *Ann Rheum Dis* 1994, **53:**30–34.
45. Yuill EA, Lum G: **Lateral epicondylosis and calcific tendonitis in a golfer: a case report and literature review.** *J Can Chiropr Assoc* 2011, **55:**325–332.
46. Bales CP, Placzek JD, Malone KJ, Vaupel Z, Arnoczky SP: **Microvascular supply of the lateral epicondyle and common extensor origin.** *J Shoulder Elbow Surg* 2007, **16:**497–501.

9

Animal study assessing safety of an acoustic coupling fluid that holds the potential to avoid surgically induced artifacts in 3D ultrasound guided operations

Asgeir S Jakola[1,2,3,4*], Arve Jørgensen[5], Tormod Selbekk[4,6], Ralf-Peter Michler[7], Ole Solheim[1,4], Sverre H Torp[8,9], Lisa M Sagberg[4], Petter Aadahl[5] and Geirmund Unsgård[1,4]

Abstract

Background: Use of ultrasound in brain tumor surgery is common. The difference in attenuation between brain and isotonic saline may cause artifacts that degrade the ultrasound images, potentially affecting resection grades and safety. Our research group has developed an acoustic coupling fluid that attenuates ultrasound energy like the normal brain. We aimed to test in animals if the newly developed acoustic coupling fluid may have harmful effects.

Methods: Eight rats were included for intraparenchymal injection into the brain, and if no adverse reactions were detected, 6 pigs were to be included with injection of the coupling fluid into the subarachnoid space. Animal behavior, EEG registrations, histopathology and immunohistochemistry were used in assessment.

Results: In total, 14 animals were included, 8 rats and 6 pigs. We did not detect any clinical adverse effects, seizure activity on EEG or histopathological signs of tissue damage.

Conclusion: The novel acoustic coupling fluid intended for brain tumor surgery appears safe in rats and pigs under the tested circumstances.

Keywords: Brain imaging, Brain tumor, Intraoperative imaging, Ultrasound

Background

For glial brain tumors the extent of resection is associated with survival [1,2]. However, extensive resection should not jeopardize function [3,4]. Tools for enhancing surgical resection of brain tumors, in particular gliomas, are increasing [4-7]. Ultrasound is currently used as a tool for providing 2D or 3D images for the purpose of tumor localization and resection control. Ultrasound has the potential to guide resections and increase resection grades, and thereby increase survival [8]. While ultrasound image quality is linked to resection grades in glioma surgery the image quality may sometimes be threatened by artifacts [9], most commonly seen towards the end of an operation, reducing the specificity [10,11]. When ultrasound is used for resection control the resection cavity is filled with saline to provide acoustic coupling between the ultrasound transducer and tissue. However, attenuation of acoustic waves is very low in saline compared to the brain and this difference in attenuation may cause artifacts that degrade the ultrasound images. Such artifacts are seen as high-intensity signals at the resection cavity wall and beyond, potentially masking a small tumor remnant, or even mimic tumor when there is none, and generally make the image interpretation more difficult (Figure 1).

This research group has developed a patent pending fluid intended for use in the resection cavity instead of saline. The effect on image quality has been tested in laboratory measurements using phantoms and fresh animal cadavers. The fluid seems to enhance ultrasound image

* Correspondence: asgeir.s.jakola@ntnu.no
[1]Department of Neurosurgery, St.Olavs University Hospital, N-7006 Trondheim, Norway
[2]MI Lab, Norwegian University of Science and Technology, Trondheim, Norway
Full list of author information is available at the end of the article

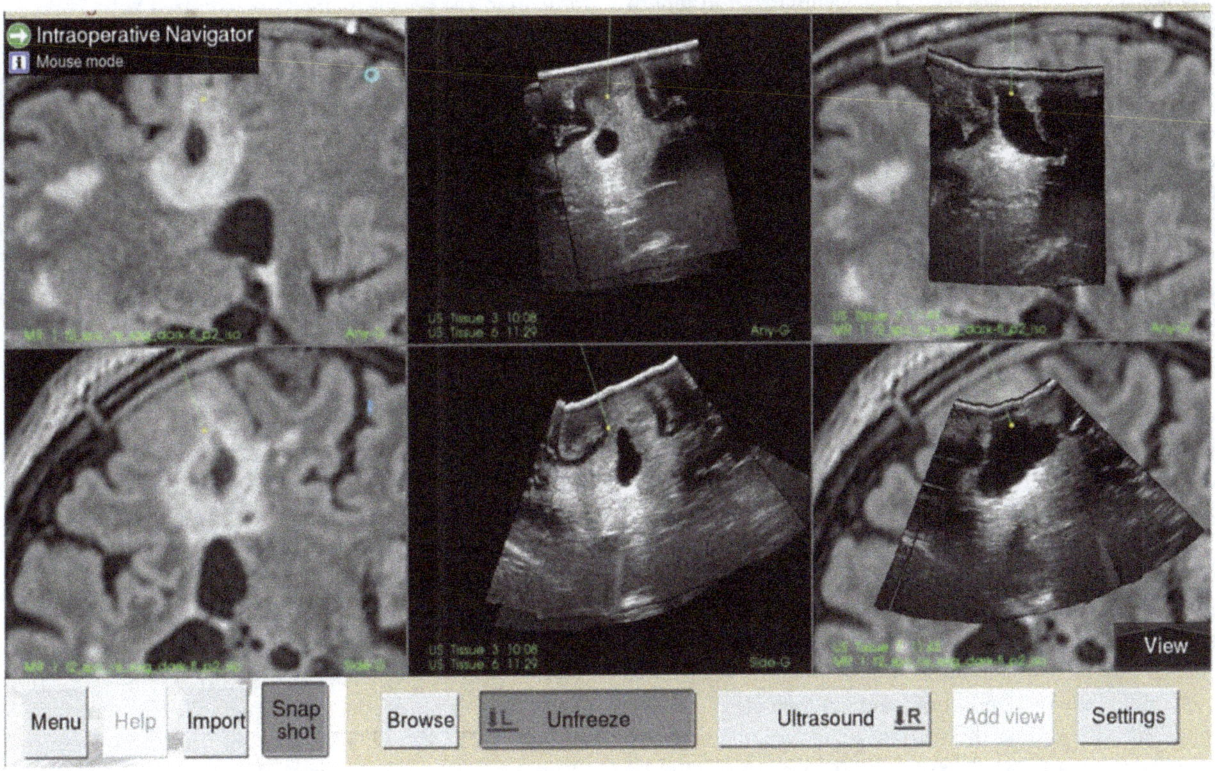

Figure 1 Ultrasound imaging during glioma resection. Screen dump from the ultrasound based neuronavigation system (SonoWand®). Images to the left are preoperative MRI demonstrating a hyperintense region suspect of diffuse glioma (above; sagittal view, below; coronal view). Images in the middle represent the corresponding ultrasound images taken intraoperatively before resection. Pictures to the right demonstrate corresponding ultrasound images approximately midway in the resection. Notice the bright-rim in the bottom of the cavity, representing an artifact, making the interpretation of hyperintense areas that could represent tumor on the images somewhat more difficult.

quality by the reduction of ultrasound artifacts around the resection cavity. We believe that the acoustic fluid will make image interpretation easier towards the end of surgery by easing delineation of normal brain tissue and tumor tissue, thus improving resection grades and improving safety.

In this two-step animal safety study we aimed to examine if the newly developed acoustic coupling fluid has any harmful effect related to its intended use.

Materials and methods

Study design

We designed a two-phased animal study with assessment in eight rats first, and if no adverse reactions were detected, pigs were to be included. Animals were successively included and no animals were excluded after the initiation of the experiments. The rat experiment was a non-randomized experimental study with each rat being its own control as the acoustic fluid was injected in one hemisphere and isotonic saline in the other. The pig experiment included six animals in a non-randomized consecutive study with no controls.

Experimental acoustic fluid

The (developed) acoustic coupling fluid is based on substances available in the pharmacy for intended use by humans. In the developed fluid we tested a pharmaceutical grade triglyceride and a pharmaceutically acceptable emulsifier and a pharmaceutically acceptable humectant. The main ingredient of the fluid we use is purified soybean oil in addition to lecithin and glycerol. These "active ingredients" is then diluted with a crystalloid solution (e.g. physiologic saline or Ringer's lactate), the more you dilute the lower the attenuation will be. From attenuation measurements in the laboratory and ultrasound imaging on fresh animal cadavers we established a certain blend of the above mentioned ingredients that should attenuate sound waves similarly as the human brain. See also Selbekk et al. [12].

Experimental animals

In the first phase of the study, acoustic fluid was injected in the frontal cortex of one randomly chosen hemisphere and control fluid in the contralateral hemisphere of eight adult female Sprague-Dawley rats (Taconic, Denmark). In the second phase, acoustic fluid was injected in the cisterna magna of six female domestic farm pigs, *Sus scrofa domesticus* (Nortura, Norway). The acclimatization length was four days for three pigs and five days for the other three pigs. One additional pig served as control for the model of assessing epileptogenicity by injecting penicillin G instead of the acoustic fluid into the cerebrospinal fluid in cisterna magna. Rats were housed in groups of three per cage in an animal facility and pigs were housed together except for the first day after the intervention when they were kept separated. Illumination was controlled on a 12:12-h light-dark cycle at room temperature 21°C and humidity 60% ± 2 SD. Animals had free access to water and a pellet rodent or pig diet.

Injection of fluid in brain parenchyma of rats

The rats were anesthetized with a gas mixture of 5% isoflurane (Abbot Scandinavia, Solna, Sweden), O_2 0.25 L · min^{-1} and N_2O 0.55 L · min^{-1}. After induction of anesthesia all rats received 0.012 mg atropine subcutaneous injection diluted in 1 mL NaCl 0.9% solution. The isoflurane concentration was adjusted down gradually to 1.8%, not faster than 0.5% each minute. The rat's head was fixed in horizontal position by a stereotactic frame. The procedure was done under sterile conditions, and an operating microscope was used during the surgical intervention. After exposing of the cranial vault, xylocain 10% was sprayed onto the surface and two 1 mm wide holes were drilled. Dura mater was carefully removed using a dura hook. The fluids were injected into the frontal lobe cortex of both hemispheres at 0.16 µL · min^{-1} by means of a 33 gauge internal cannula (C315I; Plastics One) inside a 26 gauge outer cannula (C315G; Plastics One) with the tip of the inner cannula protruding 0.9 mm out of the outer cannula. The cannula was connected by polyethylene tubing to a 25 µL Hamilton syringe in a CMA/100 microinfusion pump (Carnegie Medicine, Stockholm, Sweden). The entry point was 1.5 mm posterior to Bregma, 3.4 mm to both sides of the sagital suture, and 1.5 mm deep into the somatosensory cortex. A total volume of 1.00 µL fluid (either saline or acoustic fluid) was injected, and the cannula was retracted five minutes after each injection to prevent backflow of the fluid. The skin was sutured before the rats returned to their cages. Core temperature was maintained during the procedure using a heating pad and monitored using a rectally inserted thermometer. The equipment and procedure for injection were the same as used by Hafting et al. [13].

Subarachnoid injection of fluid in cisterna magna of pigs

The pigs were sedated with a combination of 10 mL azaperone (40 mg · mL^{-1}) and 2 mL diazepam (5 mg · mL^{-1}). Intravenous access was established via an ear vein. Just before intubation 1 mL atropin (1 mg · mL^{-1}), 5 mL ketamin (50 mg · mL^{-1}), 5 mL fentanyl (50 µg · mL^{-1}) and 5 mL thiopentothal (25 mg · mL^{-1}) were administered. After intubation the pigs remained anesthetized with 1–3% isoflurane (Abbot Scandinavia, Solna, Sweden), adjusted individually, 50% oxygen with the remaining being medical air 3 L · min^{-1} (AGA AS, Linde Healthcare, Norway). Pigs were positioned in prone position on a heating blanket with the neck flexed over the operating table to facilitate puncture of cisterna magna. Fluoroscopy was utilized for guidance in all animals. After verification of needle position in cisterna magna a total amount of 2 mL cerebrospinal fluid was collected. This equals 10% of the total CSF volume in pigs which is approximately 20 mL [14]. With the needle in place, 1 mL of the acoustic fluid was slowly injected and flushed with 1 mL of autologous cerebrospinal fluid. After the injection all animals were observed for 20 minutes while monitoring oxygen saturation and heart rate with 3-lead ECG continuously. After the observation period isoflurane was stopped. The pigs were extubated when they were capable of unassisted breathing and protection of airway.

Electroencephalography recordings in pigs

Scalp electroencephalography (EEG) was recorded throughout the procedure in all pigs. The EEG protocol we utilized equals the EEG protocol in use for children at St. Olavs Hospital. A Schwarzer ED 21 (Picker International GmbH) was used to record 12 channel EEG (longitudinal bipolar, 10-20 electrode system, two common central scalp reference electrodes were applied, the filter was 0.5–70 Hz, sensitivity 100 mV · cm^{-1}) which was digitized (Rhythm version 9, Stellate Systems) using a sampling rate equal to 200 · s^{-1} for eight minutes. Electrode placements were: Fp1-T3, T3-O1, Fp2-T4, T4-O2, Fp1-C3, C3-O1, Fp2-C4, C4-O2, T3-C3, C3-Cz, Cz-C4 and C4-T4. Subcutaneously needle electrodes were used. EEG was recorded throughout the injection procedure in all pigs. One pig served as control with the purpose to validate the model. In this pig 1 mL penicillin G (1 000 000 U · mL^{-1}, diluted in 0.9% NaCl) was injected at two time points with 20 minutes interval. After the first injection the pig developed tachycardia and generalized rhythmic fast sharp activity (Figure 2). After the second injection there was after three minutes markedly pathological EEG (generalized spikes, spike/wave and slow waves) consistent with ongoing seizure activity (Figure 3). After additional seven minutes the pig developed frequent widespread and small muscle contractions, and the pig was then euthanized according to protocol with an overdose of 10% pentobarbital.

Follow-up and assessment of animals

In rats, weight was measured prior to, right after, and nine days after the procedure. All animals, rats and pigs, had supervision at least two times daily and any abnormal behavior and signs of CNS affection after the procedure was

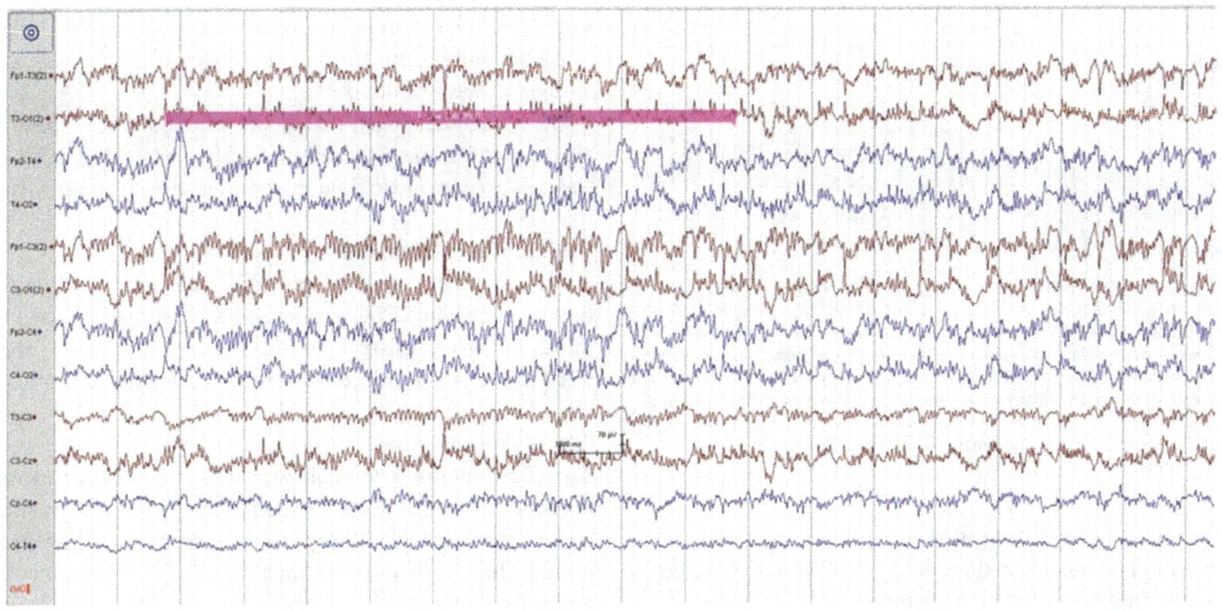

Figure 2 EEG registrations immediate after the first injection of penicillin G leading to generalized rhythmic fast sharp activity.

monitored and registered by a veterinarian. In rats, general behavior, the level of stress and activity and animal appearance like body posture and fur (bristling or not) were registered. Behavior in pigs was systematically scored twice daily to enable capturing of any abnormal behavior or negative trends (Table 1).

Brain biopsy of rats

The whole brain was acquired the ninth day after the surgical procedure. Isoflurane (Abbot Scandinavia, Solna, Sweden) was used to induce anesthesia, followed by intraperitoneal injection of an overdose of 10% pentobarbital (300 $mg \cdot kg^{-1}$). When the rats stopped breathing, the thorax was immediately opened and 100 mL phosphate-buffered saline was injected through the left cardiac ventricle while the heart was still beating, followed by 100 mL injection of 4% formalin for intravascular fixation of the brain parenchyma, a method adapted from Wideroe et al. [15]. Injection rate was set to 35 $mL \cdot min^{-1}$. An incision in the right atrium allowed solution to leave the circulation,

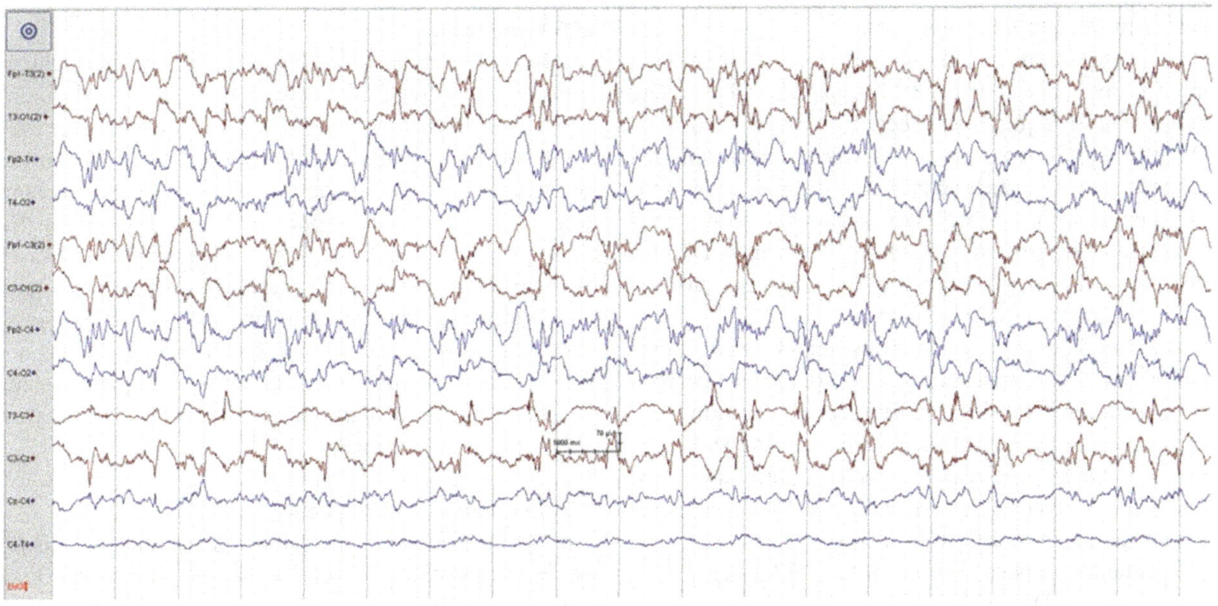

Figure 3 EEG registrations after the second injection of penicillin G leading to seizure activity.

Table 1 Scores of symptoms in pigs post-procedure

	Day 2	Day 4	Day 6	Day 8	Day 10	Day 12
Pig 1	0/12	0/12	1/12	1/12	1/12	1/12
Pig 2	0/12	1/12	0/12	0/12	0/12	0/12
Pig 3	0/12	0/12	0/12	0/12	0/12	0/12
Pig 4	1/12	2/12	0/12	0/12	0/12	0/12
Pig 5	0/12	0/12	0/12	0/12	0/12	0/12
Pig 6	2/12	2/12	1/12	0/12	0/12	0/12

The score was predefined by a veterinarian and the score was based on: appearance, behavior, nutritional status and relevant clinical signs (gait disturbances and/or seizure). For each dimension a range from 0 (normal) to 3 (markedly abnormal) was possible giving a range from 0-12 on each observation. The scores presented were from the assessment where the individual pig reached the highest sum (most symptoms). A total score of 0-3 was predefined as normal unless the pig scored 3 in one dimension (severe symptoms). A total score higher than 3 or maximal score in one dimension warranted a consult with a veterinarian.

thus avoiding volume overload and subsequent tissue damage. The head was then decapitated and embedded in 4% buffered formalin for two weeks prior to histopathological analysis.

Brain biopsy of pigs

The brain biopsies were acquired at day 13 for three pigs and at day 16 for the other three. The pigs were sedated with 2 mL stesolid (5 $mg \cdot mL^{-1}$), 4 mL azaperone (40 $mg \cdot mL^{-1}$), 14 mL ketamin (50 $mg \cdot mL^{-1}$) and later euthanized with 40 mL 10% pentobarbital. Shortly after injection a large craniectomy was performed. Sampling of dura and brain parenchyma both above and below the tentorium was performed and acquired biopsies were embedded in 4% buffered formalin. In addition, plexus choroideus were sampled in all pigs.

Assessment of histopathology

In the rat experiment the brain was cut in coronal sections (2 mm) and embedded in paraffin. From the paraffin-blocks 4 μm thick sections were cut, stained with haematoxylin-eosin, and examined microscopically. To assess processes such as gliosis, fibrosis or inflammation immunohistochemistry was performed using antibodies against lymphocytes (CD3 for T-cells and CD20 for B-cells), microglia/macrophages (CD68), and reactive astrocytes (glial fibrillary acidic protein (GFAP)).

Tissue samples of pig brain from supratentorial, infratentorial and brain stem region were fixed in buffered 4% formalin and embedded in paraffin. Paraffin-sections of 4 μm thickness were cut, stained with haematoxylin-eosin for microscopical analyses. The sections were also incubated with antibodies against GFAP, CD45 (leukocyte common antigen), and CD68 (microglial activation). The immunostaining was carried out on a DAKO Autostainer (Dako, Glostrup, Denmark). Visualization of immunoreactivity was performed with DAKO EnVision system with diaminobenzidin as chromogene. Sections were counterstained with haematoxylin. Positive controls were included in each staining run. In the negative controls the primary antibodies were omitted.

The neuropathologist (SHT) was blinded with respect to all data concerning the animal status and which side it was saline or acoustic fluid injection in the rat experiment.

Statistical considerations

As the primary end-points were qualitative in nature (animal behavior, EEG registrations, histopathology and immunohistochemistry) we only present descriptive analysis. Average is presented as mean ± standard deviation.

Ethical approval

The experimental protocols were reviewed and approved by the Norwegian Committee for Animal Experiments, and conform to the European Convention for the Protection of Vertebrate Animals Used for Experimental and other Scientific Purposes.

Results

General

The mean weight of the eight rats was 273 g ± 8 before the procedure and 267 g ± 8 after nine days post-procedure. The mean weight of the six pigs was 37 kg ± 2 before the procedure and 43 kg ± 4 at end of follow-up.

Animal behavior

In rats, no apparent discomfort or altered behavior was registered during the follow up assessment. In pigs the post-procedure behavior was scored systematically (Table 1) without detection of adverse events (score ≥ 3/12).

EEG registrations

In the six animals receiving injection of the acoustic fluid we have five EEG registrations with good quality. Median registration time was 43 minutes (range 26 – 54 minutes) with all pigs having more than 20 minutes of registration post-injection. For unknown reasons one EEG recording disappeared at attempt of storing. This pig (pig 5) did not appear any different with respect to heart rate, oxygen saturation or behavior after the procedure. The pig had an uneventful immediate recovery. In the other five pigs there were EEG recordings of good quality and there were no signs of seizure activity. Figure 4 demonstrates the pre- and post-procedure EEG in pig 3.

Histopathological assessment

No inflammation or tissue damage was seen after injection of the acoustic or control fluid in rat brain parenchyma with any of the techniques used. Figure 5 demonstrates the area of injection without any reactions. In pigs

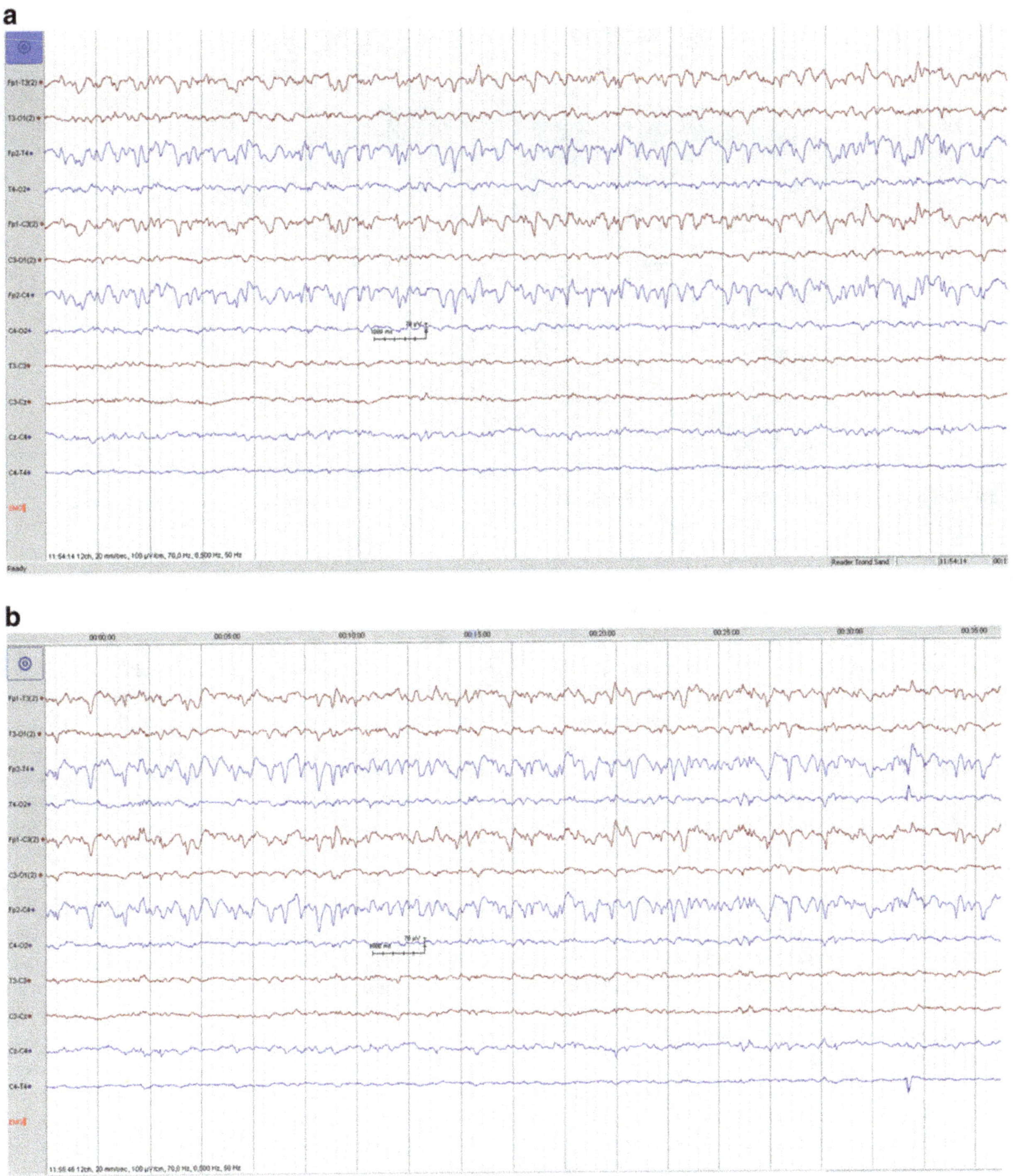

Figure 4 EEG registrations in pig 3. a) Before the procedure. Synchronous background activity 4-6 Hz with highest amplitudes in the frontotemporal region. **b)** After injection of the acoustic coupling fluid. There was no evidence of seizure activity on EEG.

microscopical analyses did not reveal any kind of inflammation, neither in meninges, nor in brain tissue or vessels. Furthermore, no gliosis or microglial response was observed after immunohistochemistry. In the brain-stem biopsy in pig 4 a small focal area was observed with a few lymphocytes, eosinophiles, macrophages and slight spongiforme changes (subtle loss of neural tissue). No neutrophile granulocytes were observed. This focal area appeared microscopically to be of a chronic character and not due to the procedure.

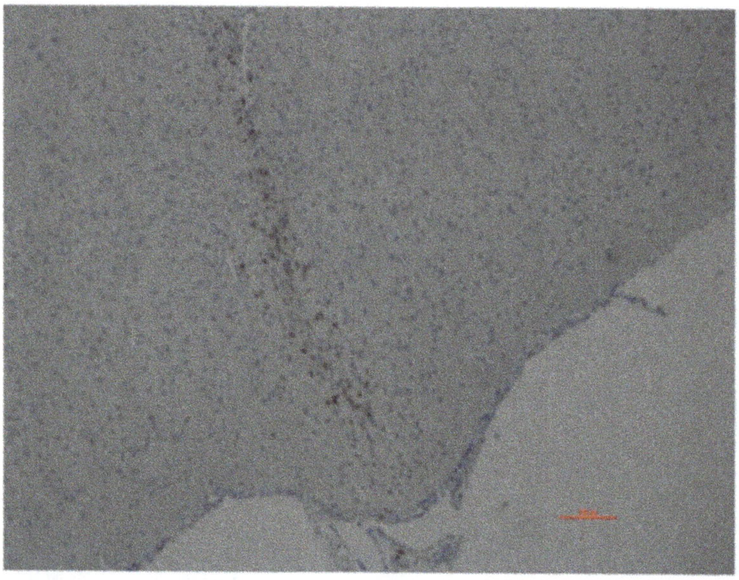

Figure 5 Histology of injection site of the acoustic fluid in rat. There was a minor macrophage response just around the needle site which is a normal reaction to brain trauma. Except from this there was no evidence of any reactions around the needle site.

Discussion

In this safety study in rats and pigs we were unable to detect adverse clinical events of the newly developed acoustic coupling fluid for improving image quality in ultrasound-guided operations. Intra-procedure EEG was also unable to demonstrate any signs of epileptogenic effects. Also, there were no signs of acute inflammation in histopathological samples.

The intention with this testing was a relevant and sophisticated administration of the acoustic fluid (intraparenchymal and subarachnoidal) in two different species. Thus, we examined a local effect in rats and a more regional effect in pigs. The administration methods were chosen to minimize procedural damage, thereby enhancing post-procedural observation. The refined assessment was important to be able to detect any subtle damage to nervous tissue or its surroundings. Also, such methods are also in line with the 3R's (refinement, reduction, replacement) in animal research.

Although no adverse events or signs of toxicity were observed in the two animal models, toxicity may be both dose-dependent and time-dependent. In rats 1 μL was injected intraparenchymal (approximately 1/2000 of the mean brain volume) and in pigs 1 mL was administered into the subarachnoid space (approximately 5% of total CSF volume) [14]. This would equal accumulation of 7.5 mL in the human CSF. Since the acoustic coupling fluid is likely to be opaque, a prerequisite for the usefulness would be 3D ultrasound imaging so that the region of interest in the ultrasound image can be retrieved. With ultrasound it is possible to update the image information several times during a brain tumor resection to follow the progression of tumor resection and to correct for brain shift [6]. Thus, repeated administration and removal of the acoustic fluid will be carried out. Acquisition of a 3D ultrasound image recording typically takes 2-3 minutes. Thereafter the coupling fluid will be removed with suction and irrigation. Topical accumulation of the fluid is unlikely since the surgeons after image acquisition would want to remove the fluid since it is opaque. Also, most of the fluid will presumably stay in the resection cavity since a horizontal craniotomy is most often attempted when brain tumor resections are facilitated by ultrasound [6]. The experience in animals is that the fluid is easily removed by suction and flushing with Ringer's solution. A potential pitfall for excessive accumulation of the fluid to levels higher than tested in the animals could be in tumors where the ventricles are opened as a result of tumor resection. This could be the case in tumors similar to the situation seen in Figure 1. In these situations special care is necessary and until further safety data is available our recommendation is that fluid should not be administered *after* opening the ventricles.

The strengths of the model are testing of both rats and pigs in addition to use of relevant application methods (intraparenchymal and subarachnoid space) with sophisticated methods and the use of EEG monitoring. However, the drugs used to sedate the pigs could possibly increase the seizure threshold and mask EEG disturbances. Also, due to the number of tested animals it remains a possibility that more rare events may have gone unnoticed. However, further animal testing for rare events or reactions due to very high doses or delayed effects was considered less relevant because of the benign profile seen in our experiments. Still, translating positive therapeutic findings or negative toxicity findings from animal to humans are naturally always subject to uncertainty due to the inherent biological differences. We decided that the potential gain of further animal testing was limited and consequently we designed a study assessing safety in selected brain tumor patients. Recently this protocol was approved by the Norwegian Medicines Agency and the local ethical committee and we are now in the beginning of a phase 1 safety study (EudraCT number 2012-005567-27).

The acoustic fluid holds potential to enhance image quality when using 3D ultrasound in brain tumor resections. We hope this will make image interpretation easier at the end of a brain tumor resection, an improvement that could be of particular importance for users with limited experience in using ultrasound guided surgery. Improved imaging near the end of the surgery could be associated with improved resection grades that again improves clinical outcome [2,4,5,16]. We now hope to translate these positive findings from simulation and the animal models to highly selected patients with suspected high-grade glioma to further evaluate the potential benefits while carefully monitor any potential adverse events.

Conclusion

We have in rats and pigs demonstrated that the newly developed acoustic coupling fluid intended for use in ultrasound-guided brain tumor surgery appears safe under the tested circumstances. We are now in the beginning of a phase 1 clinical study where different concentrations of the acoustic coupling fluid is tested in selected patients at our institution in order to assess safety and impact on ultrasound image quality.

Competing interests

Geirmund Unsgård and Tormod Selbekk have submitted a patent application with respect to the novel acoustic fluid.

Authors' contributions

ASJ: planned the experiments, carried out the animal experiments, collected data, drafted the article, submitted manuscript on behalf of authors. AJ: planned the experiments, carried out the rat experiments, revised the manuscript. TS: planned the experiments, responsible for the development of the acoustic fluid, assisted in the experiments, revised the article. RPM: assisted in the experiments, revised the article. OS: planned the experiments, revised the article. SHT: did the histopathological analysis, revised the article. LMS: planned and assisted in the experiments, revised the article. PA: planned and assisted in the experiments, revised the article. GU: planned experiments, responsible for the development of acoustic fluid, revised the article. All authors read and approved the final manuscript.

Acknowledgements

Tora Bonnevie and May-Britt Moser; the Kavli Institute and the Centre for the Biology of Memory, NTNU, for sharing their experience and equipment for injection of substances in rat brain. Sissel Brox; Department of Neurology and Clinical Neurophysiology, St.Olavs University Hospital, for recording of EEG. Oddveig Lyng; The Unit of Comparative Medicine, NTNU, for invaluable help in the pig experiment. Marianne Haugvold, Operating Room of the Future, St.Olavs University Hospital, for help in planning and logistics.

Author details

[1]Department of Neurosurgery, St.Olavs University Hospital, N-7006 Trondheim, Norway. [2]MI Lab, Norwegian University of Science and Technology, Trondheim, Norway. [3]Department of Neuroscience, Norwegian University of Science and Technology, Trondheim, Norway. [4]National Competence Centre for Ultrasound and Image-guided Therapy, Trondheim, Norway. [5]Department of Diagnostic Imaging, St.Olavs University Hospital, Trondheim, Norway. [6]Department of Medical Technology, SINTEF, Trondheim, Norway. [7]Department of Neurology and Clinical Neurophysiology, St. Olavs University Hospital, Trondheim, Norway. [8]Department of Laboratory Medicine, Children's and Women's Health, Norwegian University of Science and Technology, Trondheim, Norway. [9]Department of Pathology and Medical Genetics, St.Olavs University Hospital, Trondheim, Norway.

References

1. Stummer W, Reulen H-J, Meinel T, Pichlmeier U, Schumacher W, Tonn J-C, Rohde V, Oppel F, Turowski B, Woiciechowsky C, Franz K, Pietsch T, ALA-Glioma Study Group: **Extent of resection and survival in glioblastoma multiforme: identification of and adjustment for bias.** *Neurosurgery* 2008, **62**(3):564–576.
2. Jakola AS, Myrmel KS, Kloster R, Torp SH, Lindal S, Unsgard G, Solheim O: **Comparison of a strategy favoring early surgical resection vs a strategy favoring watchful waiting in low-grade gliomas.** *JAMA* 2012, **308**(18):1881–1888.
3. Stummer W, Tonn C Jr, Mehdorn HM, Nestler U, Franz K, Goetz C, Bink A, Pichlmeier U: **Counterbalancing risks and gains from extended resections in malignant glioma surgery: a supplemental analysis from the randomized 5-aminolevulinic acid glioma resection study.** *J Neurosurg* 2010, **114**(3):613–623.
4. Senft C, Bink A, Franz K, Vatter H, Gasser T, Seifert V: **Intraoperative MRI guidance and extent of resection in glioma surgery: a randomised, controlled trial.** *Lancet Oncol* 2011, **12**(11):997–1003.
5. Stummer W, Pichlmeier U, Meinel T, Wiestler OD, Zanella F, Reulen H-J: **Fluorescence-guided surgery with 5-aminolevulinic acid for resection of malignant glioma: a randomised controlled multicentre phase III trial.** *Lancet Oncol* 2006, **7**(5):392–401.
6. Unsgaard G, Rygh OM, Selbekk T, Müller TB, Kolstad F, Lindseth F, Hernes TAN: **Intra-operative 3D ultrasound in neurosurgery.** *Acta Neurochir* 2006, **148**(3):235–253.
7. Szelényi A, Bello L, Duffau H, Fava E, Feigl GC, Galanda M, Neuloh G, Signorelli F, Sala F: **Intraoperative electrical stimulation in awake craniotomy: methodological aspects of current practice.** *Neurosurg Focus* 2010, **28**(2):E7.
8. Saether CA, Torsteinsen M, Torp SH, Sundstrom S, Unsgard G, Solheim O: **Did survival improve after the implementation of intraoperative neuronavigation and 3D ultrasound in glioblastoma surgery? A retrospective analysis of 192 primary operations.** *J Neurol Surg A Cent Eur Neurosurg* 2012, **73**(2):73–78.
9. Solheim O, Selbekk T, Jakola AS, Unsgård G: **Ultrasound-guided operations in unselected high-grade gliomas—overall results, impact of image quality and patient selection.** *Acta Neurochir* 2010, **152**(11):1873–1886.
10. Rygh O, Selbekk T, Torp S, Lydersen S, Hernes T, Unsgaard G: **Comparison of navigated 3D ultrasound findings with histopathology in subsequent phases of glioblastoma resection.** *Acta Neurochir* 2008, **150**(10):1033–1042.
11. Gerganov VM, Samii A, Giordano M, Samii M, Fahlbusch R: **Two-dimensional high-end ultrasound imaging compared to intraoperative MRI during resection of low-grade gliomas.** *J Clin Neurosci* 2011, **18**(5):669–673.
12. Selbekk T, Jakola AS, Solheim O, Johansen TF, Lindseth F, Reinertsen I, Unsgard G: **Ultrasound imaging in neurosurgery: approaches to minimize surgically induced image artefacts for improved resection control.** *Acta Neurochir (Wien)* 2013, **155**(6):973–980.
13. Hafting T, Fyhn M, Bonnevie T, Moser MB, Moser EI: **Hippocampus-independent phase precession in entorhinal grid cells.** *Nature* 2008, **453**(7199):1248–1252.
14. Morgan CJ, Pyne-Geithman GJ, Jauch EC, Shukla R, Wagner KR, Clark JF, Zuccarello M: **Bilirubin as a cerebrospinal fluid marker of sentinel**

subarachnoid hemorrhage: a preliminary report in pigs. *J Neurosurg* 2004, **101**(6):1026–1029.

15. Wideroe M, Olsen O, Pedersen TB, Goa PE, Kavelaars A, Heijnen C, Skranes J, Brubakk AM, Brekken C: **Manganese-enhanced magnetic resonance imaging of hypoxic-ischemic brain injury in the neonatal rat.** *Neuroimage* 2009, **45**(3):880–890.
16. Smith JS, Chang EF, Lamborn KR, Chang SM, Prados MD, Cha S, Tihan T, VandenBerg S, McDermott MW, Berger MS: **Role of Extent of Resection in the Long-Term Outcome of Low-Grade Hemispheric Gliomas.** *J Clin Oncol* 2008, **26**(8):1338–1345.

10

Impact of a standardized training program on midwives' ability to assess fetal heart anatomy by ultrasound

Eric Hildebrand[1*], Madeleine Abrandt Dahlgren[2], Catarina Sved[3,4], Tomas Gottvall[1], Marie Blomberg[1] and Birgitta Janerot-Sjoberg[3,5,6,7]

Abstract

Background: Studies of prenatal detection of congenital heart disease (CHD) in the UK, Italy, and Norway indicate that it should be possible to improve the prenatal detection rate of CHD in Sweden. These studies have shown that training programs, visualization of the outflow tracts and color-Doppler all can help to speed up and improve the detection rate and accuracy. We aimed to introduce a more accurate standardized fetal cardiac ultrasound screening protocol in Sweden.

Methods: A novel pedagogical model for training midwives in standardized cardiac imaging was developed, a model using a think-aloud analysis during a pre- and post-course test and a subsequent group reflection. The self-estimated difficulties and knowledge gaps of two experienced and two beginner midwives were identified. A two-day course with mixed lectures, demonstrations and hands-on sessions was followed by a feedback session three months later consisting of an interview and check-up. The long-term effects were tested two years later.

Results: At the post-course test the self-assessed uncertainty was lower than at the pre-course test. The qualitative evaluation showed that the color Doppler images were difficult to interpret, but the training seems to have improved their ability to use the new technique. The ability to perform the method remained at the new level at follow-up both three months and two years later.

Conclusions: Our results indicate that by implementing new imaging modalities and providing hands-on training, uncertainty can be reduced and examination time decreased, but they also show that continuous on-site training with clinical and technical back-up is important.

Keywords: Color Doppler, Congenital heart disease, Detection of congenital heart defects, Fetal heart scanning, Learning program, Prenatal cardiology, Second trimester screening, Standardized training program, Ultrasound screening

Background

Congenital heart disease (CHD) is the most common congenital defect and can lead to major adverse consequences for the child. Internationally, just below 1% of all pregnancies are affected by CHD and usually there is no identifiable cause [1,2]. About half of the CHD cases are regarded as major, requiring surgery or intervention in the child's first year of life. Furthermore, about one third of the major CHD cases will have a duct-dependent anomaly, an anomaly that, if not identified before birth or recognized shortly after birth, will become a life threatening condition [3,4].

In a recently published study, the incidence of CHD in the Southeast region of Sweden was 8/1,000 fetuses/newborns whereof 3/1,000 were major. The detection rate of CHD cases was only 5% before birth if all cases were included but became 37,5% if all cases of minor CHD were excluded [5]. Similar results were found in another large Swedish study (n = 36,299) where 15% of major CHDs were detected before 22 weeks [6]. A study

* Correspondence: eric.hildebrand@lio.se
[1]Department of Obstetrics and Gynaecology, and Department of Clinical and Experimental Medicine, Linköping University, Linköping, Sweden
Full list of author information is available at the end of the article

from Trondheim in Norway reported a 46% detection rate of major CHD at the time of the 18 week routine scan [4]. Del Bianco et al. state that in Italy almost 90% of major CHD defects are detectable before birth if a full heart examination is performed at 20–24 weeks of gestation [7]. These data indicate that the Swedish prenatal detection rate of CHD has a potential for being significantly increased and that the screening performance is in need of improvement. Recognition of this situation was what led us to make this study.

Training programs have been proven effective in increasing the antenatal detection of CHD. McBrien et al. reported a rise in detection rate from 28% to 43% after a relatively simple training program was implemented in the UK [8]. Oggè et al. conducted a multicenter study in Italy, and after training the sensitivity for CHD was 65,5% with a specificity of 99,7% [9]. Allen et al. demonstrated a marked geographical difference in detection rate of structural cardiac defects in the UK, ranging from 0 to 70%, where the higher rates of detection tended to be concentrated in areas where teaching programs in cardiac scanning had been in place for some time [10]. Results from a study by Pézard et al. in France support the hypothesis that providing learning centers where screening sonographers may improve their practice will have beneficial effects [11].

In the Southeast region of Sweden all pregnant women are offered two routine ultrasound examinations as part of the official Maternity Health Care System, one at 11 to 14 gestational weeks ("first trimester") in order to assess the gestational age, and another at 18 to 20 weeks ("second trimester") to assess the anatomical features of the fetus. The screenings are performed by specially trained midwives and 30 minutes are allocated for each scan. In the first trimester screening all women are also offered a first-trimester combined risk-assessment for trisomy 21, 13 and 18 [12]. At the second trimester scan a checklist is used for anatomical assessments. Concerning the heart, the screening results are regarded as normal if the four-chamber view is accurately obtained. This criterion has been used in the screening-situation as a simple and reproducible basis for finding anomalies of the fetal heart. However, this approach has been shown to detect only a minority of heart anomalies; it does not identify anomalies affecting the outflow tracts and the great arteries [7,13]. Adding visualization of the outflow tracts to the four-chamber view has been proven to be an effective technique to detect major CHD prenatally [14]. Previous studies have shown that using a systematic approach when examining the fetal heart facilitates the confirmation of normality and also makes it easier to recognize abnormalities [10,13-16]. If color-Doppler is added to the examination, rapid screening to detect flow abnormalities of the fetal heart may be carried out [17]. This view is supported by Chaoui et al. who suggest that color-Doppler should be added to the screening for CHD in order to allow easy detection of the majority of CHD [18]. Results from a recent study by Eggebo et al. led the authors to conclude that the routine use of color Doppler in fetal heart scanning may be helpful in the detection of major CHD [19].

The aim of this study was to evaluate the possibility for introducing a more accurate fetal cardiac ultrasound screening method, based on five additional transverse views and color-Doppler, by using a novel pedagogical approach to the standardized cardiac imaging training.

Methods

A two-day course in standardized examination techniques of the fetal heart and color-Doppler was given at Linköping University Hospital. The course was designed by a group consisting of physicians and researchers specialized in fetal medicine, pediatric cardiology and clinical physiology, a specialized sonographer, and a professor of education. Four midwives from the routine ultrasound screening in the southeast region of Sweden attended the course; two were from Linköping University Hospital and two from Värnamo county hospital. Each hospital contributed one experienced midwife with more than 20 years of experience with obstetrical ultrasound and one beginner with five years or less of experience. The local ultrasound units at the hospitals were free to choose the midwives to participate as long as they met these criteria and had given their informed consent. At arrival, a pre-course test was taken by the midwives. The intent of the pre-course test was to enhance the midwives' awareness of their present level of knowledge and skills and to identify any difficulties encountered in using the new technique, as a starting point for learning. At this test, each midwife was individually presented a series of ultrasound recordings of the fetal heart visualized as cine-loops in gray-scale with or without color Doppler. The midwives were equipped with dictaphones and instructed to "think aloud" by saying how they judged the scans and what they based their judgment on [20]. They were also instructed to comment on the quality of the scans and to note if the color Doppler added significant information. In addition, the midwives filled out a paper form on which they indicated if they judged the scan to be normal or pathological and how confident they felt about the judgment. The experiences from this test were then discussed and the discussion was audio-recorded by the group of four and the course leaders. Thirty minutes were allocated for the discussion. The recording was intended to then serve as a basis for reflection and as a source indicating needs for improved knowledge and skills. Based on the results, a detailed course syllabus was created, setting forth a program that would consist of lectures on ultrasound examination of the fetal heart using color Doppler technique as well as hands-on training. The first step was for the midwives, in the presence of cardiac sonographers, to practice color-Doppler examination of children and adolescents who came to the Department of Clinical Physiology for cardiac ultrasound exams where color-Doppler is routinely used. Each midwife used two hours of training on different patients. Informed consent was given by the patients. On the second day of the course, fetal heart screening was performed on pregnant women who had reached about 20 weeks of gestation. Another individual two hours of training on different fetuses were allocated for each midwife after she had been given informed consent by each pregnant woman. For the clinical praxis the midwives were taught to record an ultrasound gray-scale-clip starting from the abdomen of the fetus and sliding in the cephalic direction; this procedure was repeated with color Doppler added. The different anatomical landmarks are described in Table 1.

With these experiences a second thirty minute group discussion session was held and digitally audio-recorded for later analysis. The course ended by having the midwives take the same individual audio-recorded and form-completion test that they had taken before starting the course.

Before leaving, the midwives were given another protocol to be used in their clinical practice until first follow-up. This protocol included documentation of their self-assessment in a four-graded scale of their confidence in performing the different steps when examining the fetal heart (Table 2). The self-assessed significance of the specific use of color Doppler was also to be documented (Table 3). Recordings of all these examinations were to be stored as clinical routine exams in the local digital image archive and databases, assuring that they would be available for future review. The time used to achieve the proper projections of the fetal heart was also noted in the protocol at each examination.

Table 1 Protocol used for standardized examination of the fetal heart

1	Position of the fetus to determine the situs
2	Cross-section of the fetal abdomen, then slide in the cephalic direction
	S: Determine the position of the stomach, inferior vena cava and the aorta
	A: Four-chamber view
	B: Outflow-tract of aorta from left ventricle
	C: Outflow tract of pulmonary artery
	D: Three vessel view and arches
3	Repeat the slide with addition of color Doppler
	A: Four-chamber view
	B: Outflow-tract of aorta from left ventricle
	C: Outflow tract of pulmonary artery
	D: Three vessel view and arches

Table 2 Self- assessed confidence to perform the method in clinical praxis

1	Uncertain
2	More uncertain than certain
3	More certain than uncertain
4	Certain

The recordings from the group discussions were transcribed and analyzed generating a number of preliminary themes. These themes then served as a basis for the formation of the interview guide for the individual interviews. After approximately three months training with the new technique, individual interviews were performed on site with each midwife. The interview guide is shown in Table 4. The interviews were recorded and transcribed word for word. The interview texts were then analyzed qualitatively, using a simple content analysis to describe the midwives' reflections on the use of what was for them a new technique. The method of content-analysis was inspired by the methodology described by Graneheim et al. [21]. The unit of analysis was the midwives' experiences of working with the new technique. Meaning units regarding the challenges were marked in the transcript. These were then sorted into three content areas; 'color', 'orientation', and 'hands-on'. Representative manifest quotations were chosen to illustrate the experienced challenges.

The ultrasound recordings from the first and last 10 exams during this three month period were reviewed and assessed by a specialist in fetal medicine and by a cardiac sonographer specialist. They graded the ability of the midwife to perform the different steps in the examination. The flow of the training program is presented in Figure 1.

Two years after the primary course, another follow up was performed. The same midwives documented 10 ultrasound examinations performed in the clinical routine in a way similar to the procedure followed during the training program. The follow up included the self-assessment concerning confidence in using the method (Table 2) and an identical review of the ultrasound

Table 3 The Significance of color Doppler for assessment of the heart anatomy

1	No significance
2	Little significance
3	Great significance
4	Crucial

Table 4 Interview guide for the individual interviews

Introduction	Questions
During the course you had the opportunity to try color Doppler.	How did you think the color-Doppler helped you to see deviations?
	How did the color affect your ability to see deviations from normal?
	How can color be used to facilitate the assessment?
	How would you compare the assessment without color and with color added?
Several of the course participants said that assessment is facilitated if they themselves perform the ultrasound examination rather than assessing images obtained by someone else.	What do you think about that?
	Is it possible to "see" with your hands? How?
During the course you were to decide whether a number of cases were normal or abnormal.	What is important for you to be able to make a good assessment?
	What do you need to be able to judge an image as normal or not?
	What do you do if you are unsure?
Several of the course participants found it difficult to make the judgment with the help of images.	What do you find that is difficult about this?
	If you look at your ability to make judgments now, compared with before the course, how has it been affected?
	How have you been able to train your ability to make judgments after the course?
If you look at the structure of the course after completing it	What do you think about that now?
	What could have been done differently and why?
If you compare your ability to use the technique now compared to before the course.	What do you think about that now?

recordings performed by the same specialists. Additionally, the midwives took a test identical to the pre-course test described above, where a series of ultrasound recordings were assessed; Dictaphones were not used, however.

The Regional Ethical Review Board in Linköping has approved the study (EPN 7–2009).

Results

Results from the 2-day initial course

The results at the pre- and post-course test were similar, 23/132 vs 21/132 incorrect answers (ns). The self-assessed uncertainty was, however, lower at the post-course test; 30/132 vs 11/132 ($p = 0.006$).

Qualitative evaluation of the think-aloud recordings, group discussions and interviews

The group discussions prior to the training showed that the use of color Doppler produced unfamiliar images that some of the midwives found difficult to interpret. *'It was all blurred, colors all over the place.'* This difficulty was also commented on in the think-aloud protocols of the pre-course test. The training seems to have enhanced the familiarity with the new technique; one of the midwives commented on the learning *'you could not kind of recognize where you were, at first, when you did not see the usual image...but you learn to kind of change your gaze, I believe...'* The importance of the hands-on training was emphasized as being critical for learning. The judgment of the scans only, as in the pre-course test, seemed, however, to deprive the midwives of some of the manual skills in identifying anatomical landmarks needed to perform the ultrasound, *'you have to do it yourself, to know exactly the positions where you are'.* This aspect was also commented on in the three months follow up interview *'you know the position of the fetal heart..but you get a totally different perception of what is up and down, left and right, when you're watching someone else doing it, when you have no idea of how they hold the probe..It is really difficult..'* Table 5 illustrates the four midwives' judgments of 33 scans in the pre- and after-course test. Each scan consisted of several views, making several judgments possible.

Results from the 3 months fetal screenings

In total, 80 examinations (20 from each midwife) were performed with the new method in the screening-

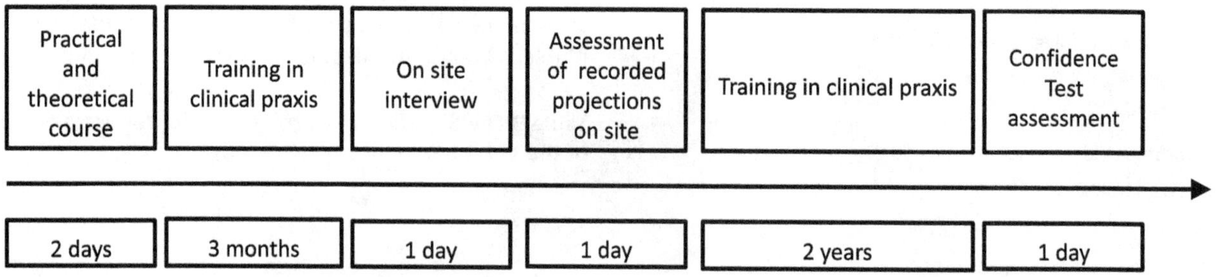

Figure 1 Flowchart of the learning program.

Table 5 Midwives' judgments of 33 scans before and after the course

Judgments	Before training	After training
No judgment made	28	29
Judgment without motivation	17	13
Judgment with motivation based on >1 view	33	36

Several judgments possible per scan.

situation three months after the course. The results are presented in Table 6. Their median self-assessed ability to technically use the new method was 3 out of 4 and the importance of color Doppler was graded 2.5 out of 4. From their self-assessment it was seen that it was possible to perform a full examination as defined in the protocol in 56/77 (73%) cases for gray-scale ultrasound registrations and in 53/77 (69%) for color Doppler registrations (ns). Data on self-assessment of the ability to perform the different steps were missing in three patients. The median time used to obtain the proper projections of the heart was four minutes (range 3–10 min).

From the specialist review of the 10 first and 10 last exams carried out by each midwife during the 3-month follow-up period with routine fetal screenings including the new method 67/80 (84%) grey scale and 52/80 (65%) color Doppler recordings were judged to be complete (ns). There were, however, large inter-individual differences in success-rate of correctly performed recordings ranging from 20/20 to 9/20 where the midwives with the longest experience had the best results.

Results from the two-year follow-up

Two years after the course the same midwives recorded 40 new ultrasound examinations of the fetal heart including the new method, 10 by each midwife. Their median self-assessed ability to technically use the new method was 4 of 4 and the importance of color Doppler was graded 3 out of 4. From their self-assessment it was seen that it was possible to perform a full examination as defined by the protocol in 33/40 (83%) cases for gray-scale and 32/40 (80%) cases for color Doppler (ns).

From the specialist review of the 40 examinations 30/40 (75%) gray scale and 33/40 (83%) color Doppler recordings were judged to be complete (Table 6).

Results from the written test were in accordance with the results from the pre- and after-course tests (ns). Nineteen out of 132 answers were incorrect corresponding to a self-assessed uncertainty in 17 out of 132 exams.

The median time used to achieve the proper projections of the fetal heart and color-Doppler recordings was 3 minutes (range 2–5 min). This was significantly shorter than at the three month follow-up.

Discussion

In the present study we describe the self-estimated difficulties and show the ability of the midwives to successfully add new ultrasound modalities to a standardized fetal ultrasound screening of the heart. By designing a short initial course based on a combination of the experience and actual needs and skills of the participants, hands-on training as advocated reduced uncertainty, but it was found that continuous on-site training with clinical and technical back-up are important.

In the present screening program in the South Eastern region of Sweden the fetal heart is considered normal if it is possible to obtain and verify a normal four-chamber view. This has, however, been proven to be highly ineffective for the detection of most CHD [5,6]. Is it possible, with a short course and further on-site training with backup, to achieve a better detection rate in a routine clinical screening situation in a low-risk population in Sweden? As noted in the introduction, the antenatal detection of CHD could be significantly increased by adding the three-vessel view [7,14,16]. McBrien et al. used a relatively simple training program to improve the detection rate for CHD from 28% pre-training to 43% in the year of training. The program included hands-on training and a refresher day where the sonographers were given a new lecture on fetal echocardiography and cases with CHD were reviewed, emphasizing the importance of continuous and repeated training [8]. Pézard et al. studied the difference between sonographers attending a training

Table 6 Self-assessment of the examinations in clinical praxis, number of correct performed examinations when assessed by specialist in fetal medicine and specialized sonographer and time spent to achieve the proper projections

	At three months	At two years	p-value
Self-assessed confidence to perform the method, median/range	3/(1–4)	4/(2–4)	-
Self-assessed significance of color-Doppler, median/range	2.5/(2–4)	3/(1–4)	-
Self-assessed correctly performed examinations in grey scale, No/out of (%)	56/77 (73%)	33/40 (83%)	0.240
Self-assessed correctly performed examinations in color Doppler, No/out of (%)	53/77 (69%)	32/40 (80%)	0.199
Specialist review: Correctly performed gray-scale examinations, No/out of (%)	67/80 (84%)	30/40 (75%)	0.251
Specialist review: Correctly performed color-Doppler examinations, No/out of (%)	52/80 (65%)	33/40 (83%)	0.047
Time spent to achieve the proper projections median/range (min)	4/(3–10)	3/(2–5)	<0.01

course and those not attending. The sensitivity vas 37% versus 16% respectively for detecting a CHD, which further strengthens the importance of continuous training [11]. However, the size of that study was small and the methods of training not specified. The possibility to use color-Doppler for additional screening for flow abnormalities in the heart seems appealing. In the new guidelines from the International Society of Ultrasound in Obstetrics and Gynecology (ISUOG) it is stated that the outflow tract and the four chamber view as a part of the screening is evidence-based. The use of color Doppler is not considered mandatory in the second trimester screening, but its use is, however, encouraged [22]. It has mainly been used to achieve additional information about already detected CHD, in particular complex cases and its use for screening is controversial [17,18]. Eggebo et al. found color-Doppler useful in the screening situation in Norway where 9/26 findings of CHD were related to the additional information given by the color.

In the present study we found that the midwives' ability to examine the fetal heart could be improved, and that their level of self-confidence could be heightened. We also found that this could be done in the normal screening program without creating time-delays. A simple 2-day course in the technique was good enough to help them begin to use the technique in standard clinical praxis, however there were inter-individual differences. These were judged to depend on the clinical experience level of the midwife although the number of participants did not allow for statistical evaluation. One possible explanation of the differences was that it was difficult to make the correct settings in the equipment and this caused the cineloops to be too short. The midwives in our study were able to acquire sufficient skills to perform the different views, especially the part in gray-scale. They found it was more difficult to perform the color-Doppler registrations, and the midwives also considered the color-Doppler to be less significant in the assessment of the heart anatomy, a view that may change with time and experience [23,24]. At the follow-up after two years in practice, the ability to perform the examination was in accordance with the results from the 3-month follow-up, suggesting that the level of skill in performing the different steps in the examination persists if it is used in every-day practice. They still considered it to be difficult to perform Color-Doppler after two years in the self-assessment, but improved when analyzing the ability to obtain the correct views. The time spent to achieve the proper projections was also shorter, indicating that use in clinical practice improves the skills in obtaining the views wanted and that it does not significantly increase the time needed to administer the exam. The results from the written test given on three occasions did not show any improvements in interpreting images. One might conclude that assessment of the images obtained with the method is a more useful method to evaluate the introduction of a new way of performing the examinations than a written test based on review of acquired ultrasound images.

The combination of qualitative and quantitative analysis used is here a strength. The qualitative methods used were content analyses of participants "think aloud" notes/protocols during a pre- and post-course test, an audio-recorded group discussion session, and the recorded interviews about using the new technique, including the self-assessment of the performance to assess the fetal heart in clinical practice. One possible improvement of this study might have been to video record the pre-and post-course test for subsequent analysis. Reviewing the recordings together with the midwives would have given them the opportunity to comment on their own way to think during the test. This might have provided us with more data for analysis. The amount of data from the interviews was also limited. A specialist in interviewing technique might have provided more data. A deeper analysis was thus not possible. Therefore a simple content analysis was performed. The quantitative methods in the study were assessment of the ultrasound recordings by specialists including number of complete recordings and the time used for obtaining the images.

In this small study with only four participants the authors contributed to the course, methods of follow up, interpretation of data and analysis of the results, which might have influenced the results. The differences in the test result before and after the course are small. There is, however, a tendency for the number of correct judgments (without giving reasons for how the judgment was reached) to decrease after training. A tendency is also seen that the number of correct judgments increases when based on one or more views.

To our knowledge this is the first time that the development of ways of reasoning during a practical course in ultrasound methodology has been described. Our experience suggests that the midwives learn, by using the new technique, to use more views as a basis for their judgments. To learn something, the learner has to discern the critical aspects of the object of learning. A condition for learning is that the learner gets to experience a variation in a dimension of that aspect, through potential alternatives [25]. The design of the training exposed the learners to a broad range of fetal heart types, which provides one of necessary conditions for learning. The midwives' reflections immediately after the training and after three months underscore the importance of hands-on training to be able to connect and integrate the experience based knowledge and skills with the new technology.

The size of the present study is a limitation but the results support the hypothesis that it is possible to add new aspects of an examination in the screening program by providing a relatively short training course. Additionally, repeated training with feed-back is needed to maintain the manual skills, obtained through experiential learning in every-day clinical practice.

Conclusions

By participating in a continuous well-structured training program the competence of the midwives could become sufficient, without significant time increase, to perform a more accurate fetal cardiac ultrasound screening by adding five additional transverse views and color-Doppler. If this method is used in the screening situation it might increase the detection of fetal cardiac defects and thereby ensure the optimal care for the affected children after birth. These encouraging results must, however, be further evaluated by including a larger number of midwives and a long term follow up of CHD detection rates.

Competing interests

The authors declare that they have no competing interests.

Authors' contributions

All authors contributed to the course, methods of follow up, interpretation of data and analysis of the results. EH, MAD and BJS planned the first protocol, EH and CS performed the assessment of the recorded ultrasound images. CS performed the interviews with the participating midwives. MAD and EH performed the qualitative evaluation of the interviews. EH and MAD drafted the original manuscript and all authors contributed in the revisions and final approval of the submitted manuscript.

Acknowledgements

The Medical Research Council of South East Sweden and the County Council of Östergötland supported the trial financially.

Author details

[1]Department of Obstetrics and Gynaecology, and Department of Clinical and Experimental Medicine, Linköping University, Linköping, Sweden. [2]Department of Medicine and Health Sciences, Faculty of Health Sciences, Linköping University, Linköping, Sweden. [3]Department of Clinical Physiology and Nuclear Medicine, University Hospital, Linköping, Sweden. [4]Department of Medicine & Health, Division of Cardiovascular medicine, Faculty of Health Sciences, Linköping University, Linköping, Sweden. [5]Department Biomedical Engineering, Linköping University, Linköping, Sweden. [6]Department of Clinical Physiology, Karolinska University Hospital, Stockholm, Sweden. [7]Department of Clinical Science, Division of Medical Imaging and Technology, Intervention and Technology, Karolinska Institutet, Stockholm, Sweden.

References

1. Mitchell SC, Korones SB, Berendes HW: **Congenital heart disease in 56,109 births: incidence and natural history.** *Circulation* 1971, **43**(3):323–332.
2. Cedergren MI, Kallen BA: **Maternal obesity and infant heart defects.** *Obes Res* 2003, **11**(9):1065–1071.
3. Hoffman JI, Kaplan S: **The incidence of congenital heart disease.** *J Am Coll Cardiol* 2002, **39**(12):1890–1900.
4. Tegnander E, Williams W, Johansen OJ, Blaas HG, Eik-Nes SH: **Prenatal detection of heart defects in a non-selected population of 30,149 fetuses–detection rates and outcome.** *Ultrasound Obstet Gynecol* 2006, **27**(3):252–265.
5. Hildebrand E, Selbing A, Blomberg M: **Comparison of first and second trimester ultrasound screening for fetal anomalies in the southeast region of Sweden.** *Acta Obstet Gynecol Scand* 2010, **89**(11):1412–1419.
6. Westin M, Saltvedt S, Bergman G, Kublickas M, Almstrom H, Grunewald C, Valentin L: **Routine ultrasound examination at 12 or 18 gestational weeks for prenatal detection of major congenital heart malformations? A randomised controlled trial comprising 36,299 fetuses.** *BJOG* 2006, 113(6):675–682.
7. del Bianco A, Russo S, Lacerenza N, Rinaldi M, Rinaldi G, Nappi L, Greco P: **Four chamber view plus three-vessel and trachea view for a complete evaluation of the fetal heart during the second trimester.** *J Perinat Med* 2006, **34**(4):309–312.
8. McBrien A, Sands A, Craig B, Dornan J, Casey F: **Impact of a regional training program in fetal echocardiography for sonographers on the antenatal detection of major congenital heart disease.** *Ultrasound Obstet Gynecol* 2010, **36**(3):279–284.
9. Ogge G, Gaglioti P, Maccanti S, Faggiano F, Todros T: **Prenatal screening for congenital heart disease with four-chamber and outflow-tract views: a multicenter study.** *Ultrasound Obstet Gynecol* 2006, **28**(6):779–784.
10. Allan L: **Prenatal diagnosis of structural cardiac defects.** *Am J Med Genet C Semin Med Genet* 2007, **145C**(1):73–76.
11. Pezard P, Bonnemains L, Boussion F, Sentilhes L, Allory P, Lepinard C, Guichet A, Triau S, Biquard F, Leblanc M, Bonneau D, Descamps P: **Influence of ultrasonographers training on prenatal diagnosis of congenital heart diseases: a 12-year population-based study.** *Prenat Diagn* 2008, **28**(11):1016–1022.
12. Nicolaides KH, Spencer K, Avgidou K, Faiola S, Falcon O: **Multicenter study of first-trimester screening for trisomy 21 in 75 821 pregnancies: results and estimation of the potential impact of individual risk-orientated two-stage first-trimester screening.** *Ultrasound Obstet Gynecol* 2005, **25**(3):221–226.
13. Sharland GK, Allan LD: **Screening for congenital heart disease prenatally. Results of a 2 1/2-year study in the South East Thames Region.** *Br J Obstet Gynaecol* 1992, **99**(3):220–225.
14. Carvalho JS, Mavrides E, Shinebourne EA, Campbell S, Thilaganathan B: **Improving the effectiveness of routine prenatal screening for major congenital heart defects.** *Heart* 2002, **88**(4):387–391.
15. Sharland G: **Routine fetal cardiac screening: what are we doing and what should we do?** *Prenat Diagn* 2004, **24**(13):1123–1129.
16. Yagel S, Cohen SM, Achiron R: **Examination of the fetal heart by five short-axis views: a proposed screening method for comprehensive cardiac evaluation.** *Ultrasound Obstet Gynecol* 2001, **17**(5):367–369.
17. Gembruch U, Chatterjee MS, Bald R, Redel DA, Hansmann M: **Color Doppler flow mapping of fetal heart.** *J Perinat Med* 1991, **19**(1–2):27–32.
18. Chaoui R, McEwing R: **Three cross-sectional planes for fetal color Doppler echocardiography.** *Ultrasound Obstet Gynecol* 2003, **21**(1):81–93.
19. Eggebo TM, Heien C, Berget M, Ellingsen CL: **Routine use of color Doppler in fetal heart scanning in a low-risk population.** *ISRN Obstet Gynecol* 2012, **2012**:496935.
20. Someren MW, Barnard YF, Sandberg JAC: *The Think Aloud Method: A Practical Guide to Modelling Cognitive Processes.* London: Academic; 1994.
21. Graneheim UH, Lundman B: **Qualitative content analysis in nursing research: concepts, procedures and measures to achieve trustworthiness.** *Nurse Educ Today* 2004, **24**(2):105–112.
22. International Society of Ultrasound in O, Gynecology, Carvalho JS, Allan LD, Chaoui R, Copel JA, DeVore GR, Hecher K, Lee W, Munoz H, Paladini D, Tutschek B, Yagel S: **ISUOG Practice Guidelines (updated): sonographic screening examination of the fetal heart.** *Ultrasound Obstet Gynecol* 2013, **41**(3):348–359.
23. Sutherland GR, Fraser AG: **Colour flow mapping in cardiology: indications and limitations.** *Br Med Bull* 1989, **45**(4):1076–1091.
24. DeVore GR, Horenstein J, Siassi B, Platt LD: **Fetal echocardiography. VII. Doppler color flow mapping: a new technique for the diagnosis of congenital heart disease.** *Am J Obstet Gynecol* 1987, **156**(5):1054–1064.
25. Pang FMMF: **On some necessary conditions of learning.** *J Learn Sci* 2006, **15**(2):193–220.

11

Validation of 3D echocardiographic volume detection of left atrium by human cadaveric casts

Jouni K. Kuusisto[1*], Vesa M. Järvinen[2] and Juha P. Sinisalo[1]

Abstract

Background: Left atrial volume is a prognostic factor in cardiac pathologies. We aimed to validate left atrial volume detection with 3D and 2D echocardiography (3DE and 2DE) by human cadaveric casts. 3DE facilitates measurement of atrial volume without geometrical assumptions or dependence on imaging angle in contrast to 2DE methods.

Methods: For method validation, six water-filled balloons were submerged in a 20-l water tank and their volumes were measured with 3DE. Seven human cadaveric left atrial casts were prepared of silicone and were transformed into ultrasound-permeable casts. Casts were imaged in the same setting, so that 3DE and 2DE of casts represented transthoracic apical view. Left ventricle analysis softwares GE 4D Auto LVQ and TomTec 4D LV-Function were used for 3DE volumetry.

Results: Balloon volumes ranged 37 to 255 ml (mean 126 ml). 3DE resulted in an excellent volumetric agreement with balloon volumes, absolute bias was – 3.7 ml (95% CI -5.9 to – 1.4). Atrial cast volumes were 38 to 94 ml (mean 56.6 ml). 3DE and 2DE volumes were excellently correlated with cast volumes (r = 0.96 to 0.99). Biases were for GE 4D LVQ -0.7 ml (95% CI -6.1 to 4.6), TomTec 4D LV-Function 3.3 ml (– 1.9 to 8.5) and 2DE 2.9 ml (– 4.0 to 9.9). 3DE resulted in lower limits of agreement and showed no volume-related bias in contrast to area-length method.

Conclusions: We conclude that measurement of human cadaveric left atrial cast volumes by 3DE is in excellent agreement with true cast volumes.

Keywords: Cardiac imaging, Echocardiography, LAV, 3DE, 2DE, Area-length method, In vitro

Background

Left atrial (LA) volume and depressed function of LA are prognostic factors of adverse cardiovascular events in cardiac pathologies, such as atrial fibrillation, heart failure and coronary artery disease [1–5], and in general population [6]. LA size can be estimated by measuring its diameter, which is associated with cardiac events, but has limited correlation to atrial volume [7]. Calculated LA volumes by two-dimensional echocardiographic (2DE) methods are stronger predictors of adverse outcomes in comparison with LA diameter or LA cross sectional area [8]. 2DE methods are recommended for the volumetric assessment in the current guideline of echocardiographic chamber quantification [9] and in recommendation of cardiac imaging in atrial fibrillation [10]. Still an underestimation of volume by 2DE methods is evident [11, 12]. Three-dimensional echocardiography (3DE) provides measure of LA volume without geometrical assumptions, which are implied in 2DE methods. Agreement of 3DE is shown to be good in comparison to cardiac magnetic resonance imaging, although there is some discrepancy in results, which might be due to various factors i.e. different imaging hardware, imaging settings and analysis algorithms. [13–15] Cardiac magnetic resonance is considered gold standard in left atrial volumetry.

Previously Chen et al. validated in vitro 3DE volume detection by excised porcine hearts for right ventricle and demonstrated superiority of 3DE over 2DE methods [16]. In 2001 Teupe et al. used 3DE to measure normal

* Correspondence: jouni.kuusisto@iki.fi
[1]Division of Cardiology, Heart and Lung Center, Helsinki University Central Hospital, Meilahti Tower Hospital, P.O. Box 340, FIN-00029 HUS Helsinki, Finland
Full list of author information is available at the end of the article

and aneurysmal left ventricles of excised pig hearts to demonstrate accuracy of 3DE volumetric method [17]. In vitro validation of cardiac MRI volume detection has been demonstrated for both human atria by human cadaveric casts [18, 19].

In this study, we imaged human cadaveric left atrial casts by 3DE and 2DE to test agreement of volumetric methods to true cast volumes measured by water displacement. We also imaged water-filled balloons to test 3DE in wider range of volumes and to validate most appropriate placement of volumetric borderline in measurements.

Methods

Materials

Six latex balloons were filled with water to represent volumes of LA both in normal physiological conditions and in left atrial enlargement. The balloons were relatively spherical in shape and their walls provided easily distinguishable ultrasound echo for analysis.

Seven human cadaveric LA casts were prepared in the Department of Forensic Medicine, Helsinki University, Finland. No fixation of cardiac tissues was used. Mitral valves and ventricular apices were removed, and the pulmonary veins were clamped. Hearts were suspended from apical portion and left hearts were filled with silicone rubber without extra filling pressure. After hardening of the silicone rubber, the casts were removed from the hearts. LA parts of the casts were separated from ventricular parts at the mitral annular level. These casts were previously used in magnetic resonance imaging studies by Järvinen and Jauhiainen in the 1990s [18, 19]. At that time, no approval of ethics committee was required and the study was approved by head of department.

For this study the silicone casts were transformed to casts made of agar-agar, as casts of silicone rubber are not permeable to ultrasound. Molds for agar-agar casts were made from latex rubber, which was applied on the primary silicone casts while they were stabilized at their mitral planes to a level surface. Four layers of latex rubber was applied on each silicone cast. Left atrial appendices were excluded at this point from the latex molds, as they are usually not included in the volumetric assessment of left atrium by transthoracic ultrasound. The latex molds were peeled from silicone casts and two further layers of latex rubber were used to shut the open left atrial appendix orifices. The latex molds were then positioned so that the mitral openings were facing upwards. A 1,5% agar-agar and water solution was prepared by heating until boiling and then poured into the latex molds at the temperature of 60 degrees centigrade. The molds were cast until the level of mitral annulus. The agar-agar casts were refrigerated overnight and then they were carefully removed from the molds (Fig. 1a).

Determination of cast and balloon volumes

True volumes of the balloons were determined by weighing the water-filled balloons, assuming one gram of weight representing one milliliter of volume. The weight of the balloons before filling with water were measured to be insignificantly low.

True volumes of the agar-agar casts were determined by volume displacement method. A vessel with an opening on its side was filled with water up to the lower level of the opening. The casts were carefully submerged in to the water and the displaced water was collected through the opening into a 100-ml measuring glass. The volume of the displaced water was assumed to be the true volume of the cast. Volumes were determined by this method before and right after imaging to detect whether the cast volumes had been affected by the immersion into water during imaging.

Imaging

GE Vivid E9 machine with 4 V probe (GE Vingmed Ultrasound AS, Horten, Norway) was used for both 3DE and 2DE imaging. The agar-agar casts were immersed in a twenty-liter tank for imaging. Water mixture with dried and crushed seeds of *Plantago ovata* was used as the imaging medium, as enhanced contrast of the water was necessary for the semi-automated volumetry softwares to function properly. Higher signal intensity of the medium than that of casts represents the relative signal intensities in the in vivo measurements where signal intensity from myocardium and other surrounding tissues is higher than from blood in the atrial cavity. Coarse cloth was placed on the bottom of the tank to attenuate reverberation. The probe was supported above the tank by a tripod so that lens of the probe was 10 mm below the water surface and orienting downwards.

The casts were stationed on a thin (diameter 3 mm) wooden support attached to a pedestal on the bottom of the tank to stabilize the cast during imaging, and the casts were positioned to represent transthoracic apical view. Mitral annular level of the cast was horizontal and thus perpendicular to ultrasound wave propagation. The orifice of left atrial appendix was positioned 60 degrees counterclockwise from the 2DE view so that the first aspect of the imaging represented the apical four chamber view. The ultrasound beam was then electronically rotated 60 degrees counterclockwise to obtain two chamber view. Zoomed 4D view was used to collect 3DE volumetric data over 4 to 6 cardiac cycles, which were defined from electrocardiogram recorded from researcher at a heat rate of 65 to 70 bpm. The gain was optimized by eye for best possible delineation. Recorded

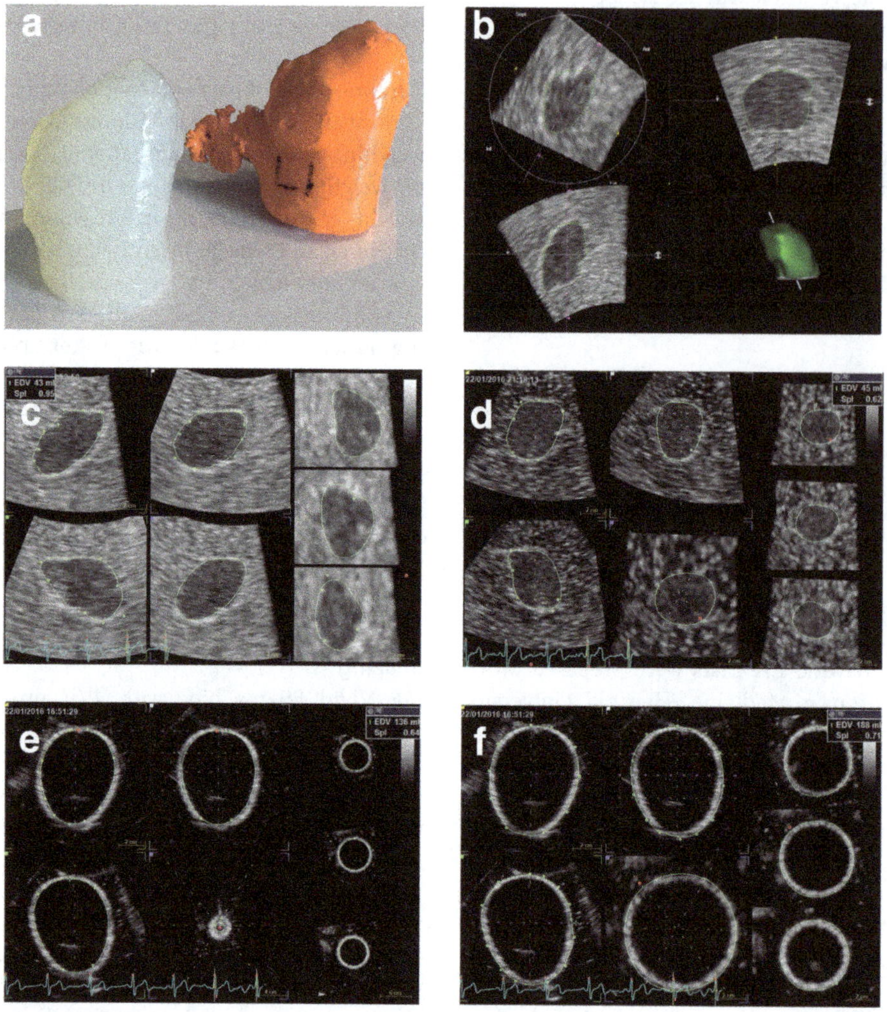

Fig. 1 a) Human cadaveric left atrial silicone cast (on right) and its transformed agar-agar cast without left atrial appendage, **b**) 3D echocardiographic volume analysis of cast no. 4 by TomTec 4D LV-Function (true volume 43 ml, measured volume 42 ml) and by **c**) GE 4D LVQ (measured volume 43 ml), **d**) cast no. 5 by GE 4d LVQ (true volume 44 ml, measured volume 45 ml), **e**) 3D volume measurement by GE 4D LVQ of a balloon with borderline on the inner aspect (true volume 140 ml, measured volume 136 ml) and **f**) on the outer aspect (measured volume 188 ml)

volume size and probe frequency were adjusted so that the volume frame rate was 35 to 50 Hz which is the typical acquisition frequency when imaging dynamic volume in vivo.

Water balloons were stationed by a thread and weight to the bottom of the tank so that the center of the balloons was approximately at 100 mm distance from the lens of the probe. 3DE images were collected similarly. No contrast enhancement agent was used during balloon imaging.

Image analysis

Image analysis was performed offline with GE EchoPAC work station software version 112.1.1 (GE Vingmed Ultrasound AS, Horten, Norway) after imaging. GE EchoPAC 4D LVQ (Figs. 1c–f) and TomTec 4D LV-Function (TomTec Imaging Systems GmbH, Unterschleissheim, Germany) (Fig. 1b) softwares were used for volume analysis. Both softwares are designed for cardiac left ventricle volume analysis, but they can also be applied for LA volumetry, as we demonstrate in this study. The researcher was blinded to the weights of the balloons and the results of volume displacement representing true volumes of balloons and casts.

There was a distinct border echo in the ultrasound images at the interface of water as medium, balloon wall, and water inside the balloon. This border echo thickness in the images was clearly greater than that of the balloon true walls (< 1 mm). To assess the most appropriate approach of volumetric measurement, the borderline was placed on the inner (Fig. 1e) and outer rims (Fig. 1f), and to the middle of this border echo by GE 4D LVQ.

Automation of TomTec software assumed the borderline to the inner aspect of the rim, so only this approach was used by TomTec software.

Measurements from the ultrasound images representing apical view during cast imaging were 1) 3DE volumetry by both softwares, 2) LA cast cross section areas from four and two chamber views and 3) the greatest length of these cross sections from middle of mitral orifice area to the roof of the atrial casts. The four and two chamber areas and their respective lengths were used to calculate approximations of volumes by biplane area-length method (A-L method) by equation $\frac{8}{3\pi} \times \frac{4ch\_area \times 2ch\_area}{length}$, where length is the shorter of the two measured lengths. Repeatability was tested for 3DE volumetry and A-L method of left atrial casts by a time interval of two weeks between repeated measurements.

Statistical and data analyses

IBM SPSS for Macintosh version 24.0 (Armonk, NY, USA) and Microsoft Excel for Mac version 15.26 (Microsoft Corporation, Redmond, WA, USA) were used for statistical and data analyses. Mean and range of true and measured volumes of balloons were determined. Paired differences of measured volumes to true volumes were calculated. Mean of these differences were considered bias. 95% confidence intervals (95% CI) for bias and limits of agreement (LOA), defined as bias ±1.96 standard deviations, were calculated. LOA represent the range in which 95% of measured volumes differ from true volumes when normal distribution is assumed. Pearson correlation coefficients and their statistical significances were calculated. The same statistical methods were applied for repeated volumetric measurements in addition to intraclass correlation coefficients and their statistical significance. Two-way mixed testing for absolute agreement was used for intraclass correlation. Bland-Altman difference plots were used to visualize data.

Results

Balloon imaging

True volumes of the water balloons ranged from 37 to 255 ml and mean volume was 126 ml. All the tested 3DE volumetric methods, including all borderline placements by GE 4D LVQ, to measure balloon volumes resulted in very high correlations to true volumes (Pearson $r > 0.999$, $p < 0.0005$). Balloon wall echo thickness was 1 to 6 mm and it was lowest in areas where ultrasound wave propagation was perpendicular to the wall balloon wall. Placement of the borderline on the inner aspect of the balloon wall echo by GE 4D LVQ resulted lowest absolute bias – 3.7 ml (95% CI -5.9 to – 1.4) and the bias did not correlate to volume (Pearson $r = -0.36$, $p = 0.481$). LOA were – 7.9 to 0.6 ml. Placement of borderline to the midline or outer aspect of the wall echo produced volume dependent overestimation of the volume and the biases were 15.5 ml (95% CI 4.7 to 26.3) and 44.2 ml (11.4 to 77.0), respectively. With TomTec software the bias was inversely related to volume resulting in greater negative bias in larger observed volumes. Mean bias was – 24,3 ml (95% CI -37.8 to – 10.8) with TomTec. As noted previously, semi-automation in TomTec software prevented precise manual adjustments to the borderline.

Cast imaging

Agar-agar cast volumes determined by volume displacement ranged from 38 to 94 ml (mean 56.6 ml). Repeated volume displacement measurements before and after imaging resulted in maximum of 2 ml difference. The measured volume displacement before the imaging was used in the later analyses.

The interface with the medium and agar-agar left atrial casts produced less prominent wall echo than with balloon imaging. As suggested most appropriate by balloon measurements, the borderline was placed closely to inner aspect of the echo representing interface of the cast and medium during 3DE volumetry and A-L method. Pearson correlation coefficients of measured volumes to true volumes for all methods were high and 95% CI of biases for these methods included zero bias. 3DE volumetric measurements with both softwares resulted in narrower limits of agreement in comparison to A-L method. With A-L method bias was positively correlated with volume (Pearson r of difference to true volume was 0.837 ($p < 0.05$)), but no statistically significant volume dependent bias was observed in 3DE methods (GE 4d LVQ $p = 0.96$ and TomTec 4d LV-Function $p = 0.24$). Measured volumes for casts, their displaced volumes and statistic characteristics are presented in Table 1 and Fig. 2a. Bland-Altman difference plots visualize the observed differences, biases and limits of agreement (Figs. 2b-d).

Repeatability

Repeated 3DE and A-L method volumetric measurements were performed to test repeatability. Both Pearson and intraclass correlation coefficients indicated very good repeatability ($r = 0.975$ to 0.982, intraclass correlation coefficients 0.967 to 0.980). Results of these measurements are depicted in Table 2. Bland-Altman charts describe the relation of measurement differences to average volumes of measurements (Figs. 3a–c).

Discussion

In this study we tested the applicability of 3D and 2D echocardiographic volumetric methods in determining volumes of human left atrial casts. To our knowledge

Table 1 3DE volumetric measurements and 2DE calculated volumes of left atrial human cadaveric casts in comparison to their true volumes

		3DE volume: GE 4D LVQ		3DE volume: TomTec LV		2DE volume	
cast no.	true volume (ml)	measured volume (ml)	difference to true volume (ml)	measured volume (ml)	difference to true volume (ml)	calculated volume (ml)	difference to true volume (ml)
1	38	36	−2	36	-2	35	−3
2	94	94	0	103	9	106	12
3	51	43	−8	50	−1	55	4
4	43	43	0	42	− 1	36	−7
5	44	45	1	50	6	40	−4
6	58	68	10	70	12	68	10
7	68	62	−6	68	0	76	8
mean (95% CI)	56.6	55.9	−0.7 (−6.1–4.6)	59.9	3.3 (−1.9–8.5)	59.5	2.9 (−4.0–9.9)
SD	19.4	20.3	5.8	22.8	5.6	26.0	7.5
range	38–94	36–94	−8–10	36–103	−2–12	35–106	−7–12
LOA			−12.1–10.6		−7.8–14.4		−11.9–17.6
r		0.959 ($p = 0.001$)		0.977 ($p = 0.0002$)		0.988 ($p = 0.00003$)	

95% CI – 95% confidence interval, 2DE volume – volume calculated by 2D echocardiographic biplane area-length method, 3DE volume: GE 4D LVQ and 3DE volume: TomTec LV – 3D echocardiographic volume measured by GE 4D LVQ and TomTec 4D LV-Function softwares, respectively, LOA – limits of agreement defined as mean ± 1.96 SD, r – Pearson correlation coefficient, SD – standard deviation

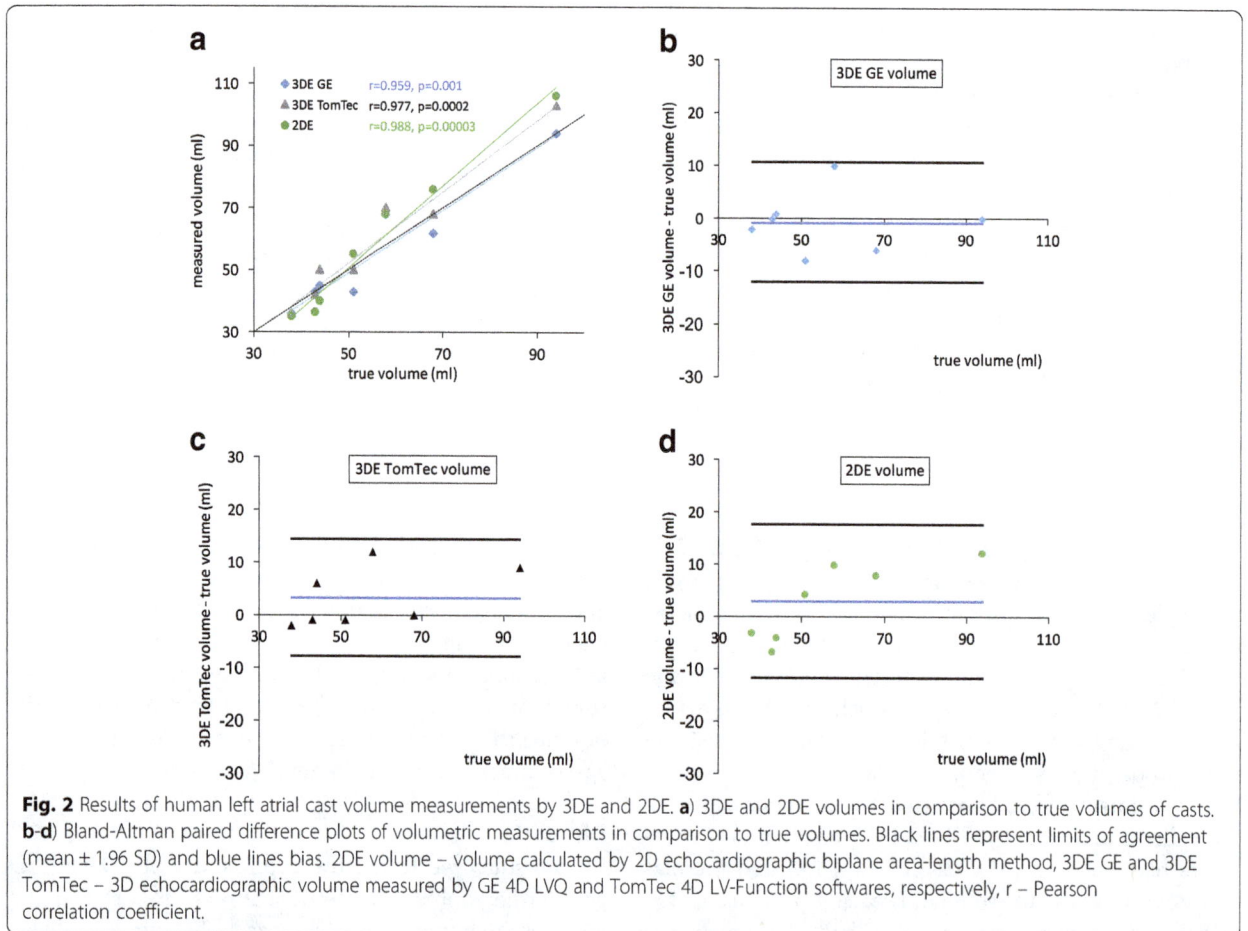

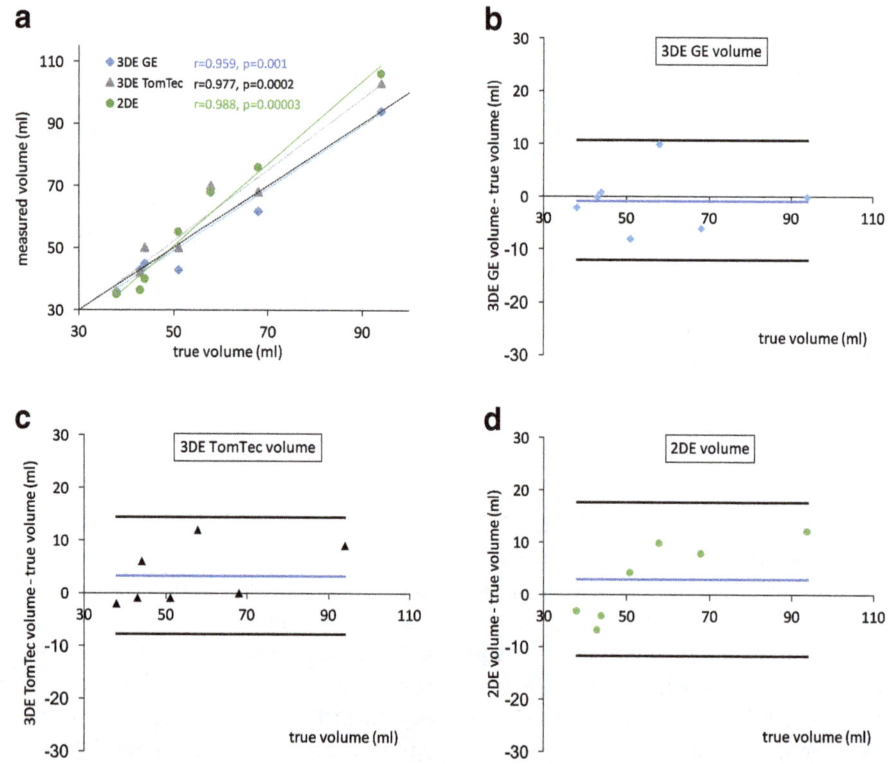

Fig. 2 Results of human left atrial cast volume measurements by 3DE and 2DE. **a**) 3DE and 2DE volumes in comparison to true volumes of casts. **b-d**) Bland-Altman paired difference plots of volumetric measurements in comparison to true volumes. Black lines represent limits of agreement (mean ± 1.96 SD) and blue lines bias. 2DE volume – volume calculated by 2D echocardiographic biplane area-length method, 3DE GE and 3DE TomTec – 3D echocardiographic volume measured by GE 4D LVQ and TomTec 4D LV-Function softwares, respectively, r – Pearson correlation coefficient.

Table 2 Repeated 3D volumetric measurements and 2D calculated volumes of left atrial human cadaveric casts

cast no.	3DE volume: GE 4D LVQ			3DE volume: TomTec LV			2DE volume		
	meas. 1 (ml)	meas. 2 (ml)	difference (ml)	meas. 1 (ml)	meas. 2 (ml)	difference (ml)	meas. 1 (ml)	meas. 2 (ml)	difference (ml)
1	36	35	−1	36	40	4	35	35	0
2	94	88	−6	103	102	−1	106	103	−3
3	43	44	1	50	59	9	55	66	11
4	43	41	−2	42	40	−2	36	33	−3
5	45	47	2	50	46	−4	40	48	8
6	68	57	−11	70	67	−3	68	68	0
7	62	60	−2	68	72	4	76	84	8
mean (95% CI)	55.9	53.1	−2.7 (−6.8–1.4)	59.9	60.9	1.0 (−3.4–5.4)	59.4	62.4	3.0 (−2.4–8.4)
SD	20.3	17.7	4.5	22.8	22.2	4.8	26.0	25.8	5.8
range	36–94	35–88	−11–2	36–103	40–102	−4–9	35–106	33–103	−3–11
LOA			−11.5–6.0			−8.3–10.3			−8.4–14.4
r	0.982, $p = 0.0001$			0.978, p = 0.0001			0.975, p = 0.0002		
ICC (95% CI)	0.967 (0.819–0.994), p = 0.00003			0.980 (0.894–0.996), $p = 0.00001$			0.972 (0.857–0.995), $p = 0.00002$		

95% CI – 95% confidence interval, 2DE volume – volume calculated by 2D echocardiographic biplane area-length method, 3DE volume: GE 4D LVQ and 3DE volume: TomTec LV – 3D echocardiographic volume measured by GE 4D LVQ and TomTec 4D LV-Function softwares, respectively, ICC – intraclass correlation coefficient, LOA – limits of agreement defined as mean ± 1.96 SD, meas. 1 and meas. 2 ¬ first and repeated measurement, r – Pearson correlation coefficient for meas. 1 and meas. 2, SD – standard deviation

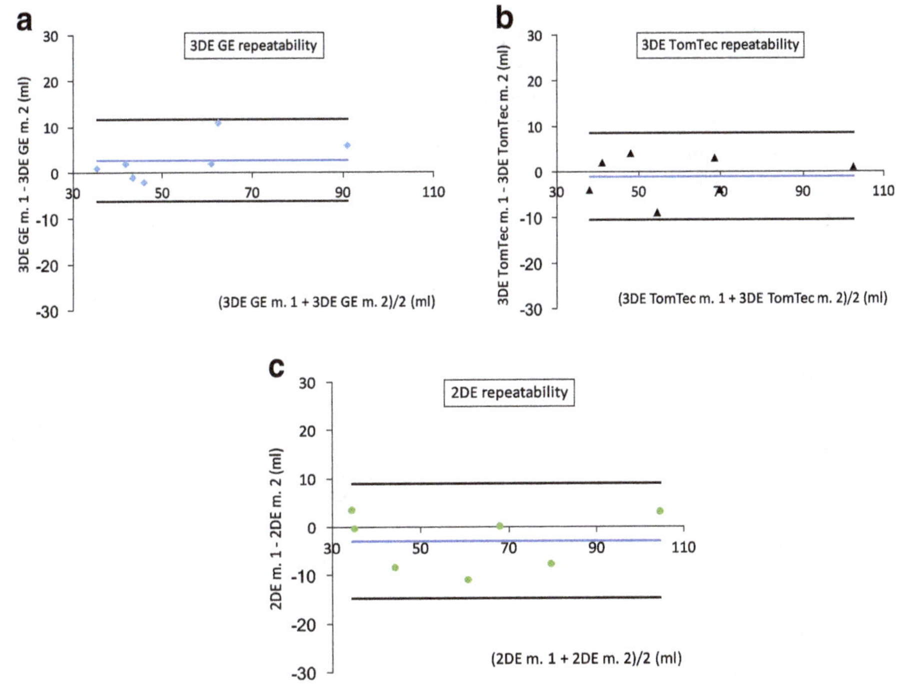

Fig. 3 Results of repeated measurements of human left atrial cast volumes. Bland-Altman paired difference plots of repeated volumetric measurements of casts in comparison to mean of measured volumes. Black lines represent limits of agreement (mean ± 1.96 SD) and blue lines mean of differences to paired averages of measured volumes. **a** 3DE GE repeatability - 3D echocardiographic repeated volume measurements by GE 4D LVQ software, **b** 3DE TomTec repeatability - 3D echocardiographic repeated volume measurements by TomTec 4D LV-Function software, **c** 2DE repeatability – repeated calculated volumes by biplane area-length method, m. 1 and m. 2 – first and repeated measurement

validation of left atrial volumetry in this setting has not been done previously. We showed that 3DE volumetry of water-filled balloons is in excellent absolute agreement with true volumes of the balloons when volumetric borderlines were placed closely on the inner aspect of the balloon wall echo. We found 3DE methods to be equally or more accurate in comparison to 2DE represented by biplane area-length method, considering lower observed limits of agreement and lack of volume dependent bias with 3DE. All methods had excellent correlation to true cast volumes and were well repeatable.

With 2DE volumetric methods there are inherent assumptions of geometrical symmetricity. With biplane area-length method an ellipsoid, and with monoplane area-length a spheroid shape is assumed. In addition to this geometrical assumption, the in vivo transthoracic apical views that are oriented along the left ventricular axis might not represent the left atrial axis. The planimetered area and length of the left atrium can thus be a misestimation resulting in an unpredictable error in estimation of the atrial volume [20]. Underestimation of volume by A-L method in comparison to cardiac magnetic resonance imaging is reported [21, 22]. With 3DE volumetry there is no need for geometrical assumptions or for orienting the echocardiographic beam along the left ventricular or atrial axis as the volume is measured along the true borders of the chamber.

Casting process and post mortem state might have affected volumes and shapes of the casts, and possible prior medical conditions of the deceased are not known. For the scope of this study we did not consider this a limitation as we aimed for volumetric validation of casts that represent the variable sizes and shapes of human left atria. Regarding some casts, areas of the interface of the cast and the medium were not explicit which at least partly contributed both to error in volumetric measurements to true volumes and repeatability. Different choice of medium or cast material could have mitigated this issue. In vitro repeatability in this study is likely better in comparison to clinical setting which has more variability in the imaging conditions.

The walls of water-filled balloons produced distinct echo lining in the images which we speculate to be at least partly due to interference of the transmitted ultrasound signal and the balloon wall. In cast imaging the interface consists of transition from contrast enhanced water to cast as a medium for ultrasound propagation which probably induces less artifacts in comparison to balloon wall. We noted, however, a less pronounced lining in the images also during cast imaging. The contrast enhanced water tended to turn less homogenous over time and stirring of the medium was required intermittently. We speculate this lining during cast imaging to consist mostly of the contrast enhanced medium, not the cast itself, giving a rationale for the placement of the volumetric borderline to inner aspect of the interface.

Conclusions

We conclude that 3DE is an accurate and feasible method to image left atrial volume in this in vitro study. Commercially available software (GE 4D LVQ and TomTec 4D LV-Function) developed for the left ventricular volume analysis can be used in the left atrial volume analysis as well.

Abbreviations

2DE: Two-dimensional echocardiography; 3DE: Three-dimensional echocardiography; 95% CI: 95% confidence interval; A-L Method: Biplane area-length method; LA: Left atrium; LOA: Limits of agreement

Acknowledgements

We are thankful for English revision to Pekka Järvinen, MSc.

Funding

Dr. Kuusisto was funded by The Education Fund, Finland.

Authors' contributions

JK and VJ performed preparation and imaging of the casts. JK analysed the data. JS, VJ and JK interpreted the data and had major contribution in writing the manuscript. All authors read and approved the final manuscript.

Consent for publication

Not applicable.

Competing interests

The authors declare that they have no competing interests.

Author details

[1]Division of Cardiology, Heart and Lung Center, Helsinki University Central Hospital, Meilahti Tower Hospital, P.O. Box 340, FIN-00029 HUS Helsinki, Finland. [2]Department of Clinical Physiology, Medical Imaging Center, Hospital District Helsinki and Uusimaa, Hyvinkää Hospital, Hyvinkää, Finland.

References

1. Gupta DK, Shah AM, Giugliano RP, Ruff CT, Antman EM, Grip LT, et al. Left atrial structure and function in atrial fibrillation: ENGAGE AF-TIMI 48. Eur Heart J. 2014. https://doi.org/10.1093/eurheartj/eht500.
2. Santos ABS, Kraigher-Krainer E, Gupta DK, Claggett B, Zile MR, Pieske B, et al. Impaired left atrial function in heart failure with preserved ejection fraction. Eur J Heart Fail. 2014. https://doi.org/10.1002/ejhf.147.
3. Pellicori P, Zhang J, Lukaschuk E, Joseph AC, Bourantas CV, Loh H, et al. Left atrial function measured by cardiac magnetic resonance imaging in patients with heart failure: clinical associations and prognostic value. Eur Heart J. 2015. https://doi.org/10.1093/eurheartj/ehu405.

4. Ristow B, Ali S, Whooley MA, Schiller NB. Usefulness of left atrial volume index to predict heart failure hospitalization and mortality in ambulatory patients with coronary heart disease and comparison to left ventricular ejection fraction (from the heart and soul study). Am J Cardiol. 2008. https://doi.org/10.1016/j.amjcard.2008.02.099.
5. Gulati A, Ismail TF, Jabbour A, Ismail NA, Morarji K, Ali A, et al. Clinical utility and prognostic value of left atrial volume assessment by cardiovascular magnetic resonance in non-ischaemic dilated cardiomyopathy. Eur J Heart Fail. 2013. https://doi.org/10.1093/eurjhf/hft019.
6. Tsang TSM, Barnes ME, Gersh BJ, Takemoto Y, Rosales AG, Bailey KR, et al. Prediction of risk for first age-related cardiovascular events in an elderly population: the incremental value of echocardiography. J Am Coll Cardiol. 2003. https://doi.org/10.1016/S0735-1097(03)00943-4.
7. Lester SJ, Ryan EW, Schiller NB, Foster E. Best method in clinical practice and in research studies to determine left atrial size. Am J Cardiol. 1999. https://doi.org/10.1016/S0002-9149(99)00446-4.
8. Tsang TSM, Abhayaratna WP, Barnes ME, Miyasaka Y, Gersh BJ, Bailey KR, et al. Prediction of cardiovascular outcomes with left atrial size. J Am Coll Cardiol. 2006. https://doi.org/10.1016/j.jacc.2005.08.077.
9. Lang RM, Badano LP, Mor-Avi V, Afilalo J, Armstrong A, Ernande L, et al. Recommendations for cardiac chamber quantification by echocardiography in adults: an update from the American Society of Echocardiography and the European Association of Cardiovascular Imaging. J Am Soc Echocardiogr. 2015. https://doi.org/10.1016/j.echo.2014.10.003.
10. Donal E, Lip GYH, Galderisi M, Goette A, Shah D, Marwan M, et al. EACVI/EHRA expert consensus document on the role of multi-modality imaging for the evaluation of patients with atrial fibrillation. Eur Heart J Cardiovasc Imaging. 2016. https://doi.org/10.1093/ehjci/jev354.
11. Kühl JT, Lønborg J, Fuchs A, Andersen MJ, Vejlstrup N, Kelbæk H, et al. Assessment of left atrial volume and function: a comparative study between echocardiography, magnetic resonance imaging and multi slice computed tomography. Int J Cardiovasc Imaging. 2012. https://doi.org/10.1007/s10554-011-9930-2.
12. Avelar E, Durst R, Rosito GA, Thangaroopan M, Kumar S, Tournoux F, et al. Comparison of the accuracy of multidetector computed tomography versus two-dimensional echocardiography to measure left atrial volume. Am J Cardiol. 2010. https://doi.org/10.1016/j.amjcard.2010.02.021.
13. Mor-Avi V, Yodwut C, Jenkins C, Kühl H, Nesser H-J, Marwick TH, et al. Real-time 3D echocardiographic quantification of left atrial volume. Multicenter Study for Validation With CMR JACC Cardiovasc Imaging. 2012. https://doi.org/10.1016/j.jcmg.2012.05.011.
14. Artang R, Migrino RQ, Harmann L, Bowers M, Woods TD. Left atrial volume measurement with automated border detection by 3-dimensional echocardiography: comparison with magnetic resonance imaging. Cardiovasc Ultrasound. 2009. https://doi.org/10.1186/1476-7120-7-16.
15. Perez de Isla L, Feltes G, Moreno J, Martinez W, Saltijeral A, de Agustin JA, et al. Quantification of left atrial volumes using three-dimensional wall motion tracking echocardiographic technology: comparison with cardiac magnetic resonance. Eur Hear J - Cardiovasc Imaging. 2014. https://doi.org/10.1093/ehjci/jeu001.
16. Chen G, Sun K, Huang G. In vitro validation of right ventricular volume and mass measurement by real-time three-dimensional echocardiography. Echocardiography. 2006. https://doi.org/10.1111/j.1540-8175.2006.00221.x.
17. Teupe C, Takeuchi M, Ram SP, Pandian NG. Three-dimensional echocardiography: in-vitro validation of a new, voxel-based method for rapid quantification of ventricular volume in normal and aneurysmal left ventricles. Int J Card Imaging. 2001. https://doi.org/10.1023/A:1010671305700.
18. Järvinen VM, Kupari MM, Hekali PE, Poutanen V-P. Assessment of left atrial volumes and phasic function using cine magnetic resonance imaging in normal subjects. Am J Cardiol. 1994. https://doi.org/10.1016/0002-9149(94)90298-4.
19. Jauhiainen T, Järvinen VM, Hekali PE, Poutanen VP, Penttilä A, Kupari M. MR gradient echo volumetric analysis of human cardiac casts: focus on the right ventricle. J Comput Assist Tomogr. 1998. https://doi.org/10.1097/00004728-199811000-00012.
20. Kebed K, Kruse E, Addetia K, Ciszek B, Thykattil M, Guile B, et al. Atrial-focused views improve the accuracy of two-dimensional echocardiographic measurements of the left and right atrial volumes: a contribution to the increase in normal values in the guidelines update. Int J Cardiovasc Imaging. 2016. https://doi.org/10.1007/s10554-016-0988-8.
21. Whitlock M, Garg A, Gelow J, Jacobson T, Broberg C. Comparison of left and right atrial volume by echocardiography versus cardiac magnetic resonance imaging using the area-length method. Am J Cardiol. 2010. https://doi.org/10.1016/j.amjcard.2010.06.065.
22. Rabbat MG, Wilber D, Thomas K, Malick O, Bashir A, Agrawal A, et al. Left atrial volume assessment in atrial fibrillation using multimodality imaging: a comparison of echocardiography, invasive three-dimensional CARTO and cardiac magnetic resonance imaging. Int J Cardiovasc Imaging. 2015. https://doi.org/10.1007/s10554-015-0641-y.

12

Sonographic swelling of pronator quadratus muscle in patients with occult bone injury

Junko Sato[1*], Yoshinori Ishii[1], Hideo Noguchi[1] and Shin-ichi Toyabe[2]

Abstract

Background: The disarranged fat stripe of the pronator quadratus muscle (PQ) on radiographs (the PQ sign) is reported to be predictive of subtle bone fractures. This study aimed to report the results of magnetic resonance imaging (MRI) study in the patients in whom bone injury was not radiographically detected around the wrist joint, and the PQ was sonographically swollen following acute trauma.

Methods: We evaluated sonographically the PQ of 55 patients who showed normal radiographs following acute trauma. The sonographic appearance of the PQ was checked on both longitudinal and transverse images. On the longitudinal image, the probe was positioned along the flexor carpi radialis tendon. For the transverse image, we adopted the image of the same level in which the PQ of the unaffected hand showed maximal thickness. The PQ was considered to be swollen with disproportionate hyperechogenicity and/or thickening compared with the unaffected side at least in one of the two images. Of the 55 patients, 25 patients whose PQ was considered to be swollen underwent MRI study. PQ thickness in millimeters was retrospectively measured on longitudinal and transverse sonographic images.

Results: Twenty-three patients (92.0%) had occult bone injury, and two adult patients (8.0%) showed only wrist joint effusion on MRI. Among these 23, the distal radius was the most frequent location of the occult bone injury (20 patients; 9 [36.0%] with an occult fracture line and 11 [44.0%] with bone bruising). In longitudinal image, the mean value of the PQ thickness of affected hands was 6.2 (3.7–9.6 mm; standard deviation [SD], 1.5) and that of unaffected hands was 4.5 (2.3–6.7 mm; SD, 1.2), respectively. In transverse image, that of dominant and nondominant hands was 7.6 (4.6–13.2 mm; SD, 2.0) and 5.5 (3.6–7.5 mm; SD, 1.1), respectively. The mean difference in PQ thickness between affected and unaffected hands was 1.7 (0.1–5.0 mm; SD, 1.1) in longitudinal image and 2.0 (0.3–6.8 mm; SD, 1.7) in transverse image.

Conclusions: Sonographic swelling of the PQ might be indicative of occult bone injury in patients with normal radiographs following acute trauma.

Keywords: Ultrasonography, Pronator quadratus, Occult bone injury, Wrist joint

Background

MacEwan [1] reported the usefulness of the radiolucent plane overlying the pronator quadratus (PQ) seen on the lateral radiograph of the distal forearm in patients with undisplaced fractures of the radius and ulna, namely the "PQ sign", which is an anterior bowing or obliteration of the stripe of fat plane paralleling between the PQ and flexor digitorum profundus muscle.

The PQ sign is visible when fluid accumulates within the PQ and the muscle becomes swollen, bulging anteriorly. The PQ occupies a distinct space without intermuscular communication in the deeper part of anterior forearm [2], and this anatomical feature seems to contribute to the appearance of the PQ sign. Moosikasuwan [3] speculated that this sign would be false-negative in such situations as the fractured level differs from the level of the PQ, the fascia covering the muscle is torn, or the radiograph is of poor quality.

Despite high sensitivity and specificity for the diagnosis of fracture in the first report of the PQ sign, with values of

* Correspondence: jun-sato@hotmail.co.jp
[1]Ishii Orthopaedic and Rehabilitation Clinic, 1089 Shimo-Oshi, Gyoda, Saitama 361-0037, Japan
Full list of author information is available at the end of the article

98% and 94%, respectively [1], subsequent studies did not always report the clinical importance of this radiographic abnormality. Zammit-Maempel et al. [4] reported only 51% of forearm fractures showed abnormal pronator fat stripe. Annamalai and Raby [5] reported that the sensitivity and specificity of the PQ sign were even less, with values of 26% and 70%, respectively in the radiographically occult fractures detected on follow-up magnetic resonance imaging (MRI). MRI seems to be the most reliable imaging modality in terms of its ability to diagnose occult bone injury; however, it is expensive and time-consuming. On the other hand, ultrasonography has great benefits in its noninvasiveness, low cost, portability and rapidity which make it easier to use in the outpatient clinic and emergency room; however, one major disadvantage of this imaging modality is the inability in qualitative diagnosis of bone marrow.

The purpose of this study was to investigate the usefulness of the sonographic PQ swelling in identifying occult bone injury following acute trauma.

Methods

Approval for this study was obtained from the institutional ethics committee of Healthcare Corporation Ashinokai, Gyoda, Saitama, Japan, and all patients were informed of study aims and procedures and signed a consent form that included a description of the protocol. In a period of 1 year, 56 consecutive patients who visited our clinic for wrist injury with a history of acute trauma within 7 days and normal initial radiographs underwent sonographic studies. All patients routinely underwent plain radiography of the wrist joint (standard dorsal-volar and lateral views) prior to the sonographic study at the initial visit to our clinic. For patients with apparent tenderness at the anatomical snuff box, we added two radiographs to check for scaphoid fracture: a dorsal-volar view with the wrist in ulnar deviation and with the thumb clenched by the other fingers, and a semipronated oblique view. The decision of additional sonographic studies depended on the presence of pain disproportionate to normal radiographs. Exclusion criteria included rheumatoid arthritis, dialysis treatment, open wounds, or a history of major hand trauma and/or major hand surgery. As a result, 55 patients were enrolled in this study, excluding one pediatric male patient with a history of a distal radius fracture on the contralateral side.

The sonographic appearance of the PQ was checked on both longitudinal and transverse images. When a probe is positioned on the volar side of the distal forearm, it allows for direct visualization of the flexor tendons and muscles, including the PQ, and the volar cortex of the radius in various planes. In the longitudinal plane, the PQ has a stippled, hypoechogenic, fusiform appearance. In the transverse plane, the two layers of the PQ (superficial and deep) are distinguished from one another by their alternating echogenicity [6]. The patients were seated with hand resting on table with elbow extended, forearm fully supinated, and wrist extended 5–10 degrees. The probe was positioned perpendicularly against the volar surface of the examined distal forearm with minimum pressure. On the longitudinal image, the probe was positioned along the flexor carpi radialis tendon (Figure 1). This image included a

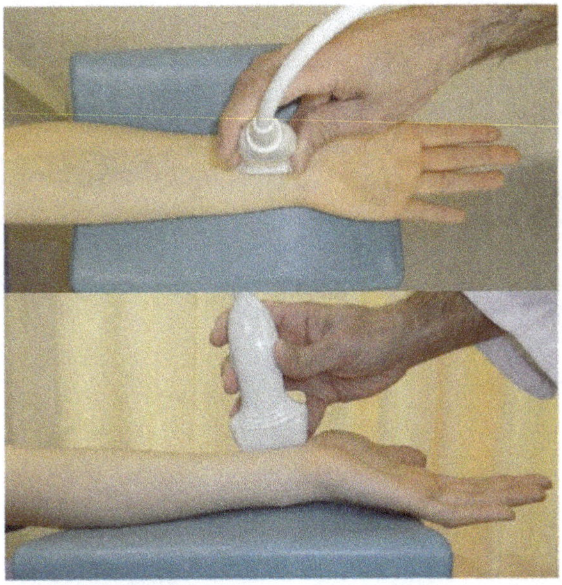

Figure 1 Position of the probe in the sonographic study on the longitudinal image.

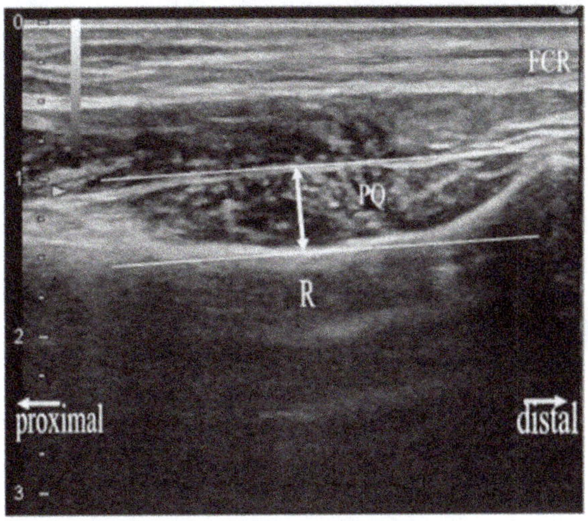

Figure 2 Sonographic longitudinal image of the examined part of the distal forearm, including anatomical reference and measurements of PQ thickness, using a 17-MHz transducer. Left hand of a 33-year-old healthy male volunteer. We referred to the line tangential to the volar concave aspect of the radius. FCR: flexor carpi radialis; PQ: pronator quadratus; R: radius; full-lined arrow: maximum thickness of the PQ.

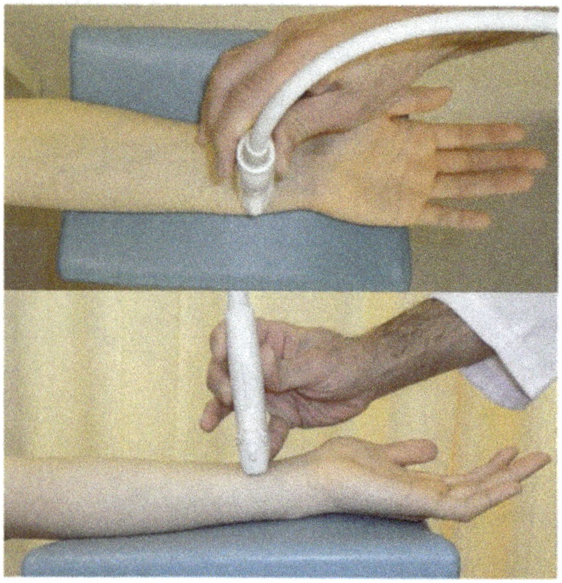

Figure 3 Position of the probe in the sonographic study on the transverse image.

longitudinal section of the flexor carpi radialis tendon, PQ, volar cortex of the radius, and, on the distal end of the image, the distal margin of the bony prominence attached to the PQ (Figure 2). For the transverse image, we initially adopted the image of the unaffected hand in which the PQ showed maximal thickness when moving the probe proximally from carpus to forearm (Figures 3 and 4). Next, we adopted the image of the affected hand at the level located the same distance from the radiocarpal joint with that of the unaffected hand. Comparisons were made with the contralateral unaffected hand. Images were created on a display showing a side-by-side comparison between affected and unaffected hands. The PQ was considered to be swollen with disproportionate hyperechogenicity and/or thickening compared with the unaffected side at least in one of the two images.

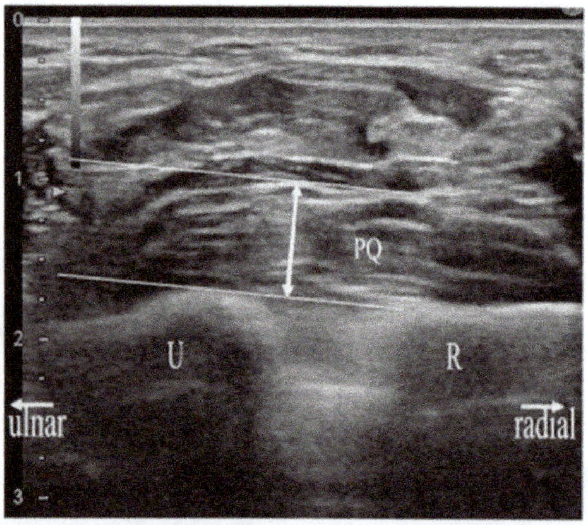

Figure 4 Sonographic transverse image of the examined part of the distal forearm, including anatomical reference and measurements of PQ thickness, using a 17-MHz transducer. Left hand of the same volunteer with Figure 2. We referred to the line tangential to the convex aspect of the ulna, which was drawn from the ulnar rim of the radius. PQ: pronator quadratus; R: radius; U: ulna; full-lined arrow: maximum thickness of PQ.

Of the 55 patients, we advised 26 whose PQ was considered to be swollen to undergo MRI to check for occult bone injury. As a result, 25 patients comprising 15 children and 10 adults underwent MRI, excluding one patient who refused a further detailed study. All patients demonstrated right-hand dominance. Affected hands included 12 right hands and 13 left hands. Sonography and MRI were performed within 3 and 5 days following trauma (mean interval, 1.0 and 2.5 days), respectively. The interval between sonography and MRI was within 5 days (mean interval, 1.4 days). In the follow-up period,

Table 1 Patients' information regarding MRI and follow-up radiography

	Period from trauma to sonography/ MRI study	Final diagnosis on MRI	Follow-up radiography occult injury detected
0 day	9/2	-	-
1 day	9/6	-	-
2 days	4/5	-	-
3 days	3/6	-	-
4 days	0/2	-	-
5 days	0/4	-	-
Distal radius contusion	-	10	-
Distal radius contusion/ capitate fracture	-	1	-
Distal radius fracture	-	6	-
Distal radius fracture/ Ulna styloid fracture	-	1	-
Distal radius fracture/ Scaphoid contusion	-	1	-
Ulna fracture	-	1	-
Scaphoid fracture	-	2	-
Scaphoid fracture	-	1	-
Joint effusion	-	2	-
Did not undergo follow-up radiography	-	-	4
1 week	-	-	3
2 weeks	-	-	2
3 weeks	-	-	10
No detected	-	-	4

The numbers of patients are described in the box.
Bold and italics indicate final diagnoses other than occult bone injury.

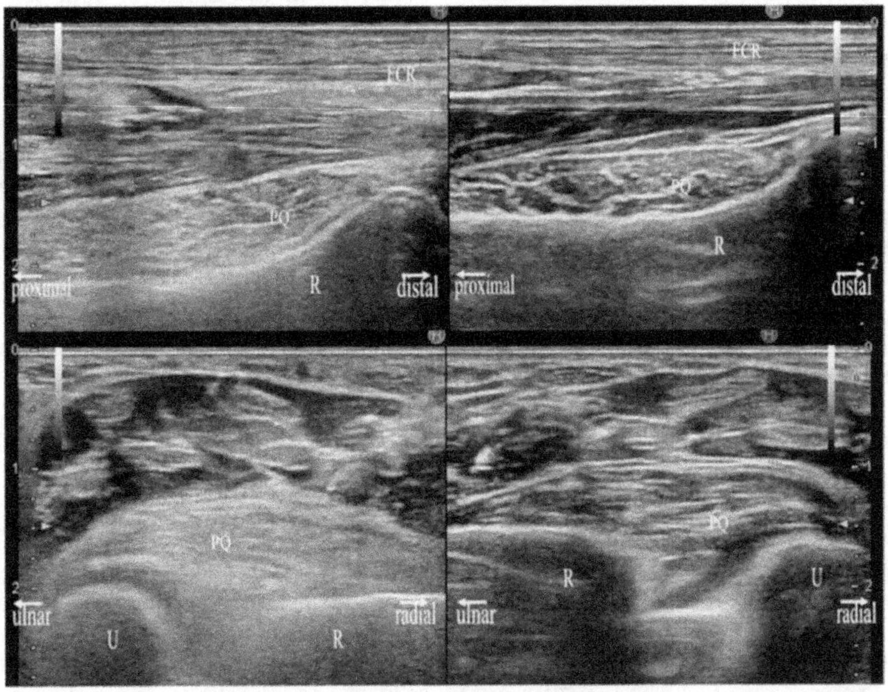

Figure 5 Sonographic images of a 71-year-old man with a diagnosis of distal radius fracture of the left hand. Sonographic images in the longitudinal (upper image) and transverse (lower image) planes were obtained using a 17-MHz transducer. Each image shows a side-by-side comparison of the right hand (right image) and left hand (left image). The PQ of the left hand is prominently thickened with hyperechogenicity. The PQ shows a convex appearance in either hand.

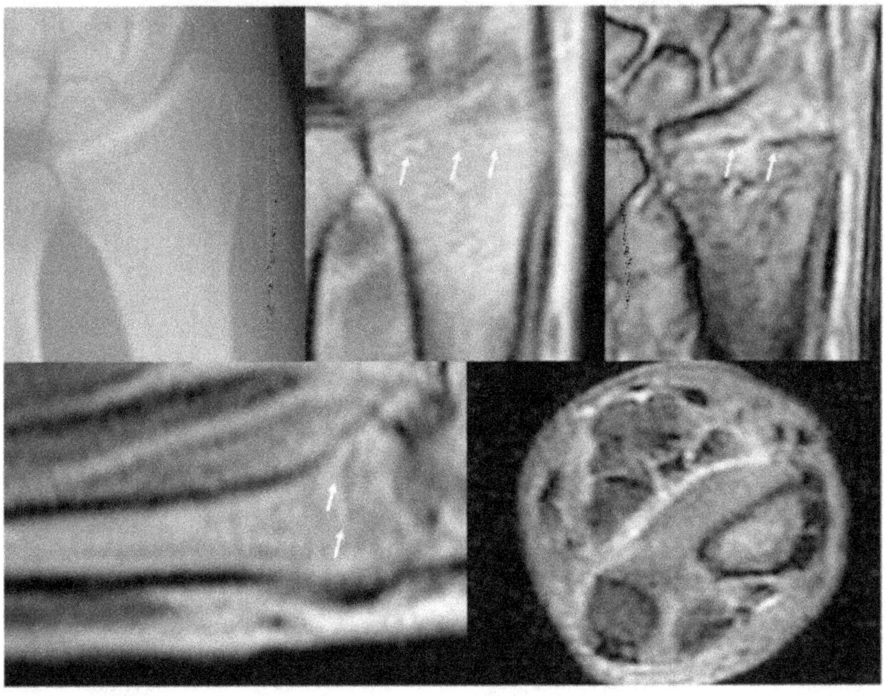

Figure 6 Radiographic, and MRI images of the same patient with Figure 5. In upper image, a plain radiograph at the initial visit (left), a PD (middle) and a T2*-weighted (right) MRI coronal image are shown. In lower image, a PD-weighted MRI sagittal image (left) and STIR MRI transverse image (right) are shown. White arrows indicate the fracture line.

we also obtained radiographs every week until 3 weeks after the initial visit to evaluate whether delayed radiographic detection was possible if occult bone injury had been detected on MRI.

On each image, the maximal dorsal-volar thickness was measured to determine whether the PQ was thickened compared with the unaffected side. Considering the correspondence to the radiographic PQ sign, we measured the maximal thickness in millimeters on the volar side at the cortical level, which seemed to mainly represent the superficial layer of the PQ in the same manner as in the previous study of normal volunteers [7] (Figures 2 and 4). On the transverse image, we referred to a line tangent to the cortical bones of the radius and ulna (Figure 4).

All sonographic studies were performed using software from the Avius ultrasound system (Hitachi Medico Co., Japan). A linear array 13.5- or 17-MHz transducer (contact area, 14 × 59 mm) was used. All MRI studies were performed using a Signa Profile EXCITE (GE Yokogawa Medical System Co., Japan); the magnetic flux density was 0.2 tesla, with a series of sagittal and coronal images in proton density (PD)-weighted, short-term T1 inversion recovery (STIR) and T2*-weighted sequences. With regard to the assessment of bone lesions on MRI, the term "fracture" was used when a line of low intensity was present on both PD-weighted and T2*-weighted images. The term "bone bruising (contusion)" was used with the presence of bone marrow edema exhibiting ill-defined low intensity on PD-weighted images and higher intensity on both STIR and T2*-weighted images without a fracture line. One senior hand surgeon with 13 years of experience in surgery and 2 years of experience in ultrasound analyzed all images. We categorized the patients into three groups according to the type of occult bone fracture; radius fracture, radius bone bruising (contusion), and other wrist fracture. We also compared the PQ thickness between each two of these groups using the Student's t-test. Results were deemed significant if $p < 0.05$.

Results

Table 1 reports patients' information regarding MRI and follow-up radiography. The patients underwent sonographic study and MRI comprised 32 men and 23 women [age, 9–80 years; mean, 26.3; standard deviation (SD), 22.8], and 15 men and 10 women [age, 10–80 years; mean, 32.64; SD, 24.8], respectively. Twenty-three patients

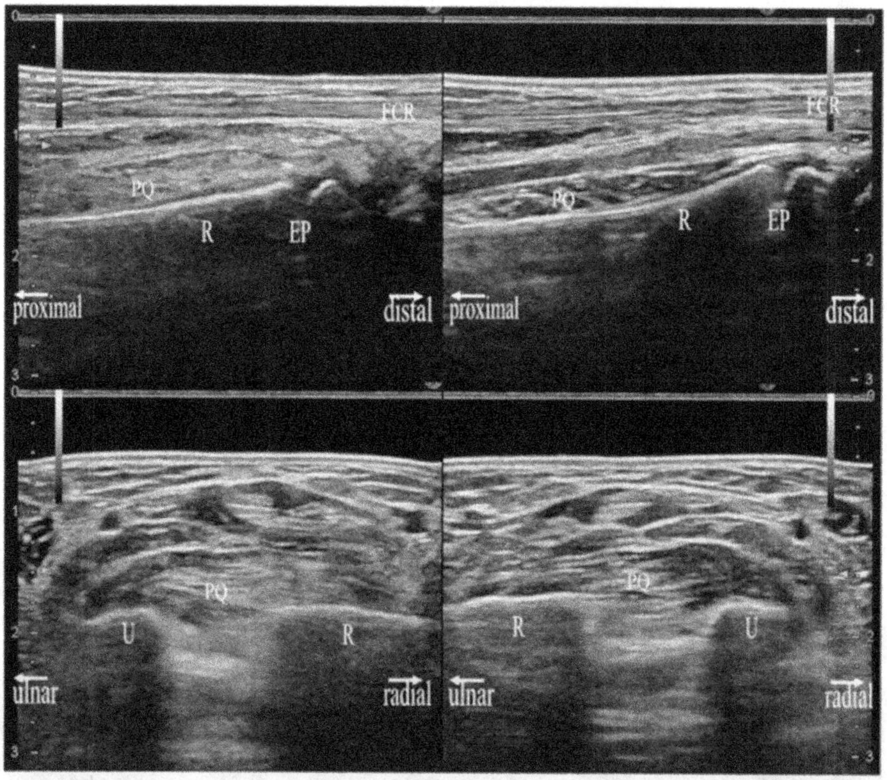

Figure 7 Sonographic images of an 11-year-old girl with a diagnosis of distal radius contusion of the left hand. Sonographic images in the longitudinal (upper image) and transverse (lower image) planes were obtained using a 17-MHz transducer. Each image shows a side-by-side comparison of the right hand (right image) and left hand (left image). The PQ of the left hand is locally thickened with hyperechogenicity on the radial side. The PQ shows a convex appearance in either hand. EP: epiphyseal plate.

(92.0%) had occult bone injury. Of these 23, the distal radius was the most frequent location for occult injury (detected in 20 patients; 9 [36.0%] with an occult fracture line (Figures 5 and 6) and 11 [44.0%] with bone bruising [contusion] (Figures 7 and 8). Two adult patients (8.0%) showed only wrist joint effusion on MRI (Figures 9 and 10). In children, all injuries detected in the distal radius were located on the proximal side of the epiphyseal line. Two patients (8.0%) had a solitary scaphoid injury, and one patient (4.0%) had a solitary ulna fracture. Four patients (16.0%) had two injured bones; they had occult radius injuries with scaphoid, capitate, or ulnar styloid injuries. In subsequent radiographs, bone injury was detected in 15 (78.9%) of 19 patients who underwent follow-up. We could not obtain the subsequent radiographs in four patients with occult bone injury because they did not visit our clinic within the follow-up period. The results of sonographic measurement of the PQ in involved patients are described in Table 2.

There was no significant difference in PQ thickness between any two groups of occult bone fracture (radius fracture vs. radius bone bruising [contusion], $p = 0.58$ in longitudinal image and $p = 0.52$ in transverse image; radius fracture vs. other wrist fracture, $p = 0.86$ in longitudinal image and $p = 0.68$ in transverse image; radius bone bruising [contusion] vs. other wrist fracture, $p = 0.82$ in longitudinal image and $p = 0.90$ in transverse image).

Discussion

The PQ is reportedly a key soft tissue in the diagnosis of radiographically undetectable fractures [1,2,4,8,9]. It is attached to the anterior aspects of the distal one-sixth of the radius and ulna and the distal radioulnar joint (DRUJ). The PQ comprises two layers: the superficial and deep layers [10,11]. Johnson and Shrewsbury [10] reported that the superficial layer was longer and wider but thinner than the deep layer, with average thicknesses of 0.2 cm for the superficial layer and 0.4 cm for the deep layer based on the dissection results of 12 forearms cross-sections made at one centimeter intervals. The superficial layer is considered to act as a prime contributor to pronation of the forearm in coordination with the pronator teres muscle [10-12]. The deep layer is active during both pronation and supination [12] and takes part in stabilizing the DRUJ by inserting onto the joint capsule [10-12]. With regard to the wrist, a 62.4% sensitivity of occult bone injuries on MRI was reported in the patients with negative radiographs and persistent pain following trauma [13], and a 40% to 65% sensitivity of scaphoid fracture on MRI was reported in the clinically suspicious patients with a normal series of plain radiographs [14,15].

The disarranged fat stripe of the PQ on radiographs (the PQ sign) is considered to be a highly predictive but low-sensitivity finding of subtle bone fractures, particularly of the distal radius and ulna [3,8], whereas Zammit-Maempel

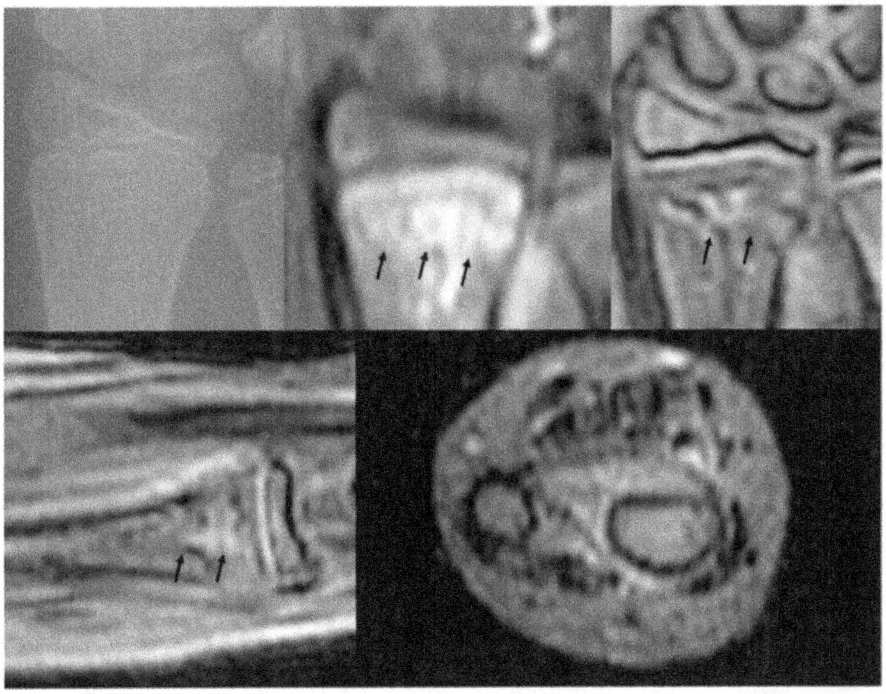

Figure 8 Radiographic, and MRI images of the same patient with Figure 7. In upper image, a plain radiograph at the initial visit (left), a STIR (middle) and a T2*-weighted (right) MRI coronal image are shown. In lower image, a T2*-weighted MRI sagittal image (left) and STIR MRI transverse image (right) are shown. Black arrows indicate the bone bruising site.

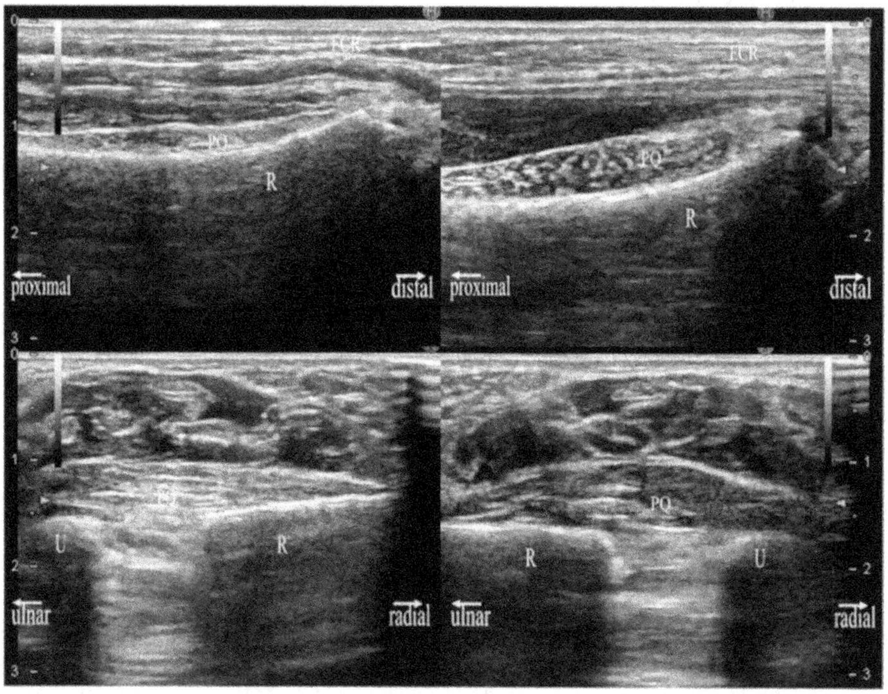

Figure 9 Sonographic images of a 59-year-old woman with a diagnosis of wrist joint effusion of the right hand. Sonographic images in the longitudinal (upper image) and transverse (lower image) planes were obtained using a 13.5-MHz transducer. Each image shows a side-by-side comparison of the right hand (right image) and left hand (left image). The PQ of the right hand is locally thickened. The PQ shows a convex appearance only in right hand.

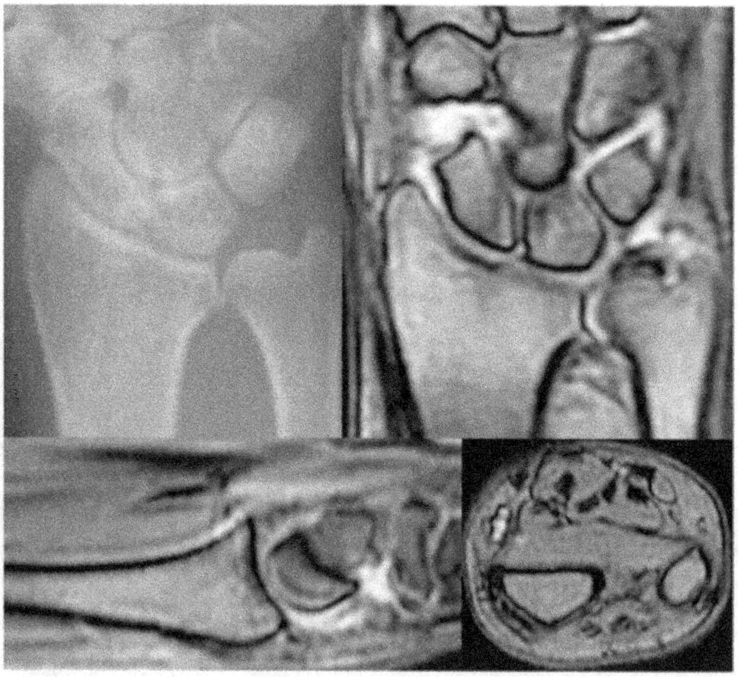

Figure 10 Radiographic, and MRI images of the same patient with Figure 9. In upper image, a plain radiograph at the initial visit (left) and a T2*-weighted (right) MRI coronal image are shown. In lower image, T2*-weighted MRI sagittal (left) and transverse (right) images are shown.

Table 2 Sonographic information of PQ, and their statistical analyses

Sonographic measurement of PQ thickness (mm)					
Longitudinal image			Transverse image		
A	UA	Difference†	A	UA	Difference†
6.2 ± 1.5	4.5 ± 1.2	1.7 ± 1.1	7.6 ± 2.0	5.5 ± 1.1	2.0 ± 1.7
(3.7 – 9.6)	(2.3 – 6.7)	(0.1 – 5.0)	(4.6 – 13.2)	(3.6 – 7.5)	(0.3 – 6.8)

PQ thicknesses are given as mean value ± standard deviation with ranges in parentheses.
A: affected hand.
UA: unaffected hand.
†Difference in PQ thickness between affected and unaffected hands.

et al. [4] reported only 51% of forearm fractures showed this sign. Annamalai and Raby [5] reported that this sign was a poor predictor of occult fractures detected on MRI in their retrospective study. Ultrasonography has distinct merits in terms of noninvasiveness and time- and cost-effectiveness, and it is best used when there is a specific clinical question regarding a well-localized abnormality [16]. Although ultrasonography is not able to make a quantitative diagnosis of bone marrow, sonographic swelling of the PQ predicted occult bone injury with high probability of 92%. Moreover, sonographic swelling of the PQ might support a recommendation for further detailed imaging studies such as MRI for the patients with normal radiographs. With regards to the thickness of the PQ, Zammit-Maempel et al. [4] measured the distance of the normal pronator fat stripe from the radius on lateral radiographs of the patients who presented with acute wrist trauma. They reported that the distance had a very wide variation with a mean value of 4.97 mm (5.72 mm in males and 4.22 mm in females) in 773 normal patients without abnormal soft tissue and/or bone injury, and that the patients with fractures of the distal radius and ulna, and distal radius had a significantly greater distance with mean values of 6.98 mm and 6.51 mm, respectively ($p < 0.01$). Sasaki et al. [8] reported the distance was less than 7 mm in 92% of 72 normal control subjects in which pronator fat shadow could be detected, and over 7 mm in 93% of 29 recent distal radius fractures under the same condition. Our results of sonographic measurement in normal subjects (unaffected hand) showed mean values of 4.5 mm in longitudinal, and 5.5 mm in transverse image.

A consensus has not been reached regarding whether occult bone injuries of the wrist should be immobilized and how long they should be immobilized. However, it is important to precisely determine the cause of symptoms and to inform patients. Actually, all four occult bone injuries in our study were contusions of the radius or scaphoid in children and could not be detected on subsequent radiographs. Even if a physician continues to check the radiographs carefully, a substantial number of occult bone injuries seem to be overlooked.

Our study has several limitations. First, our results can show only positive predictive value. We did not check the MRI of the patients with a normal sonographic appearance of the PQ. Despite economic and ethical problems, a closer study of such cases is desirable to investigate the accuracy of sonographic PQ swelling in terms of occult injury of the wrist. Second, this study might contain substantial bias in the selection of patients undergoing sonography because pain disproportionate to normal radiographs, the requirement for sonography examination, is quite examiner-subjective. We may have overlooked some patients with a swollen PQ. Third, the decision of sonographic PQ swelling depended on the comparison of the PQ thickness between affected and unaffected hands. Previous sonographic study revealed that atrophy of the PQ may be present in asymptomatic patient, and that loss in bulk of the PQ may be isolated and not related to anterior osseous neuropathy [17]. Although the authors described that it is not possible to identify or suppose a definite reason for this phenomenon, they speculated that the generic, occupational factors and anatomical variants in the innervation might be responsible. It is undeniable that atrophic PQ in the unaffected hand might be decided to be normal in our study.

Conclusions

In conclusion, sonographic swelling of the PQ might be indicative of occult bone injury in patients with normal radiographs following acute trauma. Ultrasonography might be a convenient adjunct for the decision of further detailed imaging studies in these patients as a noninvasive and portable tool that can be performed in the clinic and emergency room.

Competing interests

The authors declare that they have no competing interests.

Authors' contributions

JS designed the study, performed sonographic study, collected the data, analyzed the data and drafted manuscript. YI designed the study and approved the final manuscript. HN collected the data. ST designed the study and analyzed the data. All authors read and approved the final manuscript.

Acknowledgements

We thank Ishii Orthopaedic & Rehabilitation Clinic which paid necessary expenses for the English proofreading and the publication of this article. We also thank Edanz Editing Co., Japan, which took charge of English proofreading of this manuscript.

Author details
[1]Ishii Orthopaedic and Rehabilitation Clinic, 1089 Shimo-Oshi, Gyoda, Saitama 361-0037, Japan. [2]Division of Information Science and Biostatistics, Niigata University Graduate School of Medical and Dental Sciences, 1 Asahimachi Dori, Niigata, Niigata 951-8520, Japan.

References

1. MacEwan DW. Changes due to trauma in the fat plane overlying the pronator quadrates muscle: a radiologic sign. Radiology. 1964;82:879–86.
2. Sotereanos DG, McCarthy DM, Towers JD, Britton CA, Herndon JH. The pronator quadratus: a distinct forearm space? J Hand Surg Am. 1995;20:496–9.
3. Moosikasuwan JB. The pronator quadratus sign. Radiology. 2007;244:927–8.
4. Zammit-Maempel I, Bisset RA, Morris J, Forbes WS. The value of soft tissue signs in wrist trauma. Clin Radiol. 1988;39:664–8.
5. Annamalai G, Raby N. Scaphoid and pronator fat stripes are unreliable soft tissue signs in the detection of radiographically occult fractures. Clin Radiol. 2003;58:798–800.
6. Creteur V, Madani A, Brasseur JL. Pronator quadratus imaging. Diagn Interv Imaging. 2012;93:22–9.
7. Sato J, Ishii Y, Noguchi H, Takeda M, Toyabe S. Sonographic appearance of pronator quadratus muscle in heathy volunteers. J Ultrasound Med. 2014;33:111–7.
8. Sasaki Y, Sugioka Y. The pronator quadratus sign: its classification and diagnostic usefulness for injury and inflammation of the wrist. J Hand Surg Br. 1989;14:80–3.
9. Zimmers TE. Fat plane radiological signs in wrist and elbow trauma. Am J Emerg Med. 1984;2:526–32.
10. Johnson RK, Shrewsbury MM. The pronator quadratus in motions and in stabilization of the radius and ulna at the distal radioulnar joint. J Hand Surg Am. 1976;1:205–9.
11. Stuart PR. Pronator quadratus revisited. J Hand Surg Br. 1996;21:714–22.
12. Gordon KD, Pardo RD, Johnson JA, King GJW, Miller TA. Electromyographic activity and strength maximum isometric pronation and supination efforts in healthy adults. J Orthop Res. 2004;22:208–13.
13. Pierre-Jerome C, Moncayo V, Albastaki U, Terk MR. Multiple occult wrist bone injuries and joint effusions: prevalence and distribution on MRI. Emerg Radiol. 2010;17:179–84.
14. Brydie A, Raby N. Early MRI in the management of clinical scaphoid fracture. Br J Radiol. 2003;76:296–300.
15. Tibrewal S, Jayakumar P, Vaidya S, Ang SC. Role of MRI in the diagnosis and management of patients with clinical scaphoid fracture. Int Orthop. 2012;36:107–10.
16. Bajaj S, Pattamapaspong N, Middleton W, Teefey S. Ultrasound of the hand and wrist. J Hand Surg Am. 2009;34:759–60.
17. Tagliafico A, Perez MM, Padua L, Klauser A, Zicca A, Martinoli C. Increased reflectivity and loss in bulk of the pronator quadratus muscle does not always indicate anterior interosseous neuropathy on ultrasound. Eur J Radiol. 2013;82:526–9.

13

Cell recognition based on topological sparse coding for microscopy imaging of focused ultrasound treatment

Zhenyou Wang[1,2], Jiang Zhu[4], Yanmei Xue[3], Changxiu Song[2] and Ning Bi[1*]

Abstract

Background: Ultrasound is considered a reliable, widely available, non-invasive, and inexpensive imaging technique for assessing and detecting the development phases of cancer; both *in vivo* and *ex vivo*, and for understanding the effects on cell cycle and viability after ultrasound treatment.

Methods: Based on the topological continuity characteristics, and that adjacent points or areas represent similar features, we propose a topological penalized convex objective function of sparse coding, to recognize similar cell phases.

Results: This method introduces new features using a deep learning method of sparse coding with topological continuity characteristics. Large-scale comparison tests demonstrate that the RAW can outperform SIFT GIST and HoG as the input features with this method, achieving higher sensitivity, specificity, F1 score, and accuracy.

Conclusions: Experimental results show that the proposed topological sparse coding technique is valid and effective for extracting new features, and the proposed system was effective for cell recognition of microscopy images of theMDA-MB-231 cell line. This method allows features from sparse coding learning methods to have topological continuity characteristics, and the RAW features are more applicable for the deep learning of the topological sparse coding method than SIFT GIST and HoG.

Keywords: Topological continuity characteristics, Sparse coding, Focused ultrasound, Microscopy imaging

Background

Knowledge of cell viability, the cytoskeletal system, cell morphology, cell migration, tumor cell inhibition rate, and cell cycle (interphase, prophase, metaphase, and anaphase) are important for understanding various diseases, notably cancer [1, 2]. Changes in the cell cycle before and after drug treatment are useful for effective drug discovery research [3]. Critical to such measurements is the accurate recognition of mitotic cells in a cell culture via automated image analysis. Hundreds of thousands of living cells are recorded in time-lapse phase-contrast microscopy images or microscopy video for research studies in cancer biology and biomaterials engineering [4].

Breast cancer has accounted for approximately 30 % of all female cancers diagnosed in the European Union, and is the leading cause of female cancer deaths. Over 85,000 women (many in their reproductive and economically productive years) have succumbed to the disease [5, 6]. Traditional methods for cell recognition in microscopy images still have several limitations, although much progress has been made. However, some processes of irregular appearance, such as cell death, cytoskeletal and cell morphology changes, cell migration, and cell cycle are difficult to follow. Learning the complex relationships of the multiple states induces high computational complexity and drives the system far from the goal of real-time recognition. Hence, because of the complexity of cell behaviors and morphological variance, existing automatic systems remain limited when dealing with large volumes of time-lapse microscopy images [7, 8]. At the same time, sparse modeling is one

* Correspondence: 10253365@QQ.COM
Co-first author: Jiang Zhu
[1]School of Mathematics and Computational Science, Sun Yat-sen University, Guangzhou, P. R. China
Full list of author information is available at the end of the article

of the most successful recent signal processing paradigms, and topological features are better represented as the adjacent and similar points or areas have been extracted from the features of all points or areas. Topology of the topology sparse coding mainly simulates and describes a phenomenon and characteristics so that the adjacent neurons of the human cerebral cortex can extract a similar feature. Topological maps have features wherein adjacent points or areas correspond to adjacent points or areas in feature space, and adjacent points or areas tend to respond to similar features. Feature preference varies smoothly across the cortex, that is to say, adjacent points or areas represent similar features. These are the topological continuity properties [9].

Aapo Hyvärinen and Patrik O. Hoyer [10] have shown that this single principle of sparseness can also lead to emergence of topography and complex cell properties. Rodolphe Jenatton [11] considered an extension of this framework where the atoms are further assumed to be embedded in a tree. This is achieved using a recently introduced tree-structured sparse regularization norm, which has proven useful in several applications. The procedure has a complexity linear, or close to linear, in the number of atoms, and allows the use of accelerated gradient techniques to solve the tree-structured sparse approximation problem at the same computational cost as traditional ones, using L_1 norm. However, this method has no continuity properties for the same cell phase for different cells, and the gradient method applied here is not normal, because the L_1 norm of the non-differentiable at point zero.

In this paper, we propose a recognition method based on topological sparse coding. First, cell shape information is obtained using binarization [12]. The detected cells are then segmented via a seeded watershed algorithm [13]. After segmentation, a favorite matching plus local tree matching approach is used to track the dynamic behaviors of cell nuclei [14]. After obtaining segmented nuclei ROIs (regions of interest), each cell is represented by a region feature. Based on these results, we have designed a topological penalized convex objective function to induce sparsity and consistency constraints for dictionary learning and sparse decomposition. Finally, a support vector machine (SVM) classifier is utilized for model learning and prediction. This approach can be used to analyze the behavior of cells as extracted from a time-lapse microscopy video. For instance, we have used this analysis to identify cell phase and cell cycle progress in MDA-MB-231 cells.

Methods

The MDA-MB-231 cell line from the American Type Culture Collection (ATCC), frozen by the Cornell University Weill Medical College of The Methodist Hospital Research Institute was used. All experimental research reported in this manuscript consisted of *in vitro* experiments.

Images were acquired every 2 min for 12 h and 22 min, giving a total of 373 images per hole that were then exported from Simple PCI as 16 bit uncompressed TIFF files to 8 GB network attached storage (NAS) arrays for processing. Figure 1 shows the microscopy images the MDA-MB-231 cells.

First, cell shape information is obtained by binarization. The detected cells are then segmented via a seeded watershed algorithm. After segmentation, a favorite matching plus local tree matching approach is used to track the dynamic behaviors of the cell nuclei.

A pixel-wise intensity feature (Raw) represents the global intensity distribution of one image and implicitly contains its appearance characteristics. Histogram of Oriented Gradients (HoG) [15], Generalized Search Tree (GIST) [16], and Scale Invariant Feature Transform (SIFT) [17] are features that are widely used to represent shape characteristics, local structural information, and local visual saliency, respectively. For comparison, we extracted the pixel-wise intensity feature and three representative visual features from every nuclei [18]. After obtaining feature vectors that include information on shape and texture, they are input into deep learning process. After obtaining segmented nuclei ROIs (regions of interest), each cell is represented by a feature vector including 54 elements for the RAW, converting each candidate into a feature vector that implicitly represents the characteristics of the mitotic cell [19]. In this paper, we input the feature vectors into a topological sparse coding process.

Given a new sample and its feature $x\left(x\in R^d\right)$, The value of "d" is the vector x_i of the matrix x has "d" elements. The goal of sparse coding is to decompose it over a dictionary A, such that x = As + r, a set of N data points × in the Euclidean space R^d is written as the approximate product of a d × k dictionary A and k × N coefficients s, r is the residual. Least squares estimation (LSE), a similar model fitting procedure, is usually formulated as a minimization of the residual sum of squares to get an optimal coefficient s. However, LSE often poorly preserves both low prediction error and the high sparsity of coefficients [20]. Therefore, penalization techniques have been widely researched to improve on it. Considering the constraints of sparsity and consistency for decomposition, we designed a topological objective function for the system as follows:

$$J(A, s) = \|As - x\|_2^2 + \lambda \sum_{i,\, all\, group} \sqrt{V s_i s_i^T}. \tag{1}$$

where $\|s\|_2^2 = \Sigma_i \|s_i\|_2^2$, the s_i is the i-th row vector of the coefficient s, where V is the grouping matrix, where the group contains all of the elements of the learning set.

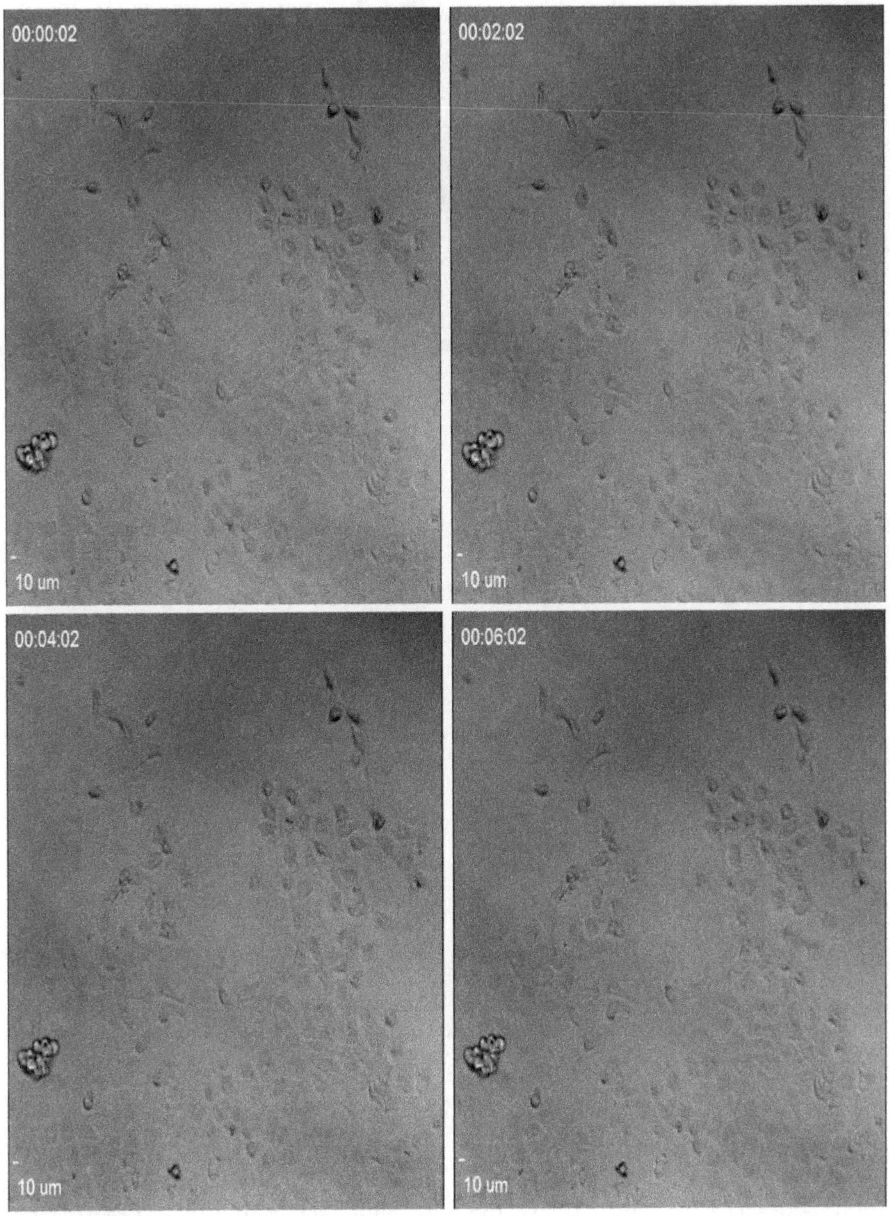

Fig. 1 Microscopy image of MDA-MB-231 cell lines. The 4 continuous images of the position 1 with sound of pressure 1Mpa for the each time 00:00:02,00:02:02,00:04:02, 00:06:02

For example, if V is 3*3 grouping matrix method, and one group begins from the 1-st row and 2-nd column, so the $\sqrt{Vs_is_i{}^T} = \sqrt{s_{12}^2 + s_{13}^2 + s_{14}^2 + s_{22}^2 + s_{23}^2 + s_{24}^2 + s_{32}^2 + s_{33}^2 + s_{34}^2}$. Small mini-batches, that is to say, we have taken learning sets into several small learning sets. Because the s_i is the i-th row vector of the coefficient s, the s_i^T is the column vector, V is the grouping matrix, so V{s_i}{s_i}^t is a value, and then the $\sqrt{Vs_is_i{}^T}$ in the J(A,s) is the $\|s\|_1$, and we have reserved the main values of the vector used by L1 norm. So the objective functions are described as "topological penalized." The objective function in Equation (1) consists of two parts, the first term penalizes the sum-of-squares difference between the reconstructed and original sample; the second term is the sparsity penalty term that is used to guarantee the sparsity of the feature set through a smaller coefficient λ values. The gradient method is not valid at point zero because L_1 norm is not differentiable at point zero. We then use $\sqrt{Vs_is_i{}^T + \varepsilon}$ that defines a smoothed topographic L_1 sparsity penalty on *s* in sparse coding instead of $\sqrt{Vs_is_i{}^T}$ on the L_1 norm smoothing, where ε is a constant.

J (A, s) is not convex if J (A, s) only includes the first term and second term, but given A, the minimum of J(A,s) to solve s is convex [21, 22]; similarly, given s, minimizing

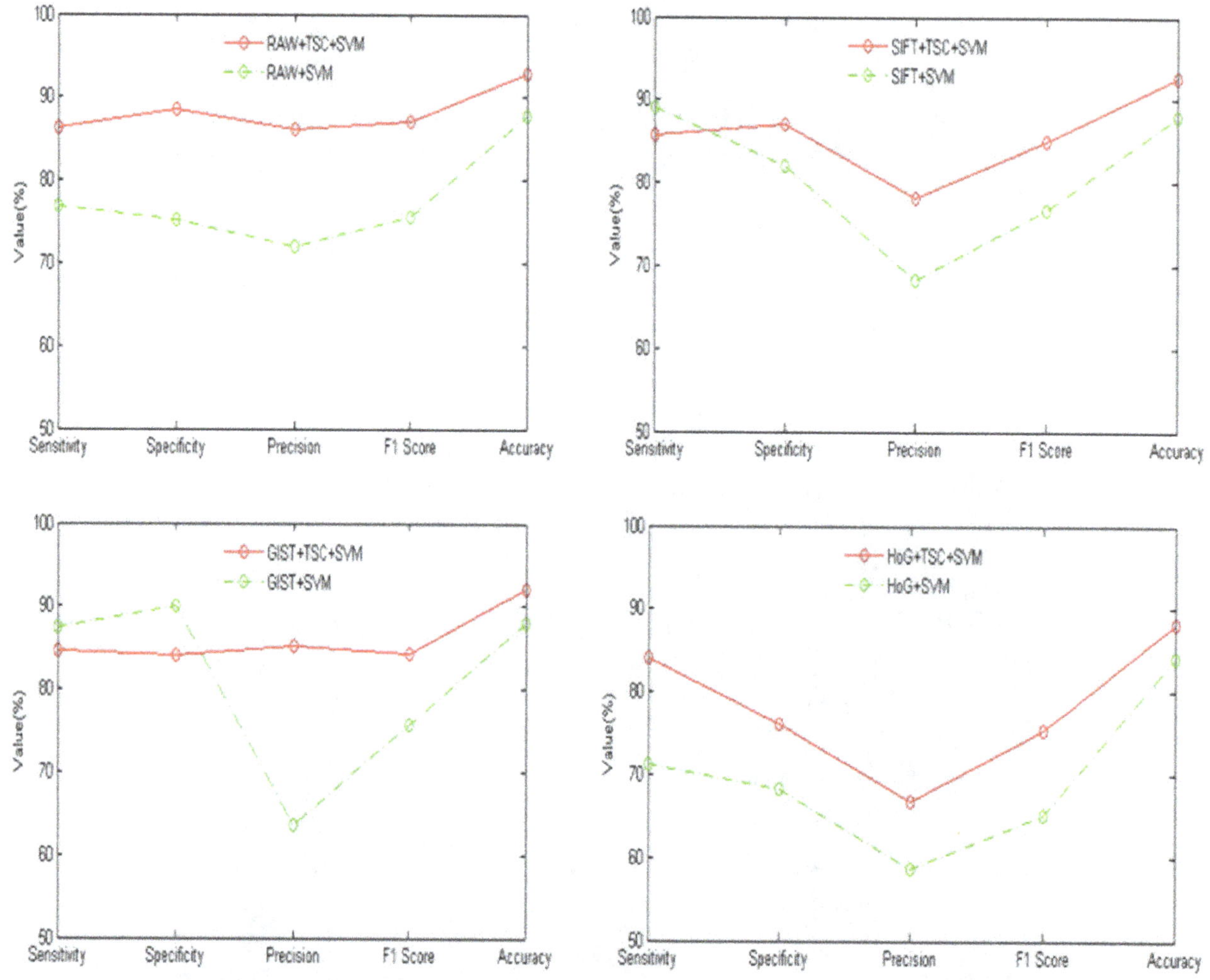

Fig. 2 Comparison with topological sparse coding deep learning or not. Red lines represents the algorithm have the deep learning step of topology sparse coding, green lines represent the algorithm don't have the deep learning step of topology sparse coding. From left to right of the first row are: RAW as input characteristics, SIFT as input characteristics. From left to right of the second row are: GIST as input characteristics, HoG as input characteristics

J(A,s) to solved A is also convex, so we add the third term, the weighted decay term with weighted decay coefficients γ into the $J(A, s)$ and then the optimization computation may use the gradient techniques. In order to achieve the following purposes: only a few coefficients values of matrix A are far greater than 0, nor that most coefficients are greater than 0. In order to solve this problem, we can make a constraint on the values of s, C is a constant.

$$\min J(A, s) = \|As - x\|_2^2 + \lambda \sum_{i,\, all\, group} \sqrt{V s_i s_i^T + \varepsilon} + \gamma \|A\|_2^2 \quad s.t \|s\|_2^2 \leq C \tag{2}$$

Assuming there are enough mitotic cell training samples such that dictionary A is over-complete, it is clear that a new mitotic cell image can be faithfully represented by a linear combination of mitotic bases contained in A. However, in reality, it is impossible to enumerate all mitotic cases for the training set. Under the sparse coding scheme, each candidate × is represented as a linear combination of bases in matrix A by coefficient s. Therefore, s explicitly reflects the relationship between x. d the bases and it can be utilized as the characteristic representation for classification. If the iterative algorithm is executed on large data sets, iteration should take a long time and this algorithm also takes a long time to reach convergence results. So we choose to run the algorithm on a mini-block, so that we can improve the speed of iteration and improve the convergence speed.

To optimize the cost function, we follow these steps:

1: Randomly initialize the A function
2: Repeat the following steps until convergence:

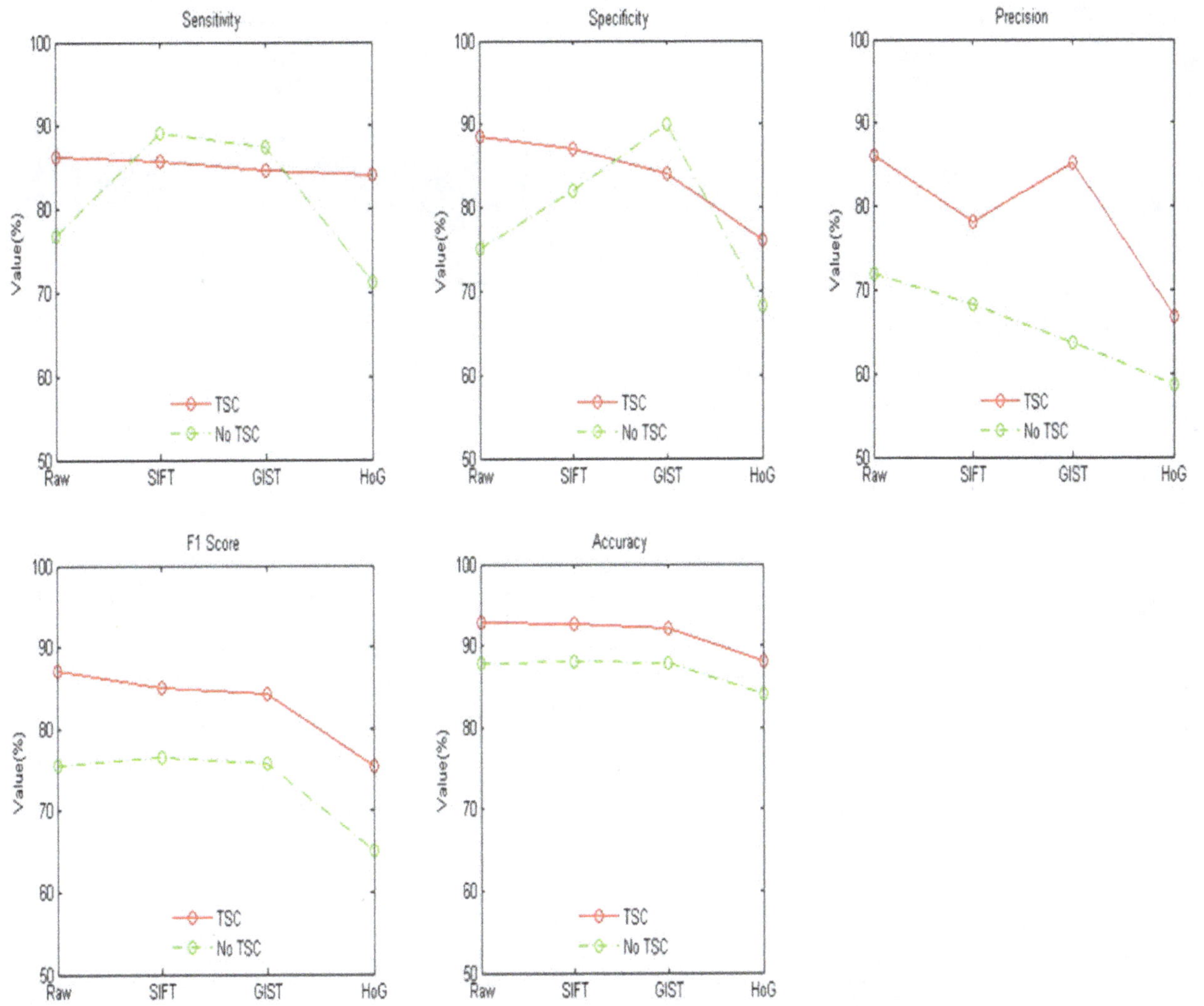

Fig. 3 Comparison with topological sparse coding deep learning or not. Red lines represents the algorithm has the deep learning step of topology sparse coding, green lines represent the algorithm does not have the deep learning step of topology sparse coding. From left to right of the first row are: sensitivity, specificity, precision. From left to right of the second row are:, F1 score, accuracy

2.1: Randomly select small mini-batches of the learning sets.
2.2: $s \leftarrow A^T x$, $s_{r,c} \leftarrow \frac{s_{r,c}}{\|A_c\|}$ where $s_{r,c}$ is the r-th feature of the c-th sample and A_c is the c-th base vector of matrix A (This is an iteration, all have taken place in the mini-batches).
2.3: Calculate s by minimizing J (A, s) according to equation 2 with gradient techniques (we have calculated the cost function J using gradient descent method (deflector for extreme values of the function), and we have obtained the s used stable point when we have fixed the A).
2.4: Obtain A such that J (A, s) is minimized according to s with gradient techniques (We have calculated the cost function J using gradient descent method (deflector for extreme values of the function). We have obtained the A used stable point when we have fixed the s).

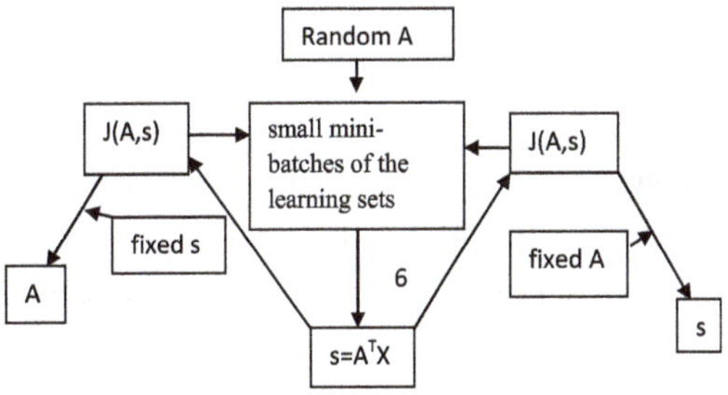

After these steps, we obtain the topological characteristic feature vectors from the same cell phase. These feature

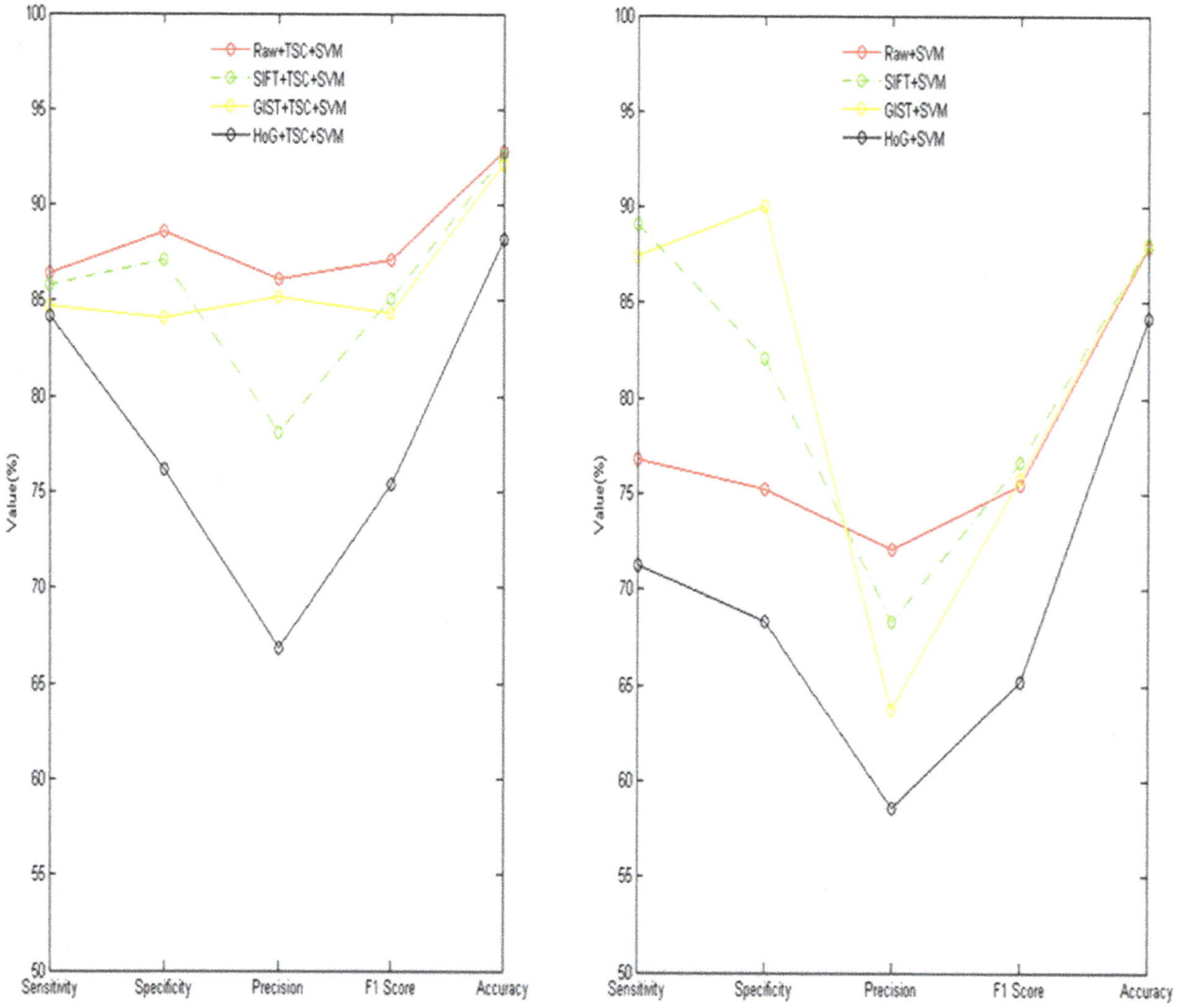

Fig. 4 Comparison of each type input characteristics.The left figure is algorithm have the deep learning step of topology sparse coding; and the right figure is algorithm don't have the deep learning step of topology sparse coding

vectors may be classified with the SVM classifier. The following diagram is the overview diagram of the algorithm.

The basic procedure for applying SVM to cell phase recognition is as follows [23]. First, the input vectors are linearly or non-linearly mapped into a feature space (possibly with a higher dimension) by selecting a relevant kernel function. In this paper, the kernel function $k(x, x') = \frac{\|x - x'\|^2}{\delta}$ is used. Then, within this feature space, an optimized linear division is sought by constructing a hyper-plane that separates the samples into four classes (interphase, prophase, metaphase, and anaphase) with the least errors and maximal margin. The SVM training process always seeks a globally optimized solution and avoids over fitting [23], hence, SVM has the ability to deal with a large number of features.

Results and discussion

We took the first 240 images of the data set as the learning set and the other 133 images for the test set. This generated a learning set consisting of 19521 nuclei and test set consisting of 10881 nuclei, where we were mainly concerned with the cell cycle phase (interphase, prophase, metaphase, and anaphase). After computation on matrix A with gradient techniques, the dimensionality

Table 1 Error rate for different approaches

	Mairal et al. [13]	Mairal et al. [13]	reWL1	RAW+TSC+SVM
approaches	(unsupervised)	(supervised)	[28] (WL1)	approache in the paper
Error rate	12.02 %	7.93 %	9.71 %	7.21 %

of x. the experiments are 54 × 19521, the dimensionality of A in the experiments are 54 × 121, the dimensionality of s. the experiments are 121 × 19,521.

To demonstrate the superiority of the proposed method for mitotic cell recognition, we evaluated the sensitivity and specificity of our experimental results. We compared the performances on the same test set for mitotic cell recognition. Let TP, TN, FP, and FN stand for the number of true positive, true negative, false positive, and false negative samples, respectively, after the completion of cell phase identification. Sensitivity is defined as: (TP/(TP + FN)), and is a statistical measure of how well-classified the positive cells are. Specificity reflects the ability to identify negative cells correctly and is defined as (TN/(TN + FP)). Precision is (TP/(TP + FP)), accuracy is ((TP + TN)/(TP + FN + FP + TN)), and the F1 score ((2 ×C precision × sensitivity)/(precision + sensitivity)) represents the overall performance of both. These are commonly-used quantitative metrics to evaluate the performance of mitotic cell recognition. λ and γ are again trade-off parameters controlling the balance between the reconstruction quality and sparsity [24, 25], when comparing the performance of different dictionary learning strategies with four visual features and different configurations, λ and γ were set to 0.1 [26, 27] and C is set to 1.

From Fig. 2, for each index of the RAW and HoG features, including sensitivity specificity precision F1 score accuracy, the classification performance with topological sparse coding deep learning was better than with none.

From Fig. 3, for precision F1 score and accuracy indexes of the RAW SIFT GIST and HoG features, the classification performance with topological sparse coding deep learning was better than with none.

From left part of Fig. 4, for each index including sensitivity specificity precision F1 score accuracy, under the condition of topological sparse coding deep learning, the classification performance used RAW feature as input feature is better than SIFT GIST and HoG features. The right part of the Fig. 4 has the same results; that is the classification performance used RAW feature as input feature is better than SIFT GIST and HoG features with no deep learning. The HoG feature performs poorer than RAW SIFT and GIST. It was thought that HoG would be the least accurate because it is not very suitable for deformable object representation in this case.

The extracting features method of topological sparse coding with topological continuity characteristics is feasible and effective for deep learning. The index of RAW with deep learning is higher than the others, implying that a pixel-wise intensity feature (RAW) represents the global intensity distribution of one image and implicitly contains its appearance characteristics. In addition, the RAW features are more applicable for deep learning of the topological sparse coding method than the SIFT, GIST, and HoG features.

Finally, we have compared our results with Mairal et al.'s unsupervised and supervised approaches [13], and sparse the coding for reWL1 [28]. The best results of these approaches are shown in Table 1. Our error rate is significantly better compared to theirs. However, it should be noted that we have used the RAW feature in all our experiments.

Conclusions

In this paper, we proposed a topological penalized convex objective function of sparse coding for the recognition of cell cycles, based on the fact that topology of the topology sparse coding mainly describes a phenomenon and characteristics that the adjacent neurons of the human cerebral cortex can extract a similar feature. This method has made the new features from the deep learning methods of sparse coding to have topological continuity characteristics. Large-scale comparison tests demonstrate that the RAW can outperform SIFT GIST and HoG, achieving higher sensitivity, specificity, F1 score, and accuracy. That is to say, the proposed topological sparse coding technique is valid and effective for the extracting of new features, and the RAW features are more applicable for the deep learning of the topological sparse coding method than SIFT GIST and HoG.

Competing interests

The authors declare that they have no competing interests.

Authors' contribution

ZY carried out the studies and drafted the manuscript. JZ participated in the design of the study, performed the experimental and statistical analysis. CS, NB conceived of the study, and participated in its design and coordination and helped to draft the manuscript. YM helped to draft and revise the manuscript. All authors read and approved the final manuscript.

Acknowledgements

We wish to thank the National Natural Science Foundation of China (Nos. 11401115, 11471012,11301276), the Project of Department of Education of Guangdong Province (No. 13KJ0396), and Science and Technology Program of Guangzhou, China (No. 2013B051000075). This work was also supported in part by the Natural Science Funds of Jiangsu Province (BK20130984).

Author details

[1]School of Mathematics and Computational Science, Sun Yat-sen University, Guangzhou, P. R. China. [2]Faculty of Applied Mathematics, Guangdong University of Technology, Guangzhou, P.R. China. [3]The School of Mathematics & Statistics, Nanjing University of Information Science Technology, Nanjing, Jiangsu, P.R. China. [4]Department of Ultrasound, Sir Run Shaw Hospital, College of Medicine ZheJiang University, Hangzhou, P.R. China.

References

1. Su H, Yin Z, Huh S, Kanade T. Cell Segmentation in Phase Contrast Microscopy Images via Semi-supervised Clustering over Optics-related Features. Med Image Anal. 2013;17:746–65.
2. Zhou X, Wong STC. Informatics challenges of High-throughput micros-copy. IEEE Signal Proc Mag. 2006;23:63–72.
3. Baguley BC, Marshall ES. *In vitro* modeling of human tumor behavior in drug discovery programmes. Eur J Canver. 2004;40:794–801.
4. Oliva A, Torralba A. Modeling the Shape of the Scene: A Holistic Representation of the Spatial Envelope. Int J Comput Vis. 2001;42(3):145–75.
5. Neel JC, Lebrun JJ. Activin and TGFβ regulate expression of the microRNA-181 family to promote cell migration and invasion in breast cancer cells. Cell Signal. 2013;25(7):1556–66.
6. Zhang Y, Duan C, Bian C, Xiong Y, Zhang J. Steroid receptor coactivator-1: A versatile regulator and promising therapeutic target for breast cancer. J Steroid Biochem Mol Biol. 2013;138:17–23.
7. Wong C, Chen AA, Behr B, Shen S. Time-lapse microscopy and image analysis in basic and clinical embryo development research. Reprod BioMed Online. 2013;26(2):120–9.
8. Brieu N, Navab N, Serbanovic-Canic J, Ouwehand WH, Stemple DL, Cvejic A, et al. Image-based characterization of thrombus formation in time-lapse DIC microscopy. Med Image Anal. 2012;16(4):915–31.
9. Olshausen B, Field D. Emergence of simple-cell receptive field properties by learning a sparse code for natural images. Nature. 1996;381(6583):607–9.
10. Hyvärinen A, Hoyer PO. A two-layer sparse coding model learns simple and complex cell receptive fields and topography from natural images. Vision Res. 2001;41(18):2413–23.
11. Jenatton R, Mairal J, Obozinski G, Bach F. Proximal Methods for Hierarchical Sparse Coding. J Mach Learn Res. 2011;12:2297–334.
12. Bradley D.M, Bagnell J.A. Differential sparse coding, in Proc. Advances in neural information processing systems(NIPS), 2008. (http://repository.cmu.edu/cgi/viewcontent.cgi?article=1043&context=robotics)
13. Mairal J, Bach F, Ponce J. Task-driven dictionary learning. IEEE Trans Pattern Anal Mach Intell. 2012;34(4):791–804.
14. Wählby C, Lindblad J, Vondrus M, Bengtsson E, Björkesten L. Algorithms for cytoplasm segmentation of fluorescence labelled cells. Anal Cell Pathol. 2002;24(2–3):101–11.
15. Lin G, Adiga U, Olson K, Guzowski JF, Barnes CA, Roysam B. A hybrid 3-D watershed algorithm incorporating gradient cues and object models for automatic segmentation of nuclei in confocal image stacks. Cytometry A. 2003;56A:23–36.
16. Yan J, Zhou X, Yang Q, Liu N, Cheng Q, Wong STC. An efficient system for optical microscopy cell image segmentation, tracking and cell phase identification. Atlanta, GA: Image Processing 2006 IEEE International Conference; 2006. p. 1917–20.
17. Memarzadeh M, Golparvar-Fard M, Niebles JC. Automated 2D detection of construction equipment and workers from site video streams using histograms of oriented gradients and colors. Autom Constr. 2013;32:24–37.
18. Lowe DG. Distinctive Image Features from Scale-Invariant Keypoints. Journal International Journal of Computer Vision. 2004;60(2):91–110.
19. Zou H, Hastie T. Regularization and variable selection via the Elastic Net. Journal of the Royal Statistical Society, Series B. 2005;67:301–20.
20. Liu AA, Li K, Kanade T. Spatiotemporal Mitosis Event Detection in Time-Lapse Phase Contrast Microscopy Image Sequences. Suntec City: Multimedia and Expo (ICME), 2010 IEEE International Conference; 2010. p. 161–6.
21. Honglak Lee, Alexis Battle, Rajat Raina, Andrew Y. Ng. Efficient sparse coding algorithms. http://robotics.stanford.edu/~hllee/nips06-sparsecoding.pdf
22. Tong T, Wolz R, Coupé P, Hajnal JV, Rueckert D. Segmentation of MR images via discriminative dictionary learning and sparse coding: Application to hippocampus labeling. Neuroimage. 2013;76(1):11–23.
23. Meng Wang, Xiaobo Zhou, Fuhai Li, Jeremy Huckins, Randall W King, Stephen T.C. Wong. Novel Cell Segmentation and Online SVM for Cell Cycle Phase Identification in Automated Microscopy.Bioinformatics. 2008;24(1):94-101.
24. Chen S, Donoho D, Saunders M. Atomicde composition by basis pursuit. SIAM J Sci Comput. 1999;20:33–61.
25. Tibshirani R. Regression shrinkage and selection via the Lasso. J R Stat Soc Ser B. 1996;67:267–88.
26. Andra's L, Zsolt P, Ga'bor S. Sparse and silent coding in neural circuits. Neurocomputing. 2012;79:115–24.
27. Chen S, Donoho D, Saunders M. Atomic decomposition by basis pursuit. SIAM J Sci Comput. 2001;43:129–59.
28. Ramirez I, Sapiro G. Universal regularizers for robust sparse coding and modeling. IEEE Trans Image Process. 2012;21(9):3850–64.

14

Cognitive tasks and cerebral blood flow through anterior cerebral arteries: a study via functional transcranial Doppler ultrasound recordings

Héloïse Bleton[1], Subashan Perera[2] and Ervin Sejdić[1]*

Abstract

Background: Functional transcanial Doppler ultrasound (fTCD) is a convenient approach to examine cerebral blood flow velocity (CBFV) in major cerebral arteries.

Methods: In this study, the anterior cerebral artery (ACA) was insonated on both sides, that is, right ACA (R-ACA) and left ACA (L-ACA). The envelope signals (the maximum velocity) and the raw signals were analyzed during cognitive processes, i.e. word-generation tasks, geometric tasks and resting state periods separating each task. Data which were collected from 20 healthy participants were used to investigate the changes and the hemispheric functioning while performing cognitive tasks. Signal characteristics were analyzed in time domain, frequency domain and time-frequency domain.

Results: Significant results have been obtained through the use of both classic/modern methods (i.e. envelope/raw, time and frequency/information-theoretic and time-frequency domains). The frequency features extracted from the raw signals highlighted sex effects on cerebral blood flow which revealed distinct brain response during each process and during resting periods. In the time-frequency analysis, the distribution of wavelet energies on the envelope signals moved around the low frequencies during mental processes and did not experience any lateralization during cognitive tasks.

Conclusions: Even if no lateralization effects were noticed during resting-state, verbal and geometric tasks, understanding CBFV in ACA during cognitive tasks could complement information extracted from cerebral blood flow in middle cerebral arteries during similar cognitive tasks (i.e. sex effects).

Keywords: Anterior cerebral arteries, Cerebral blood flow, Functional transcanial Doppler ultrasound, Signal processing

Background

Distribution patterns of cerebral blood flow can be described by neuroimaging techniques such as functional magnetic resonance imaging, single photon emission computed tomography, positron emission tomography or the xenon-clearance technique. All these methods have a high spatial resolution [1–4]. Despite their advantages, these methods restrict patient movements and usually have a low temporal resolution. The hemodynamic features of major cerebral arteries and their rapid variations in normal and pathological conditions can be characterized by functional transcanial Doppler ultrasound. Functional transcanial Doppler ultrasound (fTCD) is a non-invasive blood velocity measurement approach [5]. This technique uses the fact that cerebral perfusion is linked to neural activation which is translated into cerebral perfusion changes during cognitive tasks [6, 7]. It has a high temporal resolution due to continuous insonation of cerebral blood flow velocity. The velocity measurement is closely linked to cerebral blood flow in the event that the

*Correspondence: esejdic@ieee.org
[1]Department of Electrical and Computer Engineering, University of Pittsburgh, Pittsburgh, PA, USA
Full list of author information is available at the end of the article

diameter of cerebral arteries does not change during the insonation. Multiple studies showed that perfusion area and diameter of cerebral arteries do not change during mental processes [8–10]. Thus, blood flow velocity evolutions are due to modifications in cerebral metabolism because of cerebral activities.

fTCD has been studied during cognitive or physical tasks for both healthy participants and patients affected by neurological disorders (e.g., stroke, autism, epilepsy) [11–15]. Previous publications have examined the effects of visual perception [16, 17], auditory perception [18, 19], language processes [20, 21], spatial processes [22, 23], memory processes [24], other cognitive/mental tasks and other neurological disorders [13, 25, 26] on cerebral blood flow using fTCD. These publications pointed that the main advantages of a fTCD system include its price, easiness-to-use and its minimally stressful character [27].

fTCD is mainly used to target major cerebral arteries [28]. Usually, transducers are placed on the thinnest parts of head bone which are the acoustic windows of the skull allowing to monitor activities on cerebral arteries of the circle of Willis. The transtemporal window enables us to reach the middle (MCA), anterior (ACA) and posterior (PCA) cerebral arteries. The transforaminal window enables us to reach the basilar and the vertebral arteries; while the transorbital window reaches the ophthalmic and the internal arteries [29]. Arteries are identified by understanding the depth of insonation, the transducers position and the flow direction [30]. The most commonly insonated arteries are the ACA, the MCA and the PCA [31]. Each of these arteries supplies blood to different areas: the ACA supply to the medial regions, the MCA supply to the lateral regions and the PCA supply to the posterior basomedial regions. The MCA is most usually insonated in studies about cognitive processes [20, 32–34], as 80 % of blood to the brain is delivered by the MCA. The ACA could be also insonated during high cognitive functions such as arithmetic problems or receptive language [35–37]. As ACA are deeper than MCA [29], insonating ACA could provide complimentary information to signals acquired from MCA in order to gain further understanding of cerebral blood flow characteristics while performing mental activities [30, 38, 39].

Previous publications regarding cerebral blood flow velocities during mental stimuli on MCA highlighted the left and right hemispheric dominance introduced during the geometric task and the word-generation task respectively. However, the brain blood flow in ACA is closely linked to the activity in MCA [32, 33, 35]. In fact, lateralization in the ACA blood flow was predicted while performing cognitive processes (i.e. evolutions of cerebral blood flow velocity can be explained by the changes in the MCA during mental challenges). Moreover, handedness and sex appeared to have effects on brain response during activation periods. Distinct functioning hemispheric dominance may be foreseen according to sex and handedness [40].

Our hypothesis was that cognitive tasks affect the cerebral blood flow velocities in ACAs similarly to those changes observed in cerebral blood flow velocities in MCAs. To examine our hypothesis, we collected both raw signals and maximal velocity signals (usually called the spectral envelope signals [41]). A few fTCD studies only examined envelope signals and may lack information contained in raw signals [5, 31, 42]. Previous studies highlighted the significance of data embodied in raw signals during resting periods [43, 44]. Envelope signals are usually extracted from raw signals, which are a sum of signals corresponding to erythrocytes movement at different velocities. Raw results which are used to calculate envelope signals, may contain exhaustive information about the activation stimuli and resting-state periods.

Our major contributions include the understanding of signal patterns in various domains (time, frequency, and time-frequency) for raw and maximum velocity signals. Features from the classical analysis were examined (i.e. time and frequency approaches). We also used modern analysis characteristics from information-theoretic and time-frequency domains which have not been examined in previous studies about brain response during mental tasks [45]. Additionally, the current study complements the study of the ACA resting-state characteristics [43] and follows outcomes from MCA results during resting periods and activation stimuli (word-generation and geometric rotation tasks) [45]. These two previous papers employed the same methodology. The repercussions of sex and handedness on CBFV were also examined.

Methods

Subjects

Twenty able-bodied participants have taken part in the experiment (Males/Females = 9/11, 22.1 ± 1.86 years old; 171 ± 10.1 cm; 68.9 ± 27.3 kg). Table 1 summarizes participant demographic details. No participant had a history of heart murmurs, strokes, concussions, migraines or other brain-related injuries or neurological diseases. At first, the subjects were asked to sign the consent form approved by the University of Pittsburgh Institutional Review Board.

Table 1 Demographic information

Distribution	Male	Female	All
Age (years old)	22.3 ± 1.64	22.0±2.00	22.1±1.86
Height (cm)	180±7.26	163±5.39	171±10.1
Weight (kg)	91.6±29.3	52.6±5.89	68.9±27.3

The entire study was approved by the University of Pittsburgh Institutional Review Board.

The handedness of each participant was tested using the Edinburgh Handedness Inventory test [46]. This technique is one of the most widely used method for measuring both the direction and the degree of handedness [47, 48]. Subjects had to choose their hand preferences based on a list of activities. They could assign 1 or 2 for each activity (1 for a weak preference or 2 for a strict preference between right or left hand). The result was scored based on the formula:

$$Score = \frac{\sum X_i(R) - \sum X_i(L)}{\sum X_i(R) + \sum X_i(L)} \quad (1)$$

where $X_i(R)$ or $X_i(L)$ can take values of 0, 1 or 2 according to the domination of right/left domination. Positive score leads to right-handedness whereas negative score leads to left-handedness. This study was restricted to the analysis of handedness direction. In fact, a majority of previous publications about fTCD and brain cognitive response focused on the effects of handedness direction [35, 49, 50]. 16 subjects were right-handed (mean score of 64), 3 subjects were left-handed (mean score of -63) and one was ambidextrous. Table 2 summarizes the Edinburgh Handedness test results.

Procedure

ACA cerebral blood flow was assessed thanks to a SONARA TCD System (Carefusion, San Diego, CA, USA). Two 2 MHz transducers were placed on the left side and the right side of the skull on transtemporal windows to acquire bilateral cerebral blood flow measurements. The temporal windows are found above the zygomatic arch [38]. Transducers were fixed with a headset (5 cm in front of the ears) and were positioned to reach ACA. Additionally, the end-tidal carbon dioxide $ETCO_2$ (BCI Capnocheck Sleep Capnograph, Smiths Medical, Waukesha, Wisconsin, USA) was monitored along with respiration rate, electrocardiogram, head movement and skin conductance via a multisystem physiological data monitoring system (Nexus-X, Mindmedia, Netherlands). The $ETCO_2$ levels may have repercussions on cerebal blood flow in the ACA.

The participants were asked to complete two 15-minute cognitive parts interspersed by a 5-minute break. However, we did not collect data during these five minutes. Each 15-minute part comprises 5 mental rotation tasks, 5 word generation tasks and 5 resting conditions between each cognitive task. Each of these lasted for 45 seconds. The order of cognitive tasks was randomly assigned, but it was counterbalanced. Figures 1 and 2 illustrate the fTCD setup.

After the acquisition of R-ACA and L-ACA cerebral blood flow data in the form of audio file, information are extracted from audio files sampled at 44100 Hz. Raw data were downsampled to 8820 Hz to speed up data processing.

Table 2 Handedness information

Distribution	Right-Handed	Left-Handed	Ambidextrous
Sex	8 males, 8 females	1 male, 2 females	1 female
Average score	64	-63	0

Resting-state

During 5-minutes breaks and during the resting-state, participants were requested to remain awake, maintain a thought-free mental state and keep quiet.

Geometric rotation task

During the 45-seconds mental rotation tasks, pairs of images were randomly selected from a database constructed from 3-D cubes [51]. Pairs were displayed for 9 seconds each. Participants were asked to rotate shapes to find which ones are identical or mirror symmetrical.

Word generation task

Participants generated words silently based on letters randomly chosen and displayed at the beginning of each period. Subjects were cautioned not to vocalize any words in order to avoid any brain activations related to speech regions [52].

Feature extraction

Three common parameters in statistics were considered: standard deviation, skewness, kurtosis of the signal amplitude [53]. Statistical parameters from the envelope and the raw signals were extracted. Standard deviation of a signal estimates the spread of a distribution [53, 54]. The skewness of the amplitude distribution quantifies the asymmetry of the distribution [53, 55]. The kurtosis of a distribution evaluates the behavior of the distribution close to the boundaries [53]. These statistical features characterize signals from the right side and from the left side of ACA.

The cross-correlation coefficient at the zero lag between the L-ACA signal and the R-ACA signal was used to demonstrate whether L-ACA signal and R-ACA signal are related:

$$CC_{X_{R-ACA}/Y_{L-ACA}} = \frac{1}{N}\sum_{i=1}^{N}(x_i y_i) \quad (2)$$

where the signal $X_{R-ACA} = \{x_i\}$ and $Y_{L-ACA} = \{y_i\}$, $i = 1, \cdots, N$ are extracted from the right and the left side of the ACA.

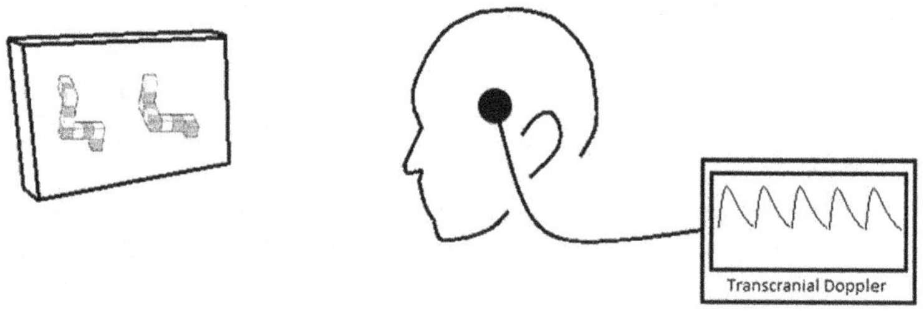

Fig. 1 Setup for the fTCD study

Information-theoretic feature

Information-theoretic features were also taken into consideration. The Lempel-Ziv complexity (LZC) and the entropy rate were extracted. These measures provide information about the complexity and the regularity of signals.

The amount of new patterns formation through finite time sequences is determined by the Lempel-Ziv complexity [56]. In fact, it estimates the predictability and the randomness of the signal [57, 58]. The Lempel-Ziv measure is often used in applications of analysis of biomedical signals [56, 59]. First, the signal amplitude is converted into a finite binary series. It is divided into 100 finite spaces defined thanks to 99 thresholds, T_h, $1 \leq h \leq 99$, $h \in \mathbb{Z}^+$. The threshold is usually chosen as the median of the signal [60]. Secondly, the quantized signal $X_1^n = \{x_1, x_2, \cdots, x_n\}$ is divided into blocks. Each block is series of successive data of length L. All block can be defined as the following formula [61]:

$$B = X_j^l = \{x_j, x_{j+1}, \cdots, x_l\}, 1 \leq j \leq l \leq n, j, l \in Z^+ \quad (3)$$

where the length L of the block is defined by $j - l + 1$. For each L, every block is tested from left to right. A counter c is defined and it increases by one unit if a block has not already appeared in previous j and l. Finally, the LZC is given as the following formula:

$$LZC = \frac{c(log_{100}c + 1)}{n} \quad (4)$$

where c denotes the final value of the counter at the end of the signal analysis and n represents the total of quantized levels in the signal.

The entropy rate ρ quantifies the regularity in a distribution [62]. First, the signal needs to be normalized to zero mean and unit variance (subtracting μ_X and dividing by σ_X) and quantized into 10 equal levels. The quantized signal $X = \{x_1, x_2, \cdots, x_n\}$ is decomposed and grouped into blocks of length L, $10 \leq L \leq 30$, which are finite series of consecutive points in the quantized signal such as $\Omega_L = \{\omega_1, \omega_2, \cdots, \omega_{n-L+1}\}$ [63].

$$\omega_i = 10^{L-1}x_{i+L-1} + 10^{L-2}x_{i+L-2} + \cdots + 10^0 x_i \quad (5)$$

where L is the length of successive series and ω_i is classified between 0 and $10^L - 1$. The Shannon entropy $S(L)$ of ω_L given the quantized signal Ω_L, where X takes discrete values ω_j with probability p_j is defined as [64]:

$$S(L) = \sum_{j=0}^{10^{L-1}} p_j l n p_j \quad (6)$$

where p_j is the approximated sample joint probability of the pattern j in Ω_L with the understanding that $\sum_{j=1}^{n-L+1} p_j = 1$ with $0 \leq p_j \leq 1$ $i = 1, \cdots, n - L + 1$. The normalized entropy rate is computed as the following formula [65, 66]:

$$N(L) = \frac{S(L) - S(L-1) + S(1)pe(L)}{S(1)} \quad (7)$$

where $pe(L)$ is the percentage of the integers in the L-dimensional phase space that appeared only once and

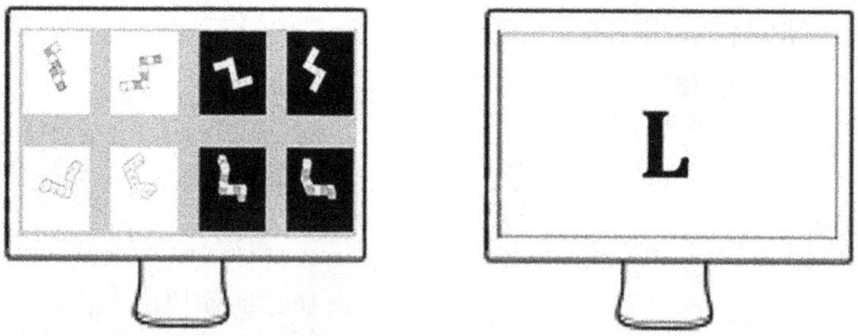

Fig. 2 A sample of the on-screen geometric and word-generation stimuli

Table 3 Time features from raw (denoted by the subscript r) and envelope (denoted by the subscript e) CBFV signals (* denotes multiplication by 10^{-3})

	Standard deviation		Skewness		Kurtosis		Cross-correlation
	R-ACA	L-ACA	R-ACA	L-ACA	R-ACA	L-ACA	
Rr	0.12 ± 0.05	0.12 ± 0.05	(-2.62 ± 0.15)*	(-0.59 ± 4.77)*	4.10 ± 2.06	4.43 ± 3.58	(5.67 ± 9.13)*
Wr	0.12 ± 0.05	0.12 ± 0.05	(-0.55 ± 9.02)*	0.89 ± 10.2)*	3.57 ± 0.90	4.26 ± 2.60	(6.96 ± 9.11)*
Gr	0.12 ± 0.04	0.12 ± 0.05	(-1.11 ± 9.38)*	(-1.26 ± 4.69)*	3.74 ± 0.95	4.42 ± 2.87	(6.50 ± 8.59)*
Re	15.9 ± 4.76	15.1 ± 5.98	1.17 ± 0.93	1.07 ± 0.58	5.95 ± 6.51	5.17 ± 2.52	0.89 ± 0.06
We	16.0 ± 4.72	15.2 ± 5.93	1.20 ± 0.90	1.13 ± 0.67	5.94 ± 6.16	5.50 ± 3.22	0.89 ± 0.06
Ge	15.9 ± 4.95	14.5 ± 5.87	1.03 ± 0.46	1.11 ± 0.63	4.74 ± 1.80	5.41 ± 2.79	0.90 ± 0.05

where $S(1)pe(L)$ is added due to the limited number of samples and the underestimation of $S(L) - S(L-1)$ for larger L. Given that the first term decreases while the second term increases with L, the goal of this method is looking for the minimum of the previous function. This minimum is an index of complexity. Finally, the regularity index ρ of the signal is defined by the following relation [66]:

$$\rho = 1 - min(N(L)) \tag{8}$$

where ρ is ranged from 0 which is equivalent to a maximal randomness to 1 which corresponds to a minimal regularity.

The cross-entropy rate quantifies the coupling of the entropy rate between two stochastic processes. It predicts data in a signal from previous and current information in another signal. Instead of making one signal normalized, both X and Y were processed (normalized, quantized and computed according to the previous method), yielding Ω_L^X and Ω_L^Y. Finally, the cross-entropy rate$\Omega_L^{X|Y}$ which represents the information rate available in one of the samples of the quantized signal x when a pattern of $L-1$ samples of the quantized signal y is established was constructed as [65]:

$$\omega_i^{X|Y} = 10^{L-1}x_{i+L-1} + 10^{L-2}y_{i+L-2} + \cdots + 10^0 y_i \tag{9}$$

The normalized cross-entropy NC of $X|Y$ is figured out as:

$$NC_{X|Y}(L) = \frac{S_{X|Y}(L) - S_Y(L-1) + S_X(1)pe_{X|Y}(L)}{S_X(1)} \tag{10}$$

where $S_X(L)$, $S_Y(L)$ and $S_{X|Y}$ represent the Shannon entropies of ω_L^X, ω_L^Y and $\omega_L^{X|Y}$. $pe_{X|Y}(L)$ is the rate of data in $\omega_L^{X|Y}$ that appeared only once and $S_X(1)pe_{X|Y}(L)$ is added due to the limited number of samples and the underestimation of $S_{X|Y}(L) - S_Y(L-1)$ for larger L. As the previous method, the goal is looking for the minimum of the previous function. The index of synchronization was used as the cross-entropy rate characteristic:

$$\Lambda_{X|Y} = 1 - min(NC_{X|Y}(L), NC_{Y|X}(L)) \tag{11}$$

where $\Lambda_{X|Y}$ is between 0 which denotes that X and Y are independent processes and 1 which proves a synchronization of X and Y.

Frequency analysis

Spectral changes of the recorded signals were examined through the peak frequency, the centroid frequency, the bandwidth of the spectrum [67, 68]. The peak frequency is associated with the maximal spectral power:

$$f_p = arg_f max\{|F_X(f)|^2\} \tag{12}$$

where $F_X(f)$ is the Fourier transform of the signal X and f_{max} in this study was 8820 Hz. The spectral centroid is defined as the center of gravity of the spectrum [69]:

$$f_c = \frac{\int_0^{f_{max}} f|F_X(f)|^2 \, df}{\int_0^{f_{max}} |F_X(f)|^2 \, df} \tag{13}$$

The bandwidth of the spectrum which represents the difference between the higher and lower frequencies of the spectrum measures the spreadness of the frequency components:

$$B = \sqrt{\frac{\int_0^{f_{max}} (f - \hat{f})^2 |F_X(f)|^2 \, ,df}{\int_0^{f_{max}} |F_X(f)|^2 \, ,df}} \tag{14}$$

The bandwidth represents the squared differences between the spectral centroid and the spectral components.

Table 4 Significant time features from raw (denoted by the subscript r) and envelope (denoted by the subscript e) CBFV signals where $p < 0.05$

Signal	ACA	Feature	Group	Group 1	Group 2
e	R-ACA	Skewness	R	M: 1.81 ± 1.09	F: 0.91 ± 0.73
e	R-ACA	Skewness	W	M: 1.50 ± 1.13	F: 0.95 ± 0.50
e	L-ACA	Skewness	G	M: 1.40 ± 0.63	F: 0.87 ± 0.62
e	R-ACA	Kurtosis	R	M: 9.21 ± 8.01	F: 4.80 ± 3.08

Table 5 Information-theoretic features from raw (denoted by the subscript r) and envelope (denoted by the subscript e) CBFV signals

	LZC		Entropy rate		Index synchronization
	R-ACA	L-ACA	R-ACA	L-ACA	
Rr	0.69 ± 0.03	0.68 ± 0.04	0.30 ± 0.14	0.35 ± 0.19	0.33 ± 0.17
Wr	0.69 ± 0.02	0.68 ± 0.03	0.28 ± 0.13	0.34 ± 0.18	0.32 ± 0.16
Gr	0.69 ± 0.02	0.68 ± 0.04	0.30 ± 0.14	0.37 ± 0.19	0.34 ± 0.17
Re	0.67 ± 0.04	0.67 ± 0.03	0.06 ± 0.07	0.04 ± 0.06	0.14 ± 0.08
We	0.67 ± 0.04	0.68 ± 0.03	0.06 ± 0.07	0.04 ± 0.06	0.14 ± 0.08
Ge	0.68 ± 0.03	0.67 ± 0.03	0.05 ± 0.05	0.04 ± 0.06	0.17 ± 0.10

Time-frequency analysis

A 10-level discrete wavelet decomposition of the signal using the discrete Meyer wavelet was calculated. The resulting decomposition is given by $W = [a_{10}\, d_{10}\, d_9\, \cdots\, d_1]$ where a_{10} is the approximation coefficients and d_k represents detail coefficients at the kth-level. The signal is observed at various frequency bands thanks to this new distribution [70]. Then, the relative energy from the approximation coefficients is defined as [71]:

$$\Xi_a = \frac{\|a_{10}\|^2}{\|a_{10}\|^2 + \sum_{k=1}^{10} \|d_k\|^2} (\%) \tag{15}$$

$$\Xi_{d_k} = \frac{\|d_k\|^2}{\|a_{10}\|^2 + \sum_{k=1}^{10} \|d_k\|^2} (\%) \tag{16}$$

where $\|.\|$ is the Euclidian norm. The relative energy which is defined by the ratio of the energy at the kth level divided by the total energy was calculated based on the wavelet transform. It denotes the distribution of energies at different frequency bands.

A wavelet entropy measures the amount of order of the signal and gives information about the distribution [71, 72]:

$$\Omega = -\Xi_{a_{10}} log_2 \Xi_{a_{10}} - \sum_{k=1}^{10} \Xi_{d_k} log_2 \Xi_{d_k} \tag{17}$$

where $\Xi_{a_{10}}$ is the relative energy. A value of Ω close to 0 demonstrates a concentration of wavelet energies in a fine band of levels even though a higher value of Ω proves an extensive band of levels (a random process).

Statistical test

To make comparisons across sex, within tasks, types of measurements and sides in a unified manner, we fitted a series of linear mixed models with each feature as the dependent variable; sex (male/female), task (geometric/verbal/resting), measurement type (raw/envelope), side (left/right) and their full multi-way interaction as independent factors; and a subject random effect to account for multiple measurements from each participants and the resulting non-independence of observations. Next, combining both sex, to make comparisons between the levels of each of the task, measurement type and side factors within the combinations of other factors, we fit a similar mixed model but only with task, measurement type, side and their interaction as independent factors. In each case, appropriately constructed means contrasts were used to estimate the pairwise means differences of interest reported here, along with their statistical significance and 95 % confidence intervals. For cross-correlation and synchronization index features which are not side specific, we employed a largely similar strategy but omitted side from the list of independent factors. SAS version 9.3 (SAS Institute, Inc., Cary, North Carolina) was used for the mixed model analysis. MATLAB (MathWorks, Natick, MA, United States) was used for feature extraction.

Results

Firstly, the effect of the end-tidal carbon dioxide level which does not influence features (ACA diameter) is not taken into consideration [73, 74], as we did not observe any relations between signal features and end-tidal carbon dioxide levels. Furthermore, participants did not exhibit any excessive head movements. Secondly, feature values for the raw and the envelope signals are displayed in tables in the form of ($mean \pm standarddeviation$) according to experimental conditions: the 45-seconds resting-state is indicated by a "R", the word-generating task is indicated by a "W" and the geometric task is indicated by a "G" in the

Table 6 Significant information-theoretic features from raw (denoted by the subscript r) and envelope (denoted by the subscript e) CBFV signals where $p < 0.05$

Signal	ACA	Feature	Group	Group 1	Group 2
e	R-ACA	LZC	R	M: 0.65 ± 0.04	F: 0.69 ± 0.04
e	L-ACA	LZC	R	M: 0.66 ± 0.03	F: 0.70 ± 0.04
e	R-ACA	LZC	W	M: 0.65 ± 0.04	F: 0.68 ± 0.03
e	L-ACA	LZC	W	M: 0.66 ± 0.04	F: 0.69 ± 0.04

Table 7 Frequency features from raw (denoted by the subscript r) and envelope (denoted by the subscript e) CBFV signals

	Spectral centroid		Peak frequency		Bandwidth	
	R-ACA	L-ACA	R-ACA	L-ACA	R-ACA	L-ACA
Rr	980 ± 193	939 ± 213	561 ± 308	564 ± 214	723 ± 116	564 ± 214
Wr	994 ± 184	950 ± 208	540 ± 239	584 ± 221	723 ± 116	696 ± 151
Gr	990 ± 192	939 ± 211	567 ± 269	527 ± 257	718 ± 120	690 ± 152
Re	13.3 ± 4.50	14.0 ± 4.30	0.36 ± 0.50	0.23 ± 0.46	13.5 ± 1.73	13.5 ± 1.43
We	13.5 ± 4.62	14.0 ± 4.30	0.38 ± 0.51	0.39 ± 0.55	13.5 ± 1.74	13.6 ± 1.47
Ge	13.5 ± 4.5	14.1 ± 4.36	0.45 ± 0.55	0.33 ± 0.51	13.5 ± 1.60	13.5 ± 1.37

tables. Using the calculated feature values, we examined the effects of lateralization, sex, handedness and tasks on the features. A, F, M, RH and LH denote "all participants", "female participants", "male participants", "right-handed participants" and "left-handed participants," respectively.

Time features

Table 3 presents time feature values for all participants in the raw and the envelope signals while Table 4 shows significant results in time domain concerning the handedness and sex effects in time domain.

No significant statistical difference was established for raw CBFV signals. On the opposite side, a few meaningful results were detected between sex on the envelope signals. Male subjects had higher skewness than female participants in R-ACA signals during resting-state ($p = 0.01$) and during verbal challenge ($p = 0.02$). A rise of skewness was noticed on the left ACA signals in the case of men during geometric task ($p = 0.02$). Additionally, larger kurtosis was observed for men on the R-ACA during the 45-seconds resting period ($p = 0.03$).

Information-theoretic features

A summary of information-theoretic feature values and statistical differences (handedness and sex effects) in information-theoretic approach are presented in Tables 5 and 6 for the raw and the envelope signals.

Multiple comparison test revealed significant results on LZC between sex on the envelope signals during resting periods and during word-generation challenges. Female had higher LZC in the R-ACA and the L-ACA signals during both periods ($p < 0.05$).

Frequency-domain features

Tables 7 and 8 present frequency feature values and significant results (handedness and sex effects) in the raw and the envelope signals.

Meaningful results were only noticed on sex in raw CBFV signals. The spectral centroid of raw R-ACA CBFV signals increased in the case of women during cognitive challenges and 45-seconds resting period ($p < 0.02$). Moreover, the bandwidth values of R-ACA was larger from female results during rest/verbal/geometric processes ($p < 0.05$).

Time-frequency features

Table 9, Fig. 3 and Fig. 4 present the wavelet entropy values and the feature values of wavelet energy decomposition for raw and the envelope signals. Table 10 shows significant results for both signals (handedness and sex effects).

The multiple comparison test revealed signal information in time-frequency domain. Sex had effects on R-ACA and L-ACA raw signals. The relative energy d_{10} of R-ACA outcomes increased in the case of women during resting state and during mental processes ($p < 0.02$), while decreasing in R-ACA and L-ACA d_7 in the case of women during rest periods and cognitive tasks ($p < 0.04$). For envelope results, cognitive challenges had some impact on R-ACA and L-ACA envelope signals in comparison with the baseline results, i.e. 45-seconds resting periods. A lower wavelet entropy was highlighted on both sides of ACA during cognitive processes ($p < 0.04$).

On the other hand, 94 % of energy were concentrated around the approximation band a_{10} for the envelope signals. Therefore, for these signals, we only considered the a_{10} level. Statistical differences in R-ACA and L-ACA a_{10} were noticed: the mental periods showed larger a_{10} than rest periods ($p < 0.02$).

Table 8 Significant frequency features from raw (denoted by the subscript r) and envelope (denoted by the subscript e) CBFV signals where $p < 0.05$

Signal	ACA	Feature	Group	Group 1	Group 2
r	R-ACA	Spectral Centroid	R	M: 855 ± 198	F: 1090 ± 225
r	R-ACA	Spectral Centroid	W	M: 913 ± 204	F: 1060 ± 181
r	R-ACA	Spectral Centroid	G	M: 896 ± 203	F: 1066 ± 192
r	R-ACA	Bandwidth	R	M: 641 ± 107	F: 734 ± 118
r	R-ACA	Bandwidth	W	M: 675 ± 137	F: 763 ± 139
r	R-ACA	Bandwidth	G	M: 665 ± 141	F: 760 ± 138

Table 9 Wavelet entropy values for raw and envelope CBFV signals

		RAW		ENVELOPE	
		R-ACA	L-ACA	R-ACA	L-ACA
Wavelet entropy	R	2.10 ± 0.23	2.12 ± 0.25	0.50 ± 0.19	0.47 ± 0.17
	W	2.07 ± 0.17	2.10 ± 0.22	0.39 ± 0.17	0.36 ± 0.16
	G	2.07 ± 0.19	2.12 ± 0.26	0.40 ± 0.18	0.35 ± 0.13

Comparison between raw and envelope signals

Results demonstrated differences between raw signals and envelope signals and showed low *p*-values except for results in Table 11.

Discussion

Raw and envelope signals were significantly different as demonstrated by the features describing their probability density functions. No effect of handedness was found on time domain features while the sex effects were exhibited on the R-ACA and L-ACA raw and envelope signals. Higher kurtosis proved that the CBFV variations are grouped around one value [75], while larger skewness highlighted higher signal assymetry [53]. R-ACA envelope signals from female participants seemed more dispersive and more symmetrical than from male subjects during the rest and verbal periods. Hence, the cerebral blood flow changed with a wider range in females than in males during resting-state and word-generation processes on the right side of ACA.

Time-domain outcomes did not reveal differences between signal characteristics during resting-state periods and during mental challenges. For example, the cross-correlation value was close to zero for raw signals implying low signal dependence in the time domain. Previous studies highlighted the dependence of signals between the two sides of MCA and the evolution of blood flow velocity during cognitive processes. Lateralization was introduced during the geometric task and the word-generation task. It was shown that there was a hemispheric lateralization due to an increase of the cerebral blood flow velocity during cognitive tasks [32, 33, 35]. The geometric task led to a dominance of R-MCA while the verbal task results in a dominance of L-MCA. Moreover, the cerebral blood flow in MCA is closely linked to the flow in ACA. Thus, an identical hemispheric dominance should be identified using results from ACA. Changes in the ACA blood flow and the possible lateralization observed in the flow can be explained by the changes in the MCA blood flow while performing cognitive processes. Nonetheless, time domain results from the current ACA study did not confirm cerebral lateralization during mental challenges.

Raw signals and envelope signals showed distinct cerebral blood flow characteristics which demonstrated the significance of extraction of envelope signals and preservation of raw signals from a statistical point of view. The envelope signals also had higher standard deviation and skewness than the raw signals. Raw signals centralized information around a value because of lower skewness and standard deviation. However, envelope signals exhibited higher cross-correlation values ($CC > 0.89$) than raw signals which proved that there was a low dependence on raw signals in the time domain.

When considering the information theoretic domain, sex effects were observed on randomness and complexity of the envelope signals. In fact, the Lempel-Ziv complexity exhibited differences between men and women. Right-sided and left-sided envelope signals from women were more complex than signals from men during resting-state period and word-generation processes. Rest periods and verbal tasks implied that the left and right ACA blood flow speed was distinguishable between men and women. Indeed, the envelope signals vary with higher fluctuations in the case of women.

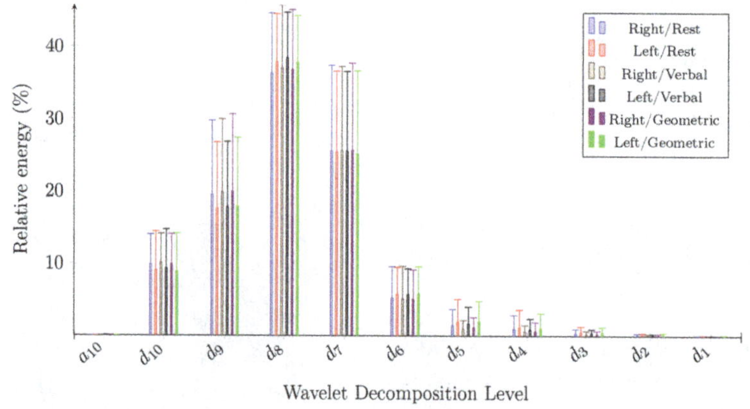

Fig. 3 The 10th level wavelet decomposition of raw signals

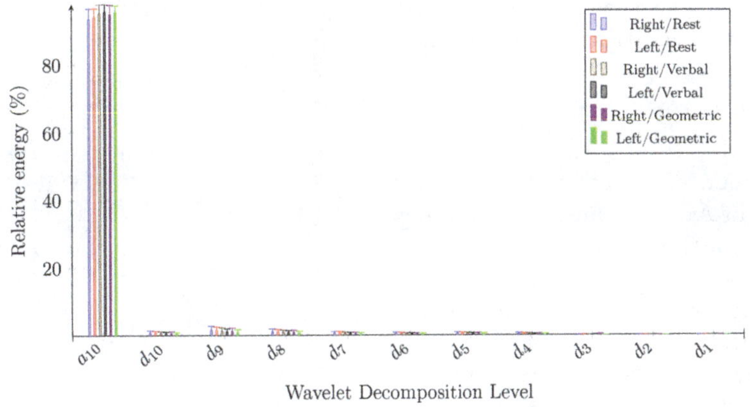

Fig. 4 The 10th level wavelet decomposition of envelope signals

In the frequency domain, raw signals exhibited higher frequency characteristics than envelope signals. As a matter of fact, envelope signals revealed a low-pass structure, while the raw signals presented a band-pass structure. When differentiating sex effects, spectral centroid frequencies and bandwidth of R-ACA raw signals from female participants had higher values than those from men during the geometric task. This finding implied an increase of right-sided blood flow above baseline was more pronounced for women than for men during geometric tasks. Sex differences during mental stimuli have been widely studied, particularly during spatial challenges. Previous publications underlined distinct hemispheric dominance seen in women and in men [40, 76, 77]. Women revealed activation of other right brain regions during geometric tasks [76]. It could be explained by two distinct strategies of task solving/the anatomical brain structure/sex hormones [78–81]. A rise of centroid frequency was also noticed during the resting-state and verbal tasks. It appeared that female subjects showed a higher right-sided CBFV baseline. These distinct baseline metabolisms may be caused by emotional brain responses (i.e. sex hormones) or by anatomical brain differences [79–82]. The frequency domain analysis did not indicate the existence of handedness-based difference.

From the time-frequency point of view, lower wavelet entropy values highlighted that right-sided and left-sided envelope signals were more ordered during cognitive periods than during 45-second resting-state periods. In addition, the rise of wavelet energy a_{10} proved that cognitive tasks led to modifications of CBFV signals comparing to resting state. Time-frequency outcomes did not expose major changes into brain functioning during mental tasks. We did not observe neither handedness nor sex effects on a_{10} values for R-ACA and L-ACA raw and envelope signals.

The uneven small number of subjects in each group may also be important limitation in the outcomes about the sex effects (i.e. 20 subjects) and handedness effects on brain response (i.e. 16 right-handed and 3 left-handed subjects). Therefore, the results obtained after analyzing comparisons between right and left-handed subjects and between male and female participants are not as pronounced. Given the low number of ambidextrous

Table 10 Significant time-frequency features from raw (denoted by the subscript r) and envelope (denoted by the subscript e) CBFV signals where $p < 0.05$

Signal	ACA	Feature	Group	Group 1	Group 2
r	R-ACA	$\Xi_{d_{10}}$	R	M: 6.92 ± 3.08	F: 11.4 ± 4.71
r	R-ACA	$\Xi_{d_{10}}$	W	M: 8.23 ± 4.05	F: 11.7 ± 3.25
r	R-ACA	$\Xi_{d_{10}}$	G	M: 7.90 ± 4.09	F: 11.7 ± 3.35
r	R-ACA	Ξ_{d_7}	R	M: 32.9 ± 12.0	F: 19.1 ± 8.02
r	L-ACA	Ξ_{d_7}	R	M: 30.3 ± 12.5	F: 21.2 ± 9.08
r	R-ACA	Ξ_{d_7}	W	M: 29.8 ± 12.2	F: 22.4 ± 9.73
r	L-ACA	Ξ_{d_7}	W	M: 29.7 ± 11.2	F: 22.1 ± 9.64
r	R-ACA	Ξ_{d_7}	G	M: 30.4 ± 12.7	F: 21.9 ± 9.97
r	L-ACA	Ξ_{d_7}	G	M: 29.5 ± 11.4	F: 21.8 ± 10.2

Table 11 Absence of statistical difference between raw and envelope CBFV signals where $p > 0.06$

Multiple	Rest periods		Verbal tasks		Geometric tasks	
	R-ACA	L-ACA	R-ACA	L-ACA	R-ACA	L-ACA
Kurtosis	A, F	A, M, F	F	A, M, F	A, M, F	A, M, F
LZC	F	A, M, F	F	A, M, F	A, M, F	A, M, F
Ξ_{d_5}	M, F	M	A, M, F	M	A, M, F	M
Ξ_{d_4}	A		A		A	
Ξ_{d_2}	M		M	M	M	
Ξ_{d_1}	A, M, F	A, M, F	A, M, F	A, M, F	A, M, F	M, F

participants (i.e. 1 ambidextrous subject), we examined the significant p-values between right and left-handed participants.

Conclusions

In this study, the evolution of the cerebral blood flow velocities in left and right ACA was investigated during three different tasks: a mental rotation task, a word generation task and resting periods between cognitive tasks. Characteristics of the raw signals and the envelope signals were analyzed in time, frequency, and time-frequency domains. Significant results have been obtained through the use of both classic/modern methods (i.e. envelope/raw, time and frequency/information-theoretic and time-frequency domains). The time and the information-theoretic results underlined modifications of shape distribution and randomness. The acquired data in the frequency domain presented a low-pass characteristic in the case of envelope signals while the raw signals presented band-pass characteristics. In the time-frequency analysis, the distribution of wavelet energies for the envelope signals was around the low frequencies during cognitive activities. Finally, differences were obtained for the raw and envelope signals based on sex effects. Distinct hemispheric functioning between men and women was highlighted during each process. A few significant statistical differences demonstrated the different brain response.

Competing interests

The authors declare that they have no competing interests.

Authors' contributions

ES conceived the experiment. HB collected and analyzed data. SP conducted the statistical analysis of the results. HB, SP and ES wrote the manuscript. All authors read and approved the final manuscript.

Acknowledgements

The work was supported by the Pittsburgh Older Americans Independence Center (NIA P30 AG024827).

Author details

[1] Department of Electrical and Computer Engineering, University of Pittsburgh, Pittsburgh, PA, USA. [2] Division of Geriatric Medicine, University of Pittsburgh, Pittsburgh, PA, USA.

References

1. Phelps ME. PET: a biological imaging technique. Neurochem Res. 1991;16(9):929–40.
2. Fiez JA. Neuroimaging studies of speech. An overview of techniques and methodological approaches. J Commun Disorders. 2001;34(6):445–54.
3. Khalil MM, Tremoleda JL, Bayomy TB, Gsell W. Molecular SPECT imaging: an overview. Int J Mol Imaging. 2011;2011(Article ID 796025):1–15.
4. Thomas DJ, Zilkha E, Redmond S, Du Boulay GH, Marshall J, Ross Russell RW, Symon L. An intravenous Xenon clearance technique for measuring cerebral blood flow. J Neurol Sci. 1979;40(1):53–63.
5. Aaslid A, Markwalder TM, Nornes H. Noninvasive transcranial Doppler ultrasound recording of flow velocity in basal cerebral arteries. J Neurosurg. 1982;57(6):769–74.
6. Deppe M, Ringelstein EB, Knecht S. The investigation of functional brain lateralization by transcranial Doppler sonography. Neuroimage. 2004;21(3):1124–46.
7. Fox PT, Raichle ME. Focal physiological uncoupling of cerebral blood flow and oxidative metabolism during somatosensory stimulation in human subjects. Proc Nat Acad Sci USA. 1986;83(4):1140–44.
8. Huber P, Handa J. Effect of contrast material, hypercapnia, hyperventilation, hypertonic glucose and papaverine on the diameter of the cerebral arteries. Angiographic determination in man. Invest Radiol. 1967;2(1):17–32.
9. Giller CA, Bowman G, Dyer H, Mootz L, Krippner W. Cerebral arterial diameters during changes in blood pressure and carbone dioxide during craniotomy. Neurosurgery. 1993;32(5):737–42.
10. Kontos HA. Validity of cerebral arterial blood flow calculations from velocity measurements. Stroke. 1989;20(1):1–3.
11. Saqqur M, Uchino K, Demchuk AM, Molina CA, Garami Z, Calleja S, Akhtar N, Orouk FO, Salam A, Shuaib A, Alexandrov AV. Site of arterial occlusion identified by transcranial Doppler predicts the response to intravenous thrombolysis for stroke. Stroke. 2007;38(3):948–54.
12. Burgin WS, Malkoff M, Felberg RA, Demchuk AM, Christou I, Grotta JC, Alexandrov AV. Transcranial Doppler ultrasound criteria for recanalization after thrombolysis for middle cerebral artery stroke. Stroke. 2000;31(5): 1128–32.
13. Knake S, Haag A, Hamer HM, Dittmer C, Bien S, Oertel WH, Rosenow F. Language lateralization in patients with temporal lobe epilepsy: a comparison of functional transcranial Doppler sonography and the Wada test. NeuroImage. 2003;19(3):1228–32.
14. Juhász C, Scheidl E, Szirmai I. Reversible focal mri abnormalities due to status epilepticus. an eeg, single photon emission computed tomography, transcranial doppler follow-up study. Electroencephalogr Clin Neurophysiol. 1998;107(6):402–7.
15. Whitehouse A, Bishop D. Cerebral dominance for language function in adults with specific language impairment or autism. Brain. 2008;131(12): 3193–200.
16. Aaslid R. The Doppler Principle Applied to Measurement of Blood Velocities in Cerebral Arteries. Vienna: Springer; 1986.
17. Conrad B, Klingelhöfer J. Dynamics of regional cerebral blood flow for various visual stimuli. Exp Brain Res. 1989;77(2):437–41.
18. Vollmer-Haase J, Finke K, Hartje W, Bulla-Hellwig M. Hemispheric dominance in the processing of J.S, Bach fugues: a transcranial Doppler sonography (TCD) study with musicians. Neuropsychologia. 1998;36(9): 857–67.
19. Evers S, Dannert J, Rödding D, Rötter G, Ringelstein EB. The cerebral haemodynamics of music perception. A transcranial Doppler sonography study. Brain. 1999;122(1):75–85.
20. Markus HS, Boland M. "Cognitive Activity" monitored by non-invasive measurement of cerebral blood flow velocity and its application to the investigation of cerebral dominance. Cortex. 1992;28(4):575–81.
21. Stroobant N, Buijs D, Vingerhoets G. Variation in brain lateralization during various language tasks: a functional transcranial Doppler study. Behav Brain Res. 2009;199(2):190–6.
22. Kelley RE, Chang JY, Suzuki S, Levin BE, Reyes-Iglesias Y. Selective increase in the right hemisphere transcranial Doppler velocity during a spatial task. Cortex. 1993;29(1):45–52.
23. Schnittger C, Johannes S, Münte TF. Transcranial Doppler assessment of cerebral blood flow velocity during visual spatial selective attention humans. Neurosci Lett. 1996;214(1):41–4.
24. Cupini LM, Matteis M, Troisi E, Sabbadini M, Bernardi G, Caltagirone C, Silvestrini M. Bilateral simultaneous transcranial Doppler monitoring of flow velocity changes during visuospatial and verbal working memory tasks. Brain. 1996;119(4):1249–53.
25. Silvestrini M, Caltagirone C, Cupini LM, Matteis M, Troisi E, Bernardi G. Activation of healthy hemisphere in poststroke recovery. A transcranial Doppler study. Stroke. 1993;24(11):1673–7.
26. Trabold F, Meyer S, Blanot PG, Carli GA, Orliaguet PA. The prognostic value of transcranial Doppler studies in children with moderate and severe head injury. Intensive Care Med. 2004;30(1):108–12.
27. Schmidt P, Krings T, Willmes K, Roessler F, Reul J, Thron A. Determination of cognitive hemispheric lateralization by "functional" Transcranial Doppler cross-validated by functional MRI. Stroke. 1999;30(5):939–45.
28. Reid JM, Spencer MP. Ultrasonic Doppler technique for imaging blood vessels. Science. 1972;176(4040):1235–6.

29. White H, Venkatesh B. Applications of transcranial Doppler in the ICU: a review. Intensive Care Med. 2006;32(7):981–4.
30. Alexandrov AV, Sloan MA, Wong LKS, Douville C, Razumovsky AY, Koroshetz M, Kaps WJ, Tegeler CH. Practice standards for transcranial Doppler ultrasound: part i– test performance. J Neuroimaging. 2007;17(1): 11–8.
31. Duschek S, Schandry R. Functional transcranial Doppler sonography as a tool in psychophysiological research. Psychophysiology. 2003;40(3): 436–54.
32. Droste DW, Harders AG, Rastogi E. A transcranial Doppler study of blood flow velocity in the middle cerebral arteries performed at rest and during mental activities. Stroke. 1989;20(8):1005–11.
33. Hartje W, Ringelstein EB, Kistinger B, Fabianek D, Willmes K. Transcranial Doppler ultrasonic assessment of middle cerebral artery blood flow velocity changes during verbal and visuospatial cognitive tasks. Neuropsychologia. 1994;32(12):1443–52.
34. Matteis M, Bivona U, Catani S, Pasqualetti P, Formisano R, Vernieri F, Troisi E. Functional transcranial Doppler assessment of cerebral blood flow velocities changes during attention tasks. Eur J Neurol. 2009;16(1):81–7.
35. Vingerhoets G, Stroobant N. Lateralization of cerebral blood flow velocity changes during cognitive task: a simultaneous bilateral transcranial Doppler study. Stroke. 1999;30(10):2152–158.
36. Kelley RE, Chang JY, Scheinman NJ, Levin BE, Duncan RC, Lee SC. Transcranial Doppler assessment of cerebral flow velocity during cognitive tasks. Stroke. 1992;23(1):9–14.
37. Vingerhoets G, Stroobant N. Reliability and validity of day-to-day blood flow velocity reactivity in a single subject: an fTCD study. Ultrasound Med Biol. 2002;2(28):197–202.
38. DeWitt LD, Wechsler LR. Transcranial Doppler. Stroke. 1988;19(7):915–21.
39. Lennihan L, Petty GW, Fink ME, Solomon RA, Mohr JP. Transcranial Doppler detection of anterior cerebral artery vasospasm. J Neurol Neurosurg Psychiat. 1993;56(8):906–9.
40. Gur R, Gur R, Obrist W, Hungerbuhler J, Younkin D, Rosen A, Skolnick B, Reivich M. Sex and handedness differences in cerebral blood flow during rest and cognitive activity. Science. 1982;217(4560):659–61.
41. Deppe M, Knecht S, Henningsen H, Ringelstein EB. Average: a Windows ®program for automated analysis of event related cerebral blood flow. J Neurosci Methods. 1997;75(2):147–54.
42. Wechsler LR, Ropper AH, Kistler JP. Transcranial Doppler in cerebrovascular disease. Stroke. 1986;17(5):905–12.
43. Huang H, Sejdić E. Assessment of resting-state blood flow through anterior cerebral arteries using transcranial Doppler recordings. Ultrasound Med Biol. 2013;39(12):2285–94.
44. Sejdić E, Kalika D, Czarnek N. An analysis of resting-state functional transcranial Doppler recordings from middle cerebral arteries. PloS ONE. 2013;8(2):55405.
45. Li M, Huang H, Boninger M, Sejdić E. An analysis of cerebral blood flow from middle cerebral arteries during cognitive tasks via functional transcranial Doppler recordings. Neurosci Res. 2014;84:19–26.
46. Oldfield RC. The assessment and analysis of handedness: The edinburgh inventory. Neuropsychologia. 1971;9(1):97–113.
47. Dragovic M. Categorization and validation of handedness using latent class analysis. Acta Neuropsychiatrica. 2004;16(4):212–8.
48. Dassonville P, Zhu X, Ugurbil K, Kim S, Ashe J. Functional activation in motor cortex reflects the direction and the degree of handedness. Proc Nat Acad Sci USA. 1997;94(25):14015–8.
49. Stroobant N, Vingerhoets G. Transcranial Doppler ultrasonography monitoring of cerebral hemodynamics during performance of cognitive tasks: a review. Neuropsychol Rev. 2000;10(4):213–31.
50. Hartje W, Ringelstein EB, Kistinger B, Fabianek D, Willmes K. Transcranial Doppler ultrasonic assessment of middle cerebral artery blood flow velocity changes during verbal and visuospatial cognitive tasks. Neuropsychologia. 1994;32(12):1443–52.
51. Peters M, Battista C. Applications of mental rotation figures of the Shepard and Metzler type and description of a mental rotation stimulus library. Brain Cogn. 2008;66(3):260–4.
52. Silvestrini M, Cupini L, Matteis M, Troisi E, Caltagirone C. Bilateral simultaneous assessment of cerebral flow velocity during mental activity. J Cereb Blood Flow Metab. 1994;14(4):643–8.
53. Papoulis A. Probability, Random Variables, and Stochastic Processes. New York: WCB/McGraw-Hill; 1991.
54. Zoubir AM, Boashash B. The bootstrap and its application in signal processing. IEEE Signal Process Mag. 1998;15(1):56–76.
55. Allen J, Coan J, Nazarian M. Issues and assumptions on the road from raw signals to metrics of frontal EEG assymetry in emotion. Biol Psychol. 2004;67(1–2):183–218.
56. Aboy M, Hornero R, Abàsolo D, Àlvarez D. Interpretation of the Lempel-Ziv Complexity measure in the context of biomedical signal Analysis. IEEE Trans Biomed Eng. 2006;53(11):2282–8.
57. Szczepański J, Amigò J, Wajnryb E, Sanchez-Vives. Characterizing spike trains with Lempel-Ziv Complexity. Neurocomputing. 2004;58–60:79–84.
58. Ahmed S, Shahjahan M, Murase K. A Lempel-Ziv Complexity-based neural network pruning algorithm. Int J Neural Syst. 2011;21(5):427–41.
59. Nagarajan R. Quantifying physiological data with Lempel-Ziv quantifying physiological data with Lempel-Ziv Complexity–Certain issues. IEEE Trans Biomed Eng. 2002;49(11):1371–3.
60. Hu J, Gao J, Principe J. Analysis of biomedical signals by the Lempel-Ziv Complexity: the effect of finite data size. IEEE Trans Biomed Eng. 2006;53(12):2606–9.
61. Lempel A, Ziv J. On the complexity of finite sequences. IEEE Trans Inform Theory. 1976;22(1):75–81.
62. Amigò J, Szczepański J, Wajnryb E, Sanchez-Vives M. Estimating the entropy rate of spike trains via Lempel-Ziv Complexity. Neural Comput. 2004;16(4):717–36.
63. Porta A, Guzzetti S, Montano N, Furlan R, Pagani M, Somers V. Entropy, entropy rate, and pattern classification as tools to typify complexity in short heart period variability series. IEEE Trans Inform Theory. 2011;48(11): 1282–91.
64. Bezerianos A, Tong S, Thakor N. Time-dependent entropy estimation of EEG rhythm changes following brain ischemia. Ann Biomed Eng. 2003;31(2):221–32.
65. Porta A, Baselli G, Lombardi F, Montano N, Malliani A, Cerutti S. Conditional entropy approach for the evaluation of the coupling strength. Biol Cybernet. 1999;81(2):119–29.
66. Porta A, Baselli G, Liberati D, Montano N, Cogliati C, Gnecchi-Ruscone T, Malliani A, Cerutti S. Measuring regularity by means of a corrected conditional entropy in sympathetic outflow. Biol Cybernet. 1998;78(1): 71–8.
67. Sejdić E, Djurović I, Jiang J. Time-frequency feature representation using energy concentration: an overview of recent advances. Digital Signal Process. 2009;19(1):153–83.
68. Lee J, Sejdić E, Steele CM, Chau T. Effects of liquid stimuli on dual-axis swallowing accelerometer signals in a healthy population. Biomed Eng Online. 2010;9(1):7.
69. Tzanetakis G, Cook P. Musical genre classification of audio signals. IEEE Trans Speech Audio Process. 2002;10(5):293–302.
70. Hilton M. Wavelet and wavelet packet compression of electrocardiograms. IEEE Trans Biomed Eng. 1997;44(5):394–402.
71. Rosso OA, Blanco S, Yordanova J, Kolev V, Figliola A, Schürmann M, Basar E. Wavelet entropy: a new tool for analysis of short duration brain electrical signals. J Neurosci Methods. 2001;105(1):65–75.
72. Robertson D, Camps O, Mayer J, Gish W. Wavelet and electromagnetic power system transients. IEEE Trans Power Delivery. 1996;11(2):1050–8.
73. Jordan J, Shannon JR, Diedrich A, Black B, Costa F, Robertson D, Biaggioni I. Interaction of carbon dioxide and sympathetic nervous system activity in the regulation of cerebral perfusion in humans. Hypertension. 2000;36(3):383–8.
74. Serrador J, Picot P, Rutt B, Shoemaker J, Bondar R. MRI measures of middle cerebral artery diameter in conscious humans during simulated orthostasis. Stroke. 2000;31(7):1672–8.
75. DeCarlo L. On the meaning and use of kurtosis. Psychol Methods. 1997;2(3):292–307.
76. Weiss E, Siedentopf C, Hofer A, Deisenhammer E, Hoptman M, Kremser C, Golaszewski S, Felber S, Fleischhacker W, Delazer M. Sex differences in brain activation pattern during a visuospatial cognitive task: a functional magnetic resonance imaging study in healthy volunteers. Neurosci Lett. 2003;344(3):169–72.
77. Gur R, Alsop D, Glahn D, Petty R, Swanson C, Maldjian J, Turetsky B, Detre J, Gee J, Gur R. An fMRI study of sex differences in regional activation to a verbal and a spatial task. Brain Lang. 2000;74(2):157–70.
78. Thomsen T, Hugdahl K, Ersland L, Barndon R, Lundervold A, Smievoll A, Roscher B, Sundberg H. Functional magnetic resonance imaging (fMRI)

study of sex differences in a mental rotation task. Med Sci Monitor. 2000;6(6):1186–96.
79. Marinoni M, Ginanneschi A, Inzitari D, Mugnai S, Amaducci L. Sex-related differences in human cerebral hemodynamics. Acta Neurologica Scandinavica. 1998;97(5):324–7.
80. Good C, Johnsrude I, Johnsrude J, Henson R, Friston K, Frackowiak S. Cerebral asymmetry and the effects of sex and handedness on brain structure: a voxel-based morphometric analysis od 465 normal adult human brains. NeuroImage. 2001;14(3):685–700.
81. Cosgrove K, Mazure C, Staley J. Evolving knowledge of sex differences in brain structure, function and chemistry. Biol Psychiat. 2007;62(8):847–55.
82. Gur R, Gur R, Mozley P, Mozley L, Resnick S, Karp J, Alavi A, Arnold S. Sex differences in regional cerebral glucose metabolism during a resting-state. Science. 1995;267(5197):528–31.

15

Imaging of thyroid tumor angiogenesis with microbubbles targeted to vascular endothelial growth factor receptor type 2 in mice

Marcello Mancini[1,2*], Adelaide Greco[3,5], Giuliana Salvatore[4], Raffaele Liuzzi[1], Gennaro Di Maro[6], Emilia Vergara[3], Gennaro Chiappetta[7], Rosa Pasquinelli[7], Arturo Brunetti[3,5] and Marco Salvatore[3]

Abstract

Background: To evaluate whether Contrast Enhanced Ultrasund (CEUS) with microbubbles (MBs) targeted to VEGFR-2 is able to characterize *in vivo* the VEGFR-2 expression in the tumor vasculature of a mouse model of thyroid cancer (Tg-TRK-T1).

Methods: Animal protocol was approved by Institutional committee on Laboratory Animal Care. Contrast-enhanced ultrasound imaging with MBs targeted with an anti-VEGFR-2 monoclonal antibody ($UCA_{VEGFR-2}$) and isotype control antibody (UCA_{IgG}) was performed in 7 mice with thyroid carcinoma, 5 mice with hyperplasia or benign thyroid nodules and 4 mice with normal thyroid. After ultrasonography, the tumor samples were harvested for histological examination and VEGFR-2 expression was tested by immunohistochemistry. Data were reported as median and range. Paired non parametric Wilcoxon's test and ANOVA of Kruskal-Wallis were used. The correlation between the contrast signal and the VEGFR-2 expression was assessed by the Spearman coefficient.

Results: The Video intensity difference (VI_D) caused by backscatter of the retained $UCA_{VEGFR-2}$ was significantly higher in mice harboring thyroid tumors compared to mice with normal thyroids ($P < 0.01$) and to mice harboring benign nodules ($P < 0.01$). No statistically significant differences of VI_D were observed in the group of mice carrying benign nodules compared to mice with normal thyroids. Moreover in thyroid tumors VI_D of retained VEGFR-2-targeted UCA was significantly higher than that of control UCA_{IgG} ($P < 0.05$). Results of immunohistochemical analysis confirmed VEGFR-2 overexpression. The magnitude of the molecular ultrasonographic signal from a VEGFR-2-targeted UCA retained by tissue correlates with VEGFR-2 expression determined by immunohistochemistry (*rho* 0.793, $P=0.0003$).

Conclusions: We demonstrated that CEUS with $UCA_{VEGFR-2}$ might be used for *in vivo* non invasive detection and quantification of VEGFR-2 expression in thyroid cancer in mice, and to differentiate benign from malignant thyroid nodules.

Keywords: Thyroid, Transgenic, High resolution ultrasound, Cancer, Contrast agent

Background

Angiogenesis is a critical determinant of tumor growth and invasion [1,2] and successful application of novel therapies that target tumor vasculature will require selection of susceptible tumors and precise evaluation of early treatment response. Vascular endothelial growth factor and its main receptor vascular endothelial growth factor receptor 2 (VEGFR-2), are overexpressed on tumor vascular endothelial cells and have been identified as targets for antiangiogenic drugs [3-10].

Papillary thyroid carcinoma (PTC) is the most common malignancy of the thyroid gland. At the molecular level PTC is characterized by genetic alterations of components of the mitogen-activated protein kinase (MAPK) pathway [11]. These include structural chromosome rearrangements affecting NTRK1 (TRK-T1) tyrosine kinase receptor that undergo in-frame recombination with various partner

* Correspondence: marcello.mancini58@gmail.com
[1]Institute of Biostructure and Bioimaging, Italian National Research Council (CNR), Naples, Italy
[2]SDN Foundation IRCCS, Naples, Italy
Full list of author information is available at the end of the article

genes [12]. Specifically, the TRK-T1 oncogene results from a paracentric inversion of chromosome 1q25 that fuses the 5′ end of the TPR (Translocated Promoter Region) to the 3′ end of NTRK1 genes generating the constitutively active and oncogenic kinase NTRK1 [12]. Transgenic mice featuring the thyroid-specific expression of TRK-T1 under the transcriptional control of the thyroid-specific bovine thyroglobulin (Tg) promoter were generated previously [13]. Twenty-three% of TRK-T1 mice of age ≤ 7 months and 78% of mice > 7 months developed thyroid nodules characterized by malignant features, such as the proliferation of follicular epithelial cells containing scant cytoplasm, mitotic figures and papillae with fibrovascular stalks [13,14].

In papillary thyroid carcinoma, increased VEGFR-2 expression correlates with an increased cancer cell proliferation assessed by Ki-67 index, with increased thyroid tumor size [15,16] and with poor prognosis [16-19]. The thyroid cancer cells of primary tumors taken from patients with metastases had an higher VEGFR-2 expression compared to cells taken from primary tumors of patients without metastases [15,16]. These observations have been suggested to be clinically useful in identifying patients who are more prone to develop metastases.

Recently, tumor angiogenesis imaging *in vivo* has been noninvasively explored using contrast enhanced ultrasound (CEUS) with microbubbles (MBs) targeted to $\alpha_v\beta_3$ integrin, endoglin, and VEGFR2 [20-24]. This technique is rapidly emerging as a noninvasive and quantitative molecular imaging modality that combines the advantages of high spatial resolution, real-time imaging, and lack of ionizing radiation and may be particularly advantageous in clinical oncology because VEGFR-2 has been implicated as marker of metastatic potential and poor prognosis in certain tumors [25-27].

Microbubbles are gas-filled echogenic US contrast agents that can be targeted to specific molecular markers by means of the attachment of appropriate ligands to the surface of the MBs. A specific characteristic of MBs is their relatively large size, which prevents them from leaking into the extravascular space. This property can be exploited for imaging by targeting the MBs to disease processes reflected on the vascular endothelial cells lining the luminal surface of capillaries and vessels, such as inflammation and angiogenesis. When these functionalized MBs are injected intravenously, they distribute throughout the whole body and attach at tissue sites expressing the targeted molecular marker, leading to a local increase of the US imaging signal. This approach allows the exclusive visualization of molecular markers of angiogenesis expressed on tumor vascular endothelial cells, have a potential clinical translation in future and should improve the ability to detect, diagnose stage, select appropriate treatments, and determine prognosis in patients with thyroid pathologies.

To our knowledge, no study has addressed the potential of targeted CEUS imaging for assessment of thyroid tumor angiogenesis *in vivo* by using MBs targeted to VEGFR-2.

This study aimed to investigate whether targeted CEUS allows noninvasive assessment of VEGFR-2 expression on tumor vascular endothelium in Tg-TRK-T1 mice, a murine model of thyroid cancer. We also investigated whether the evaluation of expression levels of VEGFR2 *in vivo* can differentiate benign from malignant nodules of the thyroid.

Methods

Animal model

Animal studies were performed in accordance with National Institutes of Health (NIH) recommendations and Animal Research Advisory Committee (ARAC) procedure [27] and the approval of the Italian Institutional animal research committee (Institutional Animal and Care Committee of the University of Naples "Federico II" and the Italian Ministry of Health). All animal procedures in this study were conducted by a veterinarian and conformed to all regulations protecting animals used for research purposes, including national guidelines [D.L. 27 Gennaio 1992, 116 Suppl. G.U 40 18 Febbraio 1992. Direttiva CEE n.609/86] as well as the protocols recommended by Workamn et al. [28].

Tg-TRK-T1 transgenic mice have been previously described [13]. From 2010 to 2011, thyroid Ultrasound was performed in 16 Tg-TRK-T1 transgenic mice model of thyroid carcinogenesis [26]. Body weight range of animals was 29–32 gr, equally distributed among male (n=9) and female (n=7). Mice were examined every six months and were sacrificed immediately after the last ultrasound scanning. At the time of the necroscopy, the age range of mice was 12–15 months.

High frequency ultrasound with targeted contrast enhanced imaging

A Vevo 770 microimaging system (Visualsonics, Toronto, Ontario, Canada) with a single element probe, center frequency of 40-MHz was used for all the examinations. The transducer has an active face of 3 mm, a lateral resolution of 68.2 μm, axial resolution of 38.5 μm, focal length of 6 mm, mechanical index 0.14, transmit power 50%, and a dynamic range 52 dB [29,30]. Precise and repeatable control over the position of the two-dimensional image plane was obtained with a rail system (Vevo Integrated Rail System II; Visualsonics). Mice were anesthetized using 1.5–2% isoflurane vaporized in oxygen (2Lt/min) on a heated stage, with constant monitoring of their body temperature, using physiological monitoring platform [31].

Hairs were removed from the area of interest (neck and the high thorax) with a depilatory cream to obtain a direct contact of the ultrasound gel to the skin of the animal minimizing ultrasound attenuation. A prewarmed gel was used to provide a coupling medium for the transducer. Real-time imaging was performed as previously described [32]. The transducer focal zone was placed at the center of the thyroid gland and nodules, when they were present. All nodules were measured in three planes, and images were recorded to document nodule location and orientation. Each examination lasted for about 30 min. All ultrasonographic assessments were performed by the same trained sonographer (A.G.) that was not aware of the tumor type and of type of MBs administered to mice.

Contrast-enhanced agent preparation and injection

The Ultrasound Contrast Agent (UCA) MicroMarker (VisualSonics, Inc, Toronto, Ontario, Canada), specifically designed for high frequency ultrasonography, was prepared and targeted according to manufacturer guidelines. These MBs have a mean diameter of 1.5 μm (range, 1–2 μm) and contain approximately 7600 molecules of streptavidin per square micrometer chemically attached to the phospholipid shell of the MBs via a polyethylene glycol spacer [22]. The contrast agent preparation protocol was designed to achieve optimal saturation of the microbubble surface with a maximal amount of antibodies while minimizing the amount of free non conjugated antibodies in the solution. A vial of the dry UCA containing 9.2×10^8 dry streptavidin-coated MBs was re-suspended in 1.2 mL of sterile saline. Then, either 30 μg of biotinylated anti-mouse VEGFR-2 antibodies (clone Avas12a1; eBioscience, San Diego,) or a biotinylated immunoglobulin G (IgG) isotype control (eBioscience, Inc, San Diego, CA) were added per vial of contrast agent to produce either a VEGFR-2-targeted ($UCA_{VEGFR-2}$) and a control UCA (UCA_{IgG}) by using biotin-streptavidin interactions, resulting in approximately 6000 ligands per square micrometer of surface area [22]. All mice were injected with two boluses of both the $UCA_{VEGFR-2}$ and UCA_{IgG} via a tail vein (injection time, 2 seconds). Each bolus containing 3.8×10^7 MBs in 0.02 mL of saline and was followed by a 0.02 mL saline flush.

To allow MBs to clear from previous injections, we waited at least 30 minutes between different bolus injections. The sequence of injections was always the same in all animals examined. The total amount injected was 80 μl.

Image acquisition and quantification

The system was set at 50% transmit power, resulting in a mechanical index of 0.14 (manufacturer specification). Images were acquired at a 20-Hz frame rate. The data were log compressed and digitized to 12 bits. Data were further compressed to 8 bits for screen display. The ultrasound probe was positioned so that the central portion of the thyroid nodule was contained within the focal zone of the ultrasound transducer. The probe position, gain settings, and midfield focus were initially optimized and maintained throughout each experiment. The goal of the ultrasonographic image acquisition and analysis protocol (Figure 1) was to differentiate the backscattered acoustic signal due to MBs retained by the tumor from the background signal of the tumor itself and MBs still freely circulating in the bloodstream. CEUS imaging was paused for 4 minutes after injection. This time allowed binding and retention of targeted MBs while awaiting wash-out of the unbound contrast agent.

After the 4-minute waiting period, approximately 300 ultrasonographic frames of the tumor were acquired at a temporal resolution of 10 seconds. A high-power ultrasound destruction sequence was then applied (20 cycles with a frequency of 10 MHz and a mechanical index of 0.59). After the destruction pulse, the system was reset with identical imaging parameters as before the destruction event, and another set of images (≈300 frames) was acquired. Image processing and quantification were performed with the software implemented in the ultrasound scanner. Image processing used in the Vevo770 system relies on 2 sets of images: a predestruction set and a postdestruction data set. The received log compressed signals were expressed in an arbitrary scale unit called Video Intensity (VI). The average VI of predestruction and postdestruction (background) sonograms was measured in a region of interest encompassing the centre of examined tumor. The difference in VI between predestruction and postdestruction ultrasonographic frames was calculated and expressed as VI difference (VI_D) that provided a relative measure of the amount of the UCA retained by the tumor and was considered to represent MBs adherent to molecular endothelial markers.

Histology and immunohistochemistry

After CEUS imaging, mice were euthanized, the thyroids were excised and immediately fixed in buffered formalin for 4 h. Tissues underwent automated processing and paraffin embedding; 5 μm sections were cut and hematoxylin and eosin stained for microscopic analysis. Thyroid tissues were classified according to the World Health Organization criteria for the evaluation of mouse thyroid tumors [33]. Briefly, thyroid was considered as normal when composed by variable-sized follicles covered by flattened monolayered epithelial cells. Hyperplastic thyroid was defined by the occurrence of small follicles with scant colloid and tall epithelial cells merging with normal areas. Follicular adenoma was defined as a well demarcated nodule with a distinct papillary and/or follicular architecture. Malignant

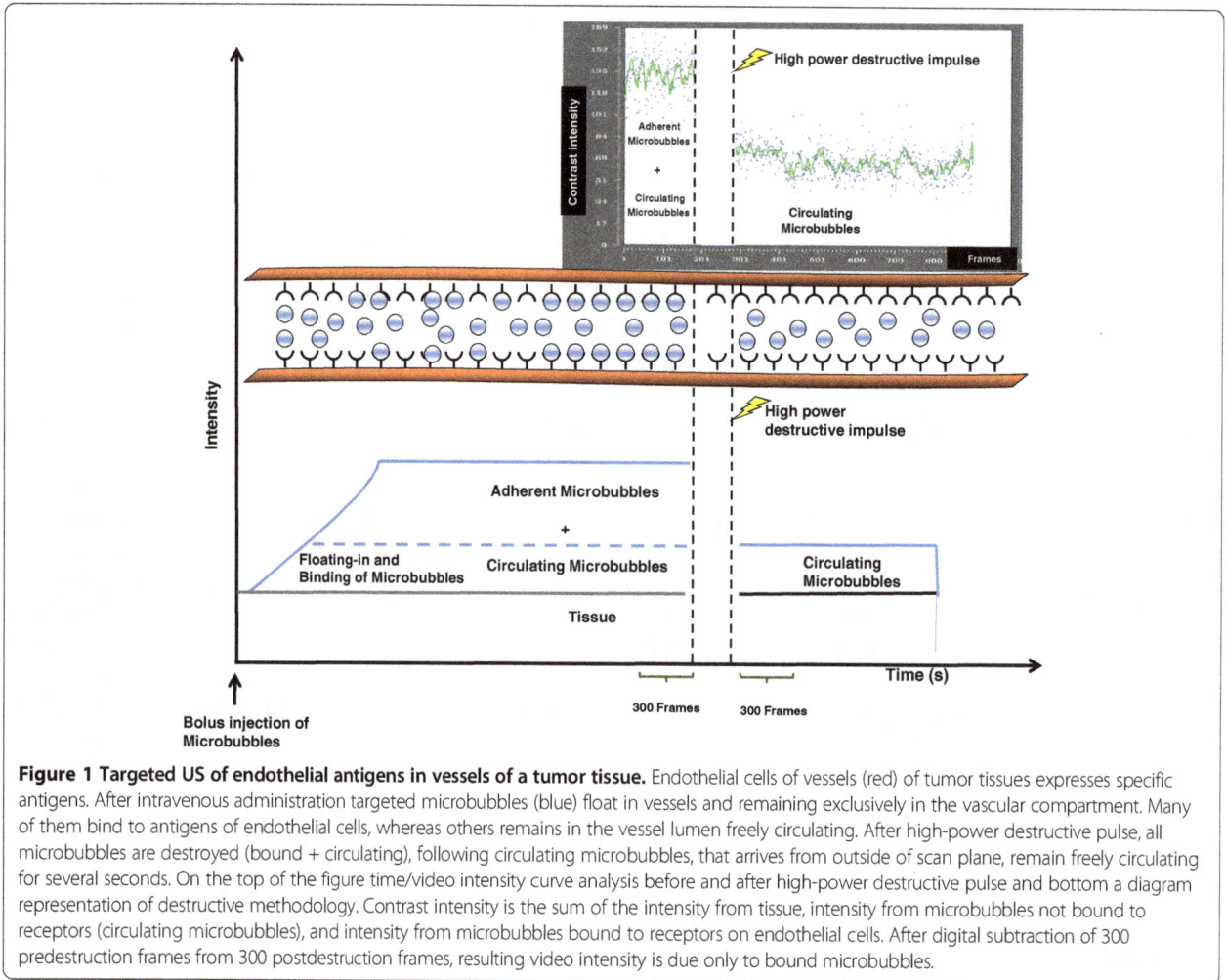

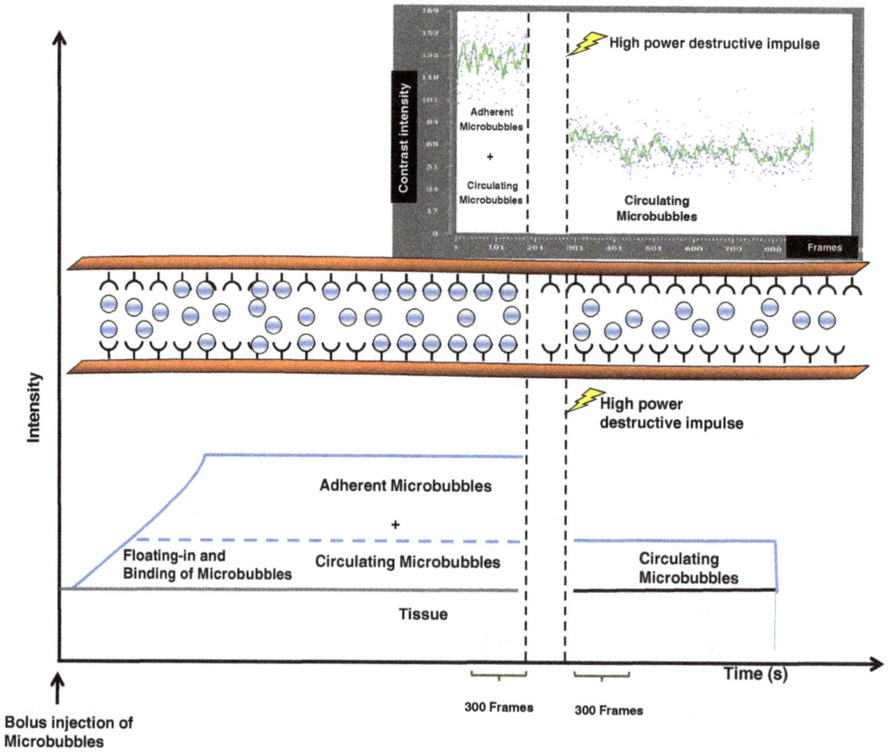

Figure 1 Targeted US of endothelial antigens in vessels of a tumor tissue. Endothelial cells of vessels (red) of tumor tissues expresses specific antigens. After intravenous administration targeted microbubbles (blue) float in vessels and remaining exclusively in the vascular compartment. Many of them bind to antigens of endothelial cells, whereas others remains in the vessel lumen freely circulating. After high-power destructive pulse, all microbubbles are destroyed (bound + circulating), following circulating microbubbles, that arrives from outside of scan plane, remain freely circulating for several seconds. On the top of the figure time/video intensity curve analysis before and after high-power destructive pulse and bottom a diagram representation of destructive methodology. Contrast intensity is the sum of the intensity from tissue, intensity from microbubbles not bound to receptors (circulating microbubbles), and intensity from microbubbles bound to receptors on endothelial cells. After digital subtraction of 300 predestruction frames from 300 postdestruction frames, resulting video intensity is due only to bound microbubbles.

lesions were defined based on the invasion of the surrounding glandular parenchyma and stroma.

To confirm expression of VEGFR-2, immunohistochemistry analysis of tumor sections was performed. Formalin-fixed and paraffin-embedded 3–5 μm sections were deparaffinized, placed in a solution of absolute methanol and 0.3% hydrogen peroxide for 30 min, and treated with blocking serum for 20 min. After blocking, slides were incubated with a mouse monoclonal anti-VEGFR-2 antibody (dilution 1:200) in a moist chamber at 4°C and processed according to standard procedures. Negative controls by omitting the primary antibody were included. Cases were scored as positive when unequivocal brown staining was observed. Immunoreactivity was expressed as the average percentage of positively stained target cells [(–): no staining (< 5% positive cells); (+): low/weak (≥ 5% - ≤ 25% positive cells); (++): medium/moderate (> 25% - < 50% positive cells); (+++): high/strong (≥ 50% positive cells)]. Score values were independently assigned by two blinded investigators (G.C. and R.P.) and a consensus was reached on all scores used for computation. All histological and immunohistochemistry studies were performed and interpreted by pathologists, who did not know the diagnosis determined by ultrasonography.

Statistical analysis

Data were reported as median and range. Paired non parametric Wilcoxon's test was used to compare data from different VI_D (UCA_{IGg} $UCA_{VEGFR-2}$). ANOVA of Kruskal-Wallis was used to compare the contrast measurements of the three groups. *Post hoc* analysis was performed using the Dunn test. The correlation between the contrast signal and the VEGFR-2 expression was assessed by the Spearman coefficient.

A $P < 0.05$ was considered statistically significant. All statistical analysis were performed with MedCalc 12.0 statistical software.

Results and discussion

Examination of the thyroid gland was performed by CEUS with $UCA_{VEGFR-2}$ and UCA_{IgG}. The UCA administration

Table 1 Quantitative video intensity for ultrasound contrast agent targeted with isotype control antibody (UCA_{IGg}) and anti-VEGFR2 monoclonal antibody (UCA_{VEGFR2})

	Normal thyroid (n.4)	Hyperplasia/Benign nodules (n.5)	Thyroid carcinoma (n.7)
Video intensity UCA_{IGg}			
Video intensity difference	11.3 (9.4-14.7)	12.2 (8.5-19.6)	19.4 (11.4-22.6)
Video intensity UCA_{VEGFR2}			
Video intensity difference	10.9 (10.3-14.9)	13.3 (10.8-15.8)	30.1 (25.1-35.6)* §

* Statistical significant difference between Thyroid carcinoma and normal thyroid or Hyperplasia/benign nodules $p<0.05$.

§ Statistical significant difference between UCA targeted with anti-VEGFR2 monoclonal antibody and isotype control antibody $p=0.0156$.

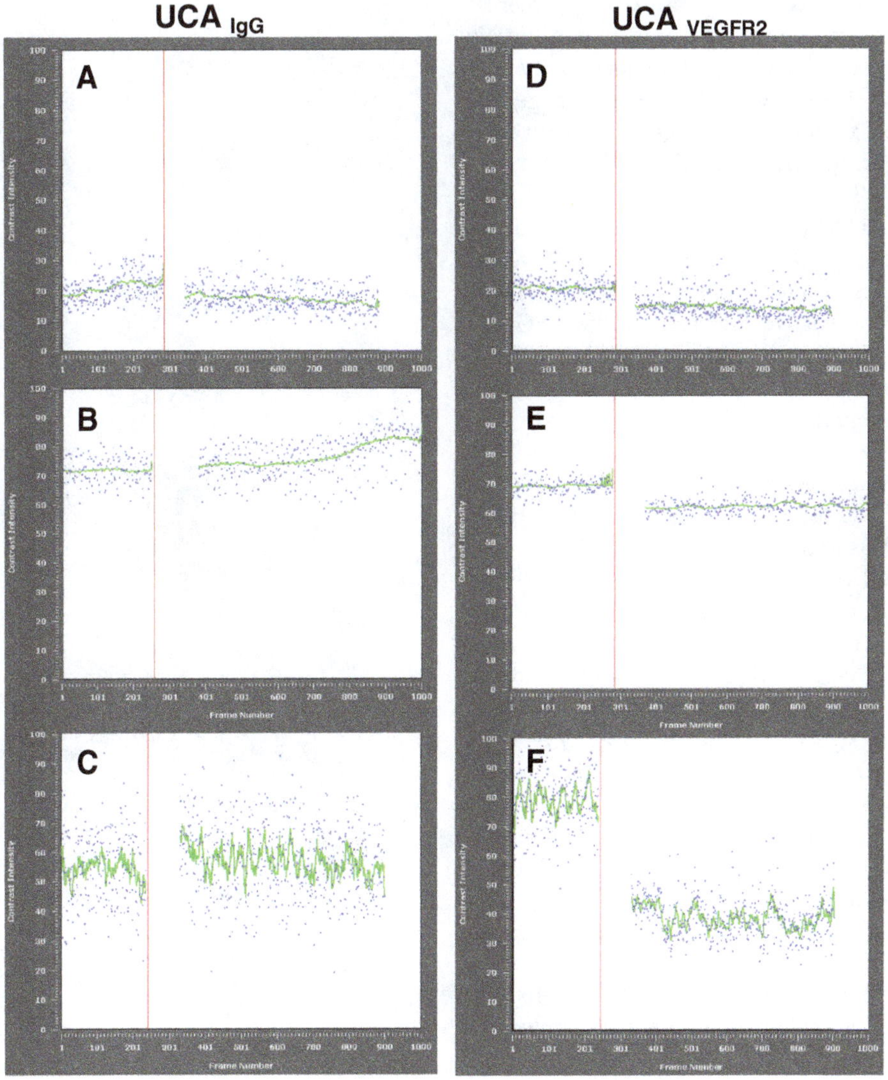

Figure 2 Video intensities curves. Predestruction and postdestruction video intensities curves for the control UCA **(A–C)** and the VEGFR2-targeted UCA **(D–F)**. The average video intensity of predestruction and postdestruction sonograms was measured and the difference in video intensity between the predestruction and postdestruction ultrasonographic frames was calculated and expressed as video intensity difference (VI_D). This value provided a relative measure of the amount of targeted microbubbles retained by the tumor. Video Intensities curves of a normal thyroid parenchyma **(A,D)**, adenoma **(B,E)** and a thyroid tumor **(C,F)**. These images show a significant difference between retention of the control and VEGFR2-targeted UCAs in a thyroid tumor.

showed no notable toxicity, and all animals recovered after US imaging without any detectable signs of distress.

At the ultrasound evaluation in 16 mice examined: in 4 the thyroid showed normal size and homogeneous echotexture of parenchyma, without nodules, and therefore classified as normal, 2 mice showed features of benign diffuse hyperplasia and 10 mice had a nodular process.

At the histological examination 4 normal thyroids, 2 hyperplasias, 3 adenomas, 7 papillary thyroid carcinoma were found, confirming Ultrasound diagnosis. The benign thyroid nodules measured 0.11–0.27 mm (median 0.17 mm) while the tumors measured 0.16–5.51 mm (median 0.54 mm).

For thyroid tumors the VI_D was significantly higher when using $UCA_{VEGFR\text{-}2}$ compared with UCA_{IgG} whereas for normal thyroids or in mice harboring benign thyroid nodules the VI_D for $UCA_{VEGFR\text{-}2}$ was equal to the VI_D for UCA_{IgG} (Table 1 and Figure 2). Median range VI_D UCA_{VEGFR2} thyroid tumors, 30.1 (range 25.1-35.6) versus VI_D UCA_{IgG} 19.4 (range 11.4-22.6) ($P < 0.01$).

Benign nodules VI_D $UCA_{VEGFR\text{-}2}$ 13.3 (range 10.8-15.8) versus $VI_D UCA_{IgG}$ 11.82 (range 8.5-19.6) (P= n.s). Normal thyroids VI_D $UCA_{VEGFR\text{-}2}$ 10.9 (range 10.3-14.9) versus VI_D in UCA_{IgG} 11.3 (9.4-14.7); (P= n.s) (Table 1). These values were used as relative measures of the VEGFR-2 over-expression within tumor vasculature and the UCA_{IgG} served as a control for demonstration of the specificity of $UCA_{VEGFR\text{-}2}$ retention.

The median difference between VI_D UCA_{IGg} and VI_D of $UCA_{VEGFR\text{-}2}$ was considered as a measure of VEGFR-2 specific binding, was 11.6 (range 9.6-19.2) VI units for thyroid carcinoma significantly higher (p=0.0037) than for normal thyroid (median 0.3, range −1.57-1.32) and hyperplasia/benign nodules (median 2.3 range −3.8-3.0).

Figure 2 shows representative VI curves of a thyroid malignant nodule, normal thyroid and benign nodule imaged with the $UCA_{VEGFR\text{-}2}$ and UCA_{IgG}. There was a moderately intense signal from the $UCA_{VEGFR\text{-}2}$ retained by the tumor (Figure 2F). The corresponding images for the UCA_{IgG} showed no retention of MBs in the tumor (Figure 2C). The $UCA_{VEGFR\text{-}2}$ in the vascular bed of benign nodules and normal thyroids showed very low retention in $UCA_{VEGFR\text{-}2}$ (Figure 2D-E).

After CEUS imaging, mice were subjected to general anesthesia and than euthanized.

In the group of examined animals the greatest $UCA_{VEGFR\text{-}2}$ Video Intensity for normal or benign thyroid nodules was 15.8 units while the lowest $UCA_{VEGFR\text{-}2}$ Video Intensity for carcinomas was 25.1 units. Therefore, we propose a cut-off value of 20 VI units to discriminate normal or benign nodules from malignant thyroid, that may be verified using a larger number of subjects.

To confirm expression of VEGFR-2, immunohistochemistry analysis of tumor sections was performed (Figure 3).

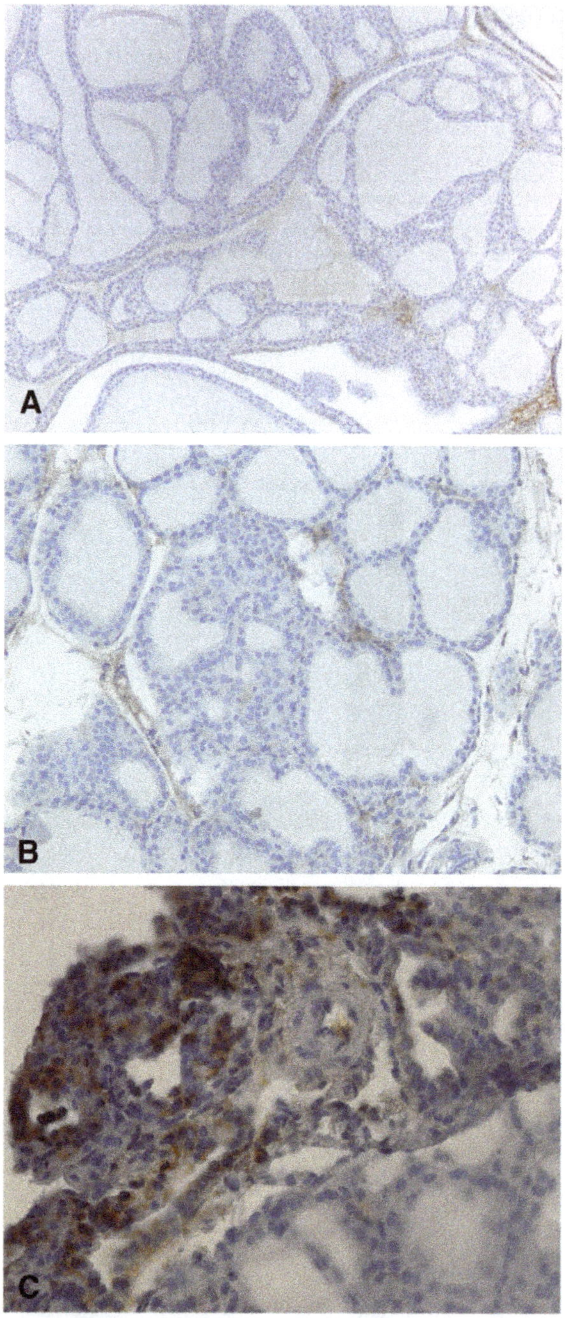

Figure 3 Representative microphotographs of immunohistochemistry analysis of murine thyroid stained with antibodies against VEGFR type 2 receptor. Brown color indicate presence of VEGFR2. Low grade expression of VEGFR-2 in normal thyroid **(A)**, in thyroid adenoma **(B)** and high grade expression in thyroid carcinoma **(C)**.

The strength of the ultrasound signal from the $UCA_{VEGFR\text{-}2}$ was significantly correlated with the level of actual VEGFR-2 expression (*rho* 0.793, P=0.0003) (Figure 4).

In this study we have evaluated the expression levels of a well-described tumor angiogenic marker i.e. VEGFR-2

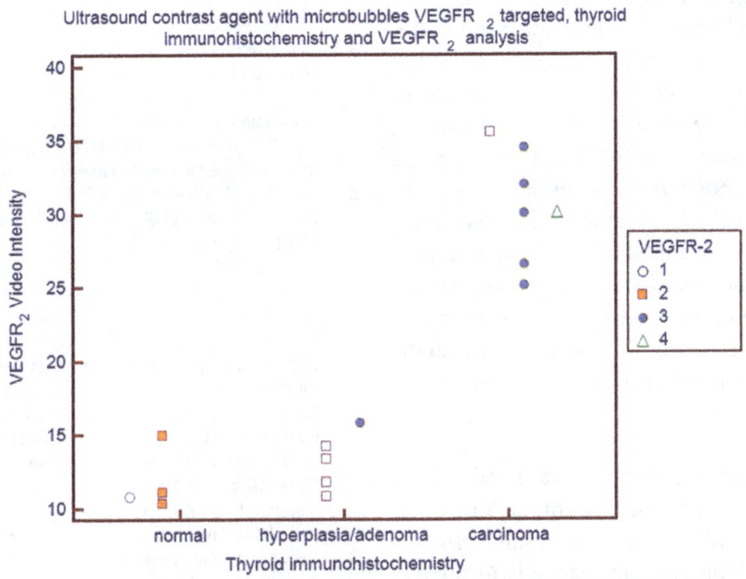

Figure 4 Video Intensity Difference of VEGFR-2 targeted microbubbles and expression of VEGFR-2 determined by Immunohistochemistry expressed as the average percentage of positively stained cells in normal thyroids, in hyperplasia/adenoma and in carcinomas [white dot: no staining (< 5% positive cells); orange square: low/weak (≥ 5% - ≤ 25% positive cells); blue dot: medium/moderate (> 25% - < 50% positive cells); triangle: high/ strong (≥ 50% positive cells)]. The correlation was assessed by the Spearman coefficient.

in a mouse model of thyroid tumor (Tg-TRK-T1) compared with normal or benign tumors and whether targeted CEUS allows assessment of this marker noninvasively. The *in vivo* binding of the VEGFR-2 targeted UCA in thyroid tumors was substantially higher compared with control UCA. This difference in retention affirmed the specificity of a VEGFR-2- conjugated UCA for endothelial targeting. The UCA-IgG was higher in the tumors than in the benign thyroid nodules and normal thyroids, however the difference was not significant. Therefore targeting with VEGFR2 was necessary for differentiating a malignant tumor from a benign nodule. Vascular endothelial growth factor receptor 2 (VEGFR-2) is one of the best-characterized molecular marker of tumor angiogenesis [34-37]. It is overexpressed on tumor vascular endothelial cells in several solid tumors, including breast [38,39], ovarian [40,41], pancreatic [42] and thyroid cancer [19] and it is considered an important factor in tumor angiogenesis. VEGFR-2 is an endothelium-specific receptor tyrosine kinase that is activated by VEGF A. Activation of the VEGF/VEGFR-2 pathway triggers multiple signaling networks that result in endothelial cell survival, mitogenesis, migration, differentiation, and vascular permeability [43]. Insights into the expression levels of tumor angiogenic markers during the progression of cancer, could be of great importance in developing novel molecular imaging strategies aimed at visualization of tumor angiogenesis markers that are overexpressed in particular in early stage cancer for screening purposes.

The *in vivo* US imaging signals of the injected targeted UCA was correlated with results from immunochemistry analysis of VEGFR-2 expression and this positive correlation suggested that targeted contrast-enhanced US imaging could be used to monitor expression levels of angiogenic markers noninvasively (Figure 4). Thus retention of a VEGFR-2-targeted UCA is a more specific as *in vivo* marker for the level of VEGFR-2 expression than for the quantification of tumor vascularity.

The ability to visualize and quantify tumor angiogenesis may allow screening and detecting cancer at an early stage and antiangiogenic treatment monitoring in patients [34].

Targeted-CEUS is a promising non invasive molecular imaging approach that allows *in vivo* assessment of molecular markers of tumor angiogenesis [44-48]. The number of attached MBs depends on various factors, including the extent of tumor vascularization, physical forces that translate the freely circulating contrast MBs to the vessel wall, and the affinity of the binding ligand to the molecular targets, as well as the expression level of the molecular targets on tumor vessels [47-52].

Our study has several limitations. Molecular imaging of VEGFR-2 expression was performed in developed tumors (0.16–5.51 mm in diameter) in which it is very likely that the receptor is expressed at more. Thus, the usefulness and accuracy of VEGFR-2-targeted UCA imaging at earlier stages of tumor development needs to be evaluated.

A 2-dimensional image acquisition method was used, and it is very difficult to know whether ultrasound scans perfectly correspond with the region subjected to histological examination. Studies carried out in 3D mode could ensure greater correspondence between quantitative ultrasonographic assessment of VEGFR-2 expression and results of immunochemical analysis.

The small animal Vevo770 US system for dedicated small-animal imaging used in our study for MBs detection operates on received signals that undergo log-compression prior to image display. Log-compressed gray scale image values referred as "Video Intensity" can produce inaccurate estimation of perfusion user and instrument-dependent.

Conclusions

The results of our study suggests that targeted CEUS imaging allows a non-invasive assessment of VEGFR-2 expression levels in thyroid *in vivo*. The results provide further insights into the biology of angiogenesis in thyroid tumors and may help in defining promising imaging targets for both early cancer detection and antitumor therapies.

Competing interests

The authors declared that they have no competing interests.

Authors' contributions

MM conception and design of the study, analysis and interpretation of data, drafting the manuscript supervision of research group. AG carried out ultrasound studies, conception and design of the study, analysis and interpretation of data, and drafting of the manuscript. GS animal models, analysis and interpretation of data, drafting of the manuscript. RL design of the study, statistical analysis, interpretation of data. GDM collection of data, animal models. EV ultrasound studies, analysis of data. GC collection of data, animal models. RP collection of data, animal models. AB conceived of the study, and participated in its design and coordination and helped to draft the manuscript. MS conceived of the study, and participated in its design and coordination and helped to draft the manuscript. All authors read and approved the final manuscript.

Acknowledgements

We thank Massimo Santoro for the TG-TRK-T1 mice.

Disclosure summary

The authors have nothing to disclose.
This study was supported by:
MIUR FIRB Prot. RBNE08E8CZ MERIT program.
Associazione Italiana per la Ricerca sul Cancro (AIRC).

Author details

[1]Institute of Biostructure and Bioimaging, Italian National Research Council (CNR), Naples, Italy. [2]SDN Foundation IRCCS, Naples, Italy. [3]Dipartimento di Scienze Biomediche Avanzate, Università degli Studi di Napoli "Federico II", 80131 Naples, Italy. [4]Dipartimento di Studi delle Istituzioni e dei Sistemi Territoriali, Università degli Studi di Napoli "Parthenope", Naples, Italy. [5]CEINGE-Biotecnologie Avanzate s.c.a.\r.l., Naples, Italy. [6]Dipartimento di Biologia e Patologia Cellulare e Molecolare, Università degli Studi di Napoli "Federico II", 80131 Naples, Italy. [7]Functional Genomic Unit, Istituto Nazionale Tumori G. Pascale, Naples, Italy.

References

1. Klener P: **Angiogenesis as part of the tumor "ecosystem" and possibilities to influence it.** *Klin Onkol* 2010, **23**(1):14–20.
2. Pandya NM, Dhalla NS, Santani DD: **Angiogenesis–a new target for future therapy.** *Vascul Pharmacol* 2006, **44**(5):265–274.
3. Sato Y: **Molecular diagnosis of tumor angiogenesis and anti-angiogenic cancer therapy.** *Int J Clin Oncol* 2003, **8**(4):200–206.
4. Sitohy B, Nagy JA, Dvorak HF: **Anti-VEGF/VEGFR therapy for cancer: reassessing the target.** *Cancer Res* 2012, **72**(8):1909–1914.
5. Kojic KL, Kojic SL, Wiseman SM: **Differentiated thyroid cancers: a comprehensive review of novel targeted therapies.** *Expert Rev Anticancer Ther* 2012, **12**(3):345–357.
6. Bertolini F, Marighetti P, Martin-Padura I, Mancuso P, Hu-Lowe DD, Shaked Y, D'Onofrio A: **Anti-VEGF and beyond: shaping a new generation of anti-angiogenic therapies for cancer.** *Drug Discov Today* 2011, **16**(23–24):1052–1060.
7. Turner HE, Harris AL, Melmed S, Wass JA: **Angiogenesis in endocrine tumors.** *Endocr Rev* 2003, **24**(5):600–603.
8. Warram JM, Sorace AG, Saini R, Umphrey HR, Zinn KR, Hoyt K: **A triple-targeted ultrasound contrast agent provides improved localization to tumor vasculature.** *J Ultrasound Med* 2011, **30**:921–931.
9. Ramsden JD, Buchanan MA, Egginton S, Watkinson JC, Mautner V, Eggo MC: **Complete inhibition of goiter in mice requires combined gene therapy modification of angiopoietin, vascular endothelial growth factor, and fibroblast growth factor signaling.** *Endocrinology* 2005, **146**(7):2895–2902.
10. Nagura S, Katoh R, Miyagi E, Shibuya M, Kawaoi A: **Expression of vascular endothelial growth factor (VEGF) and VEGF receptor-1 (Flt-1) in Graves disease possibly correlated with increased vascular density.** *Hum Pathol* 2001, **32**(1):10–17.
11. Nikiforov YE, Nikiforova MN: **Molecular genetics and diagnosis of thyroid cancer.** *Nat Rev Endocrinol* 2011, **7**(10):569–580.
12. Greco A, Miranda C, Pierotti MA: **Rearrangements of NTRK1 gene in papillary thyroid carcinoma.** *Molecular and cellular endocrinology* 2010, **321**:44–49.
13. Russell JP, Powell DJ, Cunnane M, Greco A, Portella G, Santoro M, Fusco A, Rothstein JL: **The TRK-T1 fusion protein induces neoplastic transformation of thyroid epithelium.** *Oncogene* 2000, **19**:5729–5735.
14. Kim CS, Zhu X: **Lessons from mouse models of thyroid cancer.** *Thyroid* 2009, **19**:1317–1331.
15. Klein M, Catargi B: **VEGF in physiological process and thyroid disease.** *Ann Endocrinol* 2007, **68**(6):438–448.
16. Góth MI, Hubina E, Raptis S, Nagy GM, Tóth BE: **Physiological and pathological angiogenesis in the endocrine system.** *Microsc Res Tech* 2003, **60**(1):98–106.
17. Salajegheh A, Smith RA, Kasem K, Gopalan V, Nassiri MR, William R, Lam AK: **Single nucleotide polymorphisms and mRNA expression of VEGF-A in papillary thyroid carcinoma: potential markers for aggressive phenotypes.** *Eur J Surg Oncol* 2011, **37**(1):93–99.
18. Turner HE, Nagy Z, Gatter KC, Esiri MM, Harris AL, Wass JA: **Angiogenesis in pituitary adenomas and the normal pituitary gland.** *J Clin Endocrinol Metab* 2000, **85**(3):1159–1162.
19. Risau W: **Angiogenic growth factors.** *Prog Growth Factor Res* 1990, **2**(1):71–79.
20. Ellegala DB, Leong-Poi H, Carpenter JE, Kaul S, Shaffrey ME, Sklenar J, Lindner JR: **Imaging tumor angiogenesis with contrast ultrasound and microbubbles targeted to alpha(v)beta3.** *Circulation* 2003, **108**:336–341.
21. Korpanty G, Carbon JG, Grayburn PA, Fleming JB, Brekken RA: **Monitoring response to anticancer therapy by targeting microbubbles to tumor vasculature.** *Clin Cancer Res* 2007, **13**:323–330.
22. Willmann JK, Paulmurugan R, Chen K, Gheysens O, Rodriguez-Porcel M, Lutz AM, Chen IY, Chen X, Gambhir SS: **US imaging of tumor angiogenesis with microbubbles targeted to vascular endothelial growth factor receptor type 2 in mice.** *Radiology* 2008, **2**:508–518.
23. Lee DJ, Lyshchik A, Huamani J, Hallahan DE, Fleischer AC: **Relationship between retention of a vascular endothelial growth factor receptor 2 (VEGFR2)-targeted ultrasonographic contrast agent and the level ofVEGFR2 expression in an in vivo breast cancer model.** *J Ultrasound Med* 2008, **27**(6):855–866.
24. Delorme S, Krix M: **Contrast-enhanced ultrasound for examining tumor biology.** *Cancer Imaging* 2006, **6**:148–152.
25. Klasa-Mazurkiewicz D, Jarząb M, Milczek T, Lipińska B, Emerich J: **Clinical significance of VEGFR-2 and VEGFR-3 expression in ovarian cancer patients.** *Pol J Pathol* 2011, **62**(1):31–40.
26. Büchler P, Reber HA, Büchler MW, Friess H, Hines OJ: **VEGF-RII influences the prognosis of pancreatic cancer.** *Ann Surg* 2002, **236**(6):738–749.

27. Office of Animal Care and Use (OACU) of the National Institutes of Health (NIH): **Animal Research Advisory Committee (ARAC).** http://oacu.od.nih.gov/ARAC/.
28. Workman P, Aboagye EO, Balkwill F, Balmain A, Bruder G, Chaplin DJ, Double JA, Everitt J, Farningham DAH, Glennie MJ, Kelland LR, Robinson V, Stratford IJ, Tozer GM, Watson S, Wedge SR, Eccles SA: **An ad hoc committee of the National Cancer Research Institute. Guidelines for the welfare and use of animals in cancer research.** *Br J Cancer* 2010, **102:**1555–1577.
29. Zhou YQ, Foster FS, Qu DW, Zhang M, Harasiewicz KA, Adamson SL: **Applications for multifrequency ultrasound biomicroscopy in mice from implantation to adulthood.** *Physiol Genomics* 2002, **10**(2):113–126.
30. Greco A, Mancini M, Gargiulo S, Gramanzini M, Claudio PP, Brunetti A, Salvatore M: **Ultrasound biomicroscopy in small animal research: applications in molecular and pre-clinical imaging.** *Journal of Biomedicine and Biotechnology* 2012, **Article ID 519238:**14.
31. The Australian and New Zealand Council for the Care of Animals in Research and Teaching Ltd (ANZCCART): Australia: The University of Adelaide. http://www.adelaide.edu.au/ANZCCART/publications/.
32. Mancini M, Vergara E, Salvatore G, Greco A, Troncone G, Affuso A, Liuzzi R, Salerno P, Scotto di Santolo M, Santoro M, Brunetti A, Salvatore M: **Morphological ultrasound micro-imaging of thyroid in living mice.** *Endocrinology* 2009, **150**(10):4810–4815.
33. Jokinen MP, Botts S: **WHO International Agency for Researchon Cancer.** In *Pathology of tumours in laboratory animals: tumours of the mouse Vol 2.* 2nd edition. Edited by Turusob VS, Mohr U. Lyon, France: IARC Scientific Publication; 1994:565–594.
34. Palmowski M, Huppert J, Ladewig G, Hauff P, Reinhardt M, Mueller MM, Woenne EC, Jenne JW, Maurer M, Kauffmann GW, Semmler W, Kiessling F: **Molecular profiling of angiogenesis with targeted ultrasound imaging: early assessment of antiangiogenic therapy effects.** *Mol Cancer Ther* 2008, **7**(1):101–109.
35. Hodivala-Dilke K: **Alphavbeta3 integrin and angiogenesis: a moody integrin in a changing environment.** *Curr Opin Cell Biol* 2008, **20**(5):514–519.
36. Ferrara N: **Vascular endothelial growth factor: basic science and clinical progress.** *Endocr Rev* 2004, **25**(4):581–611.
37. ten Dijke P, Goumans MJ, Pardali E: **Endoglin in angiogenesis and vascular diseases.** *Angiogenesis* 2008, **11**(1):79–89.
38. Sledge GW Jr, Rugo HS, Burstein HJ: **The role of angiogenesis inhibition in the treatment of breast cancer.** *Clin Adv Hematol Oncol* 2006, **4**(10 Suppl 21):1–10.
39. Khosravi Shahi P, Soria Lovelle A, Pérez Manga G: **Tumoral angiogenesis and breast cancer.** *Clin Transl Oncol* 2009, **11**(3):138–142.
40. Gómez-Raposo C, Mendiola M, Barriuso J, Casado E, Hardisson D, Redondo A: **Angiogenesis and ovarian cancer.** *Clin Transl Oncol* 2009, **11**(9):564–571.
41. Bednarek W, Mazurek M, Cwiklińska A, Barczyński B: **Expression of selected angiogenesis markers and modulators in pre-, peri- and postmenopausal women with ovarian cancer.** *Ginekol Pol* 2009, **80**(2):93–98.
42. Saif MW: **Primary pancreatic lymphomas.** *JOP* 2006, **7**(3):262–273.
43. Hicklin DJ, Ellis LM: **Role of the vascular endothelial growth factor pathway in tumor growth and angiogenesis.** *J Clin Oncol* 2005, **23**(5):1011–1027.
44. Lindner JR: **Microbubbles in medical imaging: current applications and future directions.** *Nat Rev Drug Discov* 2004, **3**(6):527–532.
45. Willmann JK, van Bruggen N, Dinkelborg LM, Gambhir SS: **Molecular imaging in drug development.** *Nat Rev Drug Discov* 2008, **7**(7):591–607.
46. Pysz MA, Foygel K, Rosenberg J, Gambhir SS, Schneider M, Willmann JK: **Antiangiogenic cancer therapy: monitoring with molecular US and a clinically translatable contrast agent (BR55).** *Radiology* 2010, **256**(2):519–527.
47. Willmann JK, Kimura RH, Deshpande N, Lutz AM, Cochran JR, Gambhir SS: **Targeted contrast-enhanced ultrasound imaging of tumor angiogenesis with contrast microbubbles conjugated to integrin-binding knottin peptides.** *J Nucl Med* 2010, **51**(3):433–440.
48. Lindner JR, Song J, Xu F, Klibanov AL, Singbartl K, Ley K, Kaul S: **Noninvasive ultrasound imaging of inflammation using microbubbles targeted to activated leukocytes.** *Circulation* 2000, **102**(22):2745–2750.
49. Sorace AG, Saini R, Mahoney M, Hoyt K: **Molecular ultrasound imaging using a targeted contrast agent for assessing early tumor response to antiangiogenic therapy.** *J Ultrasound Med* 2012, **31**(10):1543–1550.
50. Willmann JK, Cheng Z, Davis C: **Targeted microbubbles for imaging tumor angiogenesis: assessment of whole-body biodistribution with dynamic micro-PET in mice.** *Radiology* 2008, **249:**212–219.
51. Klibanov AL, Rasche PT, Hughes MS, Wojdyla JK, Galen KP, Wible JH Jr, Brandenburger GH: **Detection of individual microbubbles of ultrasound contrast agents: imaging of free-floating and targeted bubbles.** *Invest Radiol* 2004, **39**(3):187–195.
52. Lucidarme O, Kono Y, Corbeil J, Choi SH, Golmard JL, Varner J, Mattrey RF: **Angiogenesis: noninvasive quantitative assessment with contrast-enhanced functional US in murine model.** *Radiology* 2006, **239**(3):730–739.

In silico simulation of liver crack detection using ultrasonic shear wave imaging

Erwei Nie[1], Jiao Yu[2*], Debaditya Dutta[3] and Yanying Zhu[2]

Abstract

Background: Liver trauma is an important source of morbidity and mortality worldwide. A timely detection and precise evaluation of traumatic liver injury and the bleeding site is necessary. There is a need to develop better imaging modalities of hepatic injuries to increase the sensitivity of ultrasonic imaging techniques for sites of hemorrhage caused by cracks. In this study, we conduct an in silico simulation of liver crack detection and delineation using an ultrasonic shear wave imaging (USWI) based method.

Methods: We simulate the generation and propagation of the shear wave in a liver tissue medium having a crack using COMSOL. Ultrasound radio frequency (RF) signal synthesis and the two-dimensional speckle tracking algorithm are applied to simulate USWI in a medium with randomly distributed scatterers. Crack detection is performed using the directional filter and the edge detection algorithm rather than the conventional inversion algorithm. Cracks with varied sizes and locations are studied with our method and the crack localization results are compared with the given crack.

Results: Our pilot simulation study shows that, by using USWI combined with a directional filter cum edge detection technique, the near-end edge of the crack can be detected in all the three cracks that we studied. The detection errors are within 5%. For a crack of 1.6 mm thickness, little shear wave can pass through it and the far-end edge of the crack cannot be detected. The detected crack lengths using USWI are all slightly shorter than the actual crack length. The robustness of our method in detecting a straight crack, a curved crack and a subtle crack of 0.5 mm thickness is demonstrated.

Conclusions: In this paper, we simulate the use of a USWI based method for the detection and delineation of the crack in liver. The in silico simulation helps to improve understanding and interpretation of USWI measurements in a physical scattered liver medium with a crack. This pilot study provides a basis for improved insights in future crack detection studies in a tissue phantom or liver.

Keywords: Ultrasonic shear wave imaging, Liver crack, Speckle tracking, Directional filter, Edge detection

Background

The liver is one of the most commonly injured organs in abdominal trauma [1] and liver trauma is responsible for significant mortality [2]. A timely detection and precise evaluation of hepatic injury and bleeding site is necessary because the injury, if undetected, may progress to a more severe state, and even be life-threatening. Imaging hepatic injured site (a.k.a. laceration or crack) with conventional B-mode ultrasound may be difficult [3–5] because the injured area usually appears hypo-echoic on the sonogram due to hemorrhage. Unlike tumor masses, which have good contrast resulting from highly heterogeneous echotexture, cracks in homogeneous soft tissues lack the necessary contrast. It becomes notoriously difficult to detect when the crack in the liver is juxtaposed. There is a need to develop better imaging modalities for hepatic injuries to be integrated into a bedside ultrasound imaging system to increase the sensitivity of ultrasonic imaging techniques for sites of hemorrhage caused by cracks. This paper aims to present a method for detecting the liver crack (or bleeding site) using an ultrasonic shear wave imaging (USWI) based technique.

USWI has been found to be a valuable noninvasive tool for studying the elastic properties of biological tissue. It relies on accurate estimates of tissue motion

* Correspondence: yujiaojoy@hotmail.com
[2]College of Science, Liaoning Shihua University, Fushun, People's Republic of China
Full list of author information is available at the end of the article

between frame-to-frame deformations of the tissue. For USWI, the shear wave is generated by pushing the tissue remotely with an ultrasound transducer, and with the same transducer, the tissue deformation during shear wave propagation is recorded in real-time ultrasonic images [6, 7]. Usually afterwards, the shear wave post-processing in shear wave elasticity imaging uses inversion algorithms to reconstruct shear modulus and acquire the tissue elasticity distribution.

In this study, we conduct an in silico simulation of the ultrasonic shear wave imaging of the crack in a liver tissue model by using the ultrasound RF signal synthesis and speckle tracking technique. Different from the post-processing for the shear wave elasticity imaging, the crack localization in this study is implemented by applying a directional filter and edge detection algorithm rather than recovering the elasticity map. We will discuss the crack detection with our method. To the best of our knowledge, study using shear wave imaging based method for liver trauma has been rarely reported and very little is known about the usefulness of USWI for an improved identification of hepatic injured site. The current study is performed to improve understanding and interpretation of USWI measurements in a scattered liver medium with a crack.

Methods

Finite element simulation

Assuming liver is a purely elastic solid, a two-dimensional (2-D) homogeneous and isotropic tissue medium (5.0 × 5.0 cm^2) was constructed using a finite element (FE) package (COMSOL). Structural Mechanics Module was used for this study. At the center of the liver medium, a rectangular (3.8 cm × 0.05 cm) excitation rod was created, and a uniform plane shear wave was produced by oscillating the rod vertically with one cycle of a 100 Hz low frequency harmonic vibration. As the shear wave propagated sideways away from the center, the tissue medium was displaced along the axial direction.

The liver medium with the following characteristics was simulated: density ρ_1=1.2 × 10^3 kg/m^3, Poisson's ratio v_1=0.499, and Young's modulus E_1=6 kPa [8, 9]. The Young's modulus value corresponds to a shear elasticity of about 2 kPa, which is appropriate for the liver, based on the earlier literature [10–12]. The crack was 3.2 cm in depth, inclined downward from the upper surface at an angle of 15 degrees from the vertical direction. The crack was located between x = 1.354 cm and x = 1.519 cm at the top, with a uniform thickness of 1.6 mm (horizontal thickness was 1.65 mm). The medium between the two edges within the crack had a density of ρ_0=1.06 × 10^3 kg/m^3, Poisson's ratio of v_0=0.499, and Young's modulus of E_0=0.005 Pa, to mimic the blood [13]. The boundary conditions were assumed to be: free at the top surface of the liver tissue and the boundary of the excitation rod; fixed at the bottom surface boundary of the liver tissue; roller at the other surfaces (left, right boundaries) and the crack boundary [9, 14]. A mapped mesh with triangular elements was employed (altogether, 26,808 elements). Figure 1 shows the schematic diagram of the FE mesh of the simulation model. A time-dependent analysis was performed. With a frame rate acquisition of 5000 frames/s, the simulation was run from 0 ms to 21.0 ms with a time step of 0.2 ms, over 106 frames. Spatial and temporal profiles of propagating shear waves were recorded. The recorded time-varying axial displacements were subsequently processed in MATLAB (MathWorks Inc., USA). To avoid the influence of the boundaries and reduce unnecessary computations, only data located in the region of interest, with the X coordinate between 0 and 25 mm and Y coordinate between 0 and 50 mm, were exported and processed. The output axial displacement data is a three-dimensional matrix (200 × 400 × 106), which indicates the data containing 106 frames and divided into 200 and 400 units in the X and Y directions, respectively.

Ultrasound RF signal simulation

The ultrasonic A-lines of the tissue are generated using a 2-D linear scattering model to simulate the actual ultrasonic shear wave imaging [15]. The transducer center frequency is set at 5 MHz, with the axial component of the transducer point spread function (PSF) having a 50% half-power relative bandwidth and the lateral component of the PSF having a full width at half maximum of 0.5 mm [16]. Figure 2 shows the axial and lateral components of the transducer PSF.

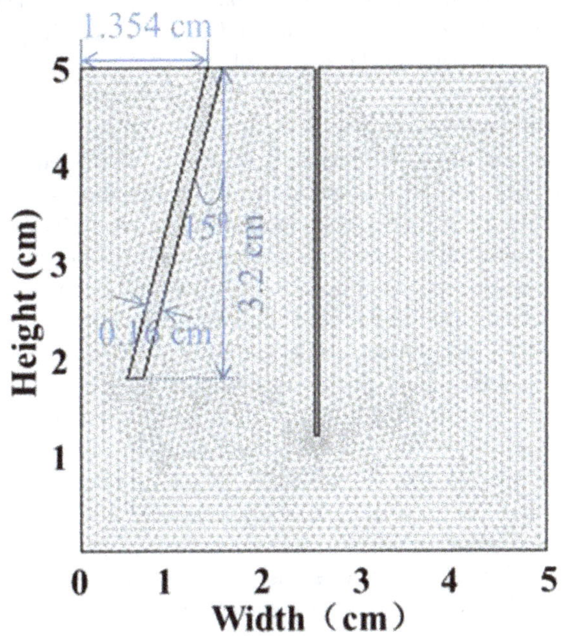

Fig. 1 Schematic diagram of FE mesh of the simulation model

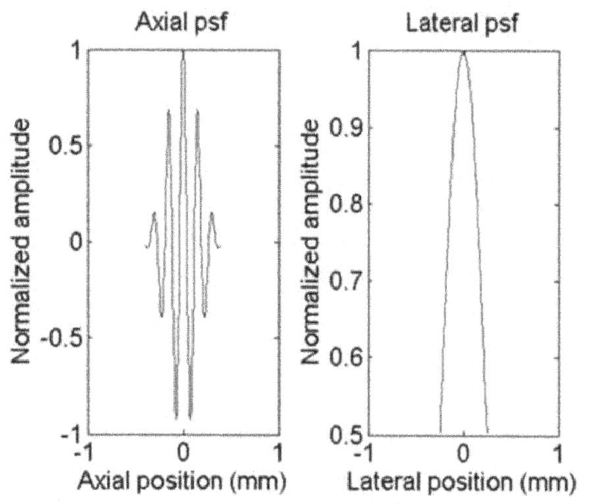

Fig. 2 The axial and lateral components of the transducer PSF

Each frame of digital RF data was then produced with a 40 MHz sampling frequency by convolving the 2-D PSF with the ultrasound scattering function. The scattering function was defined as the random distribution of ultrasound scatterers over the entire tissue area. For each time step of the FE simulation, the displacement of each scatterer was interpolated from the nodal solution and added to the pre-deformed coordinates to obtain the deformed scattering function. The speed of sound in soft tissue was assumed to be 1540 m/s. The scatter density was set as six scatterers per wavelength [14, 17]. Each RF image with a size of 5.0 cm × 2.5 cm (corresponding to 2596 axial samples × 256 beams) was generated at each time step of the deformation [9, 18]. The ratio of the mean envelope amplitude over the standard deviation in the B-scan image gives a value of 2.3, which means that the simulation produced fully developed speckle [19].

Phase-sensitive 2-D speckle tracking

After ultrasonic RF signal synthesis, a phase-sensitive correlation-based 2-D speckle tracking algorithm was applied to the RF data to estimate the displacement between the frames [20]. Frame-to-frame axial and lateral displacements were estimated from the position of the maximum correlation coefficient from the cross-correlation on the baseband complex signals derived from the RF data.

The ultrasound speckle size was estimated to be 0. 270 mm in the axial direction and 0.586 mm in the lateral direction from the 2-D correlation function of the baseband signals. The search kernel of the speckle tracking was set to be about the ultrasound speckle size for optimal displacement estimation with minimum variance [20]. Axial displacements were then refined using the phase zero-crossing of the complex correlation functions. To enhance the signal-to-noise ratio with reasonable spatial resolution, the adjacent correlation functions were filtered using 0.781 mm (lateral) by 0.308 mm (axial) separable Hanning filter. The search region was 0.781 mm in both dimensions. The frame-to-frame axial displacements were then accumulated over the entire 105 frames reference to the original geometry, to estimate the total displacement [21]. With the accumulation of frames, the displacement SNR was enhanced by reducing any uncorrelated errors in the axial displacement estimates [20].

Crack localization without reconstructing the elasticity map

Unlike shear wave elastography, which applies the conventional local inversion technique for mapping tissue elasticity, the crack localization in this study is implemented by applying a directional filter and image processing without the conventional elasticity reconstruction.The axial displacement data, from 2-D speckle tracking after the ultrasound RF signal simulation, and directly from the FE simulation, are both processed using the directional filter. The directional filter was previously used [22–24] in the pre-processing of shear modulus reconstruction to suppress the artefact in the shear velocity estimation caused by the reflected shear wave. In the present work, the reflected shear wave becomes a "signal" rather than a "noise." The directional filter decomposes the plane shear wave propagation in the [*k*,*w*] domain by performing a fast Fourier transform on the axial displacement data at all depths and then extracting the first and third quadrants, followed by the second and fourth quadrants, separately, to conduct the inverse fast Fourier transform [24]. In this way, the original shear wave was separated into its incident and reflected shear wave parts. By computing the absolute value of the displacement for each frame in the reflected wave and then accumulating over the entire imaging period, the total reflected wave field amplitude was estimated. Finally, the edge detection algorithm (Sobel method) was applied to the accumulated reflected wave magnitude image to find the crack. The detected crack locations, using speckle tracking and FE simulation, are compared to the given crack location and the relative errors are evaluated.

Detection of cracks with different sizes and contours

Two supplementary studies were carried out investigating detection of cracks with different sizes and contours. In one study, the crack was reduced to 0.5 cm in depth and 0.5 mm in thickness, with the shape and direction unchanged. The crack was located between x = 1.467 cm and x = 1.519 cm at the top, with the right edge remained immovable but shortened. In another study, we considered a crack with a curved edge. The crack was made from a segment of the intersection of two circles. The two circles are of the same radius (4.5 cm), with centers located at the same height (5 cm) but different horizontal positions (x = − 3.146 cm, x = − 2.

981 cm). The crack was still located between $x = 1.354$ cm and $x = 1.519$ cm at the top, but 1.8 cm in height. Following the same procedure as described above, the slimmer crack and the curved crack were studied for crack detection to gain an understanding of the robustness of our method.

Results

Figure 3 shows the axial displacement images during the shear wave propagation in the liver-mimicking medium. The shear wave speed observed from the movie is about 1.3 m/s, which is consistent with the expected value from the known Young's modulus of 6 kPa for a purely elastic medium ($c = \sqrt{E/(3\rho)}$), thus, the wavelength is 1.3 cm. From Fig. 3, we can see that the shear wave is largely reflected when arriving at the crack, with a minimal portion passing though the crack and continuing to travel forward, despite the fact that the crack thickness is much smaller than (about 1/10 of) the shear wavelength. Subject to the fluid–solid interface influence (Scholte wave) [25], the waveform close to the top of the images is slightly deformed.

Figure 4 shows the use of the directional filtering algorithm for the displacement data obtained from speckle tracking at 16.6 ms. The use of the directional filter (Fig. 4b) separates the incident and reflected waveforms (at 16.6 ms), in comparison with the unfiltered wave (at 16.6 ms) in Fig. 4a, which makes the observation of the shear wave more intuitive.

Figure 5 shows the crack localization after the use of the directional filter. Figure 5a, c give the accumulated reflected wave amplitude over the entire 105 and 106 frames for imaging using speckle tracking and FE simulation, respectively. Compared with the FE simulation, the displacement data obtained using the speckle tracking method is underestimated. Figure 5b, d display the crack localization result after the use of the edge detection algorithm on the accumulated reflected wave amplitude image in Fig. 5a, c. Two oblique lines with equal length are detected in Fig. 5d. By referring to Fig. 5c, we know that the oblique line on the left in Fig. 5d is the boundary, while the oblique on the right in Fig. 5d is the artefact caused by the reflection of the shear wave. The detected oblique line on the left corresponds to the right edge of the given crack, and the left edge is not detected. In Fig. 5b, the detected crack edge is in the form of point distributions. Despite being discontinuous, the contour can still be visualized and matches generally well with the result in Fig. 5d. The detected crack depth is 3.09 cm and 3.08 cm in Fig. 5b, d, respectively, in comparison with the given depth of 3.2 cm.

Figures 6 and 7 present the crack localization for the curved crack and slimmer crack, respectively, by using the same method as in Fig. 5. In both figures, the crack is well detected and localized using USWI. The detected crack depth is 1.79 cm and 0.45 cm for the curved crack and slimmer crack, in comparison with the given depth of 1.8 cm and 0.5 cm, respectively. The slimmer crack, located close to the upper surface, gives the largest error, 0.5 mm, in the depth estimation.

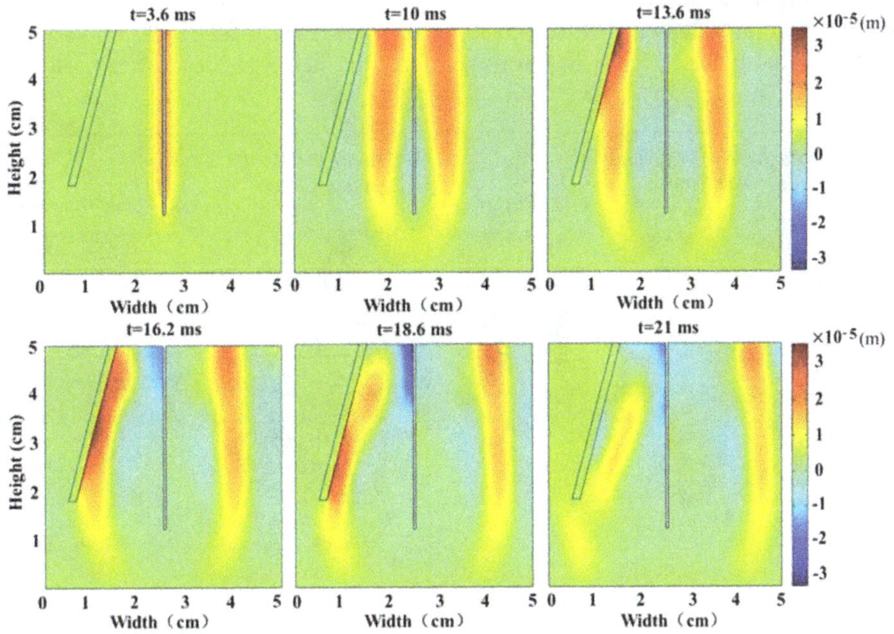

Fig. 3 The axial displacement images during the shear wave propagation in the liver-mimicking medium

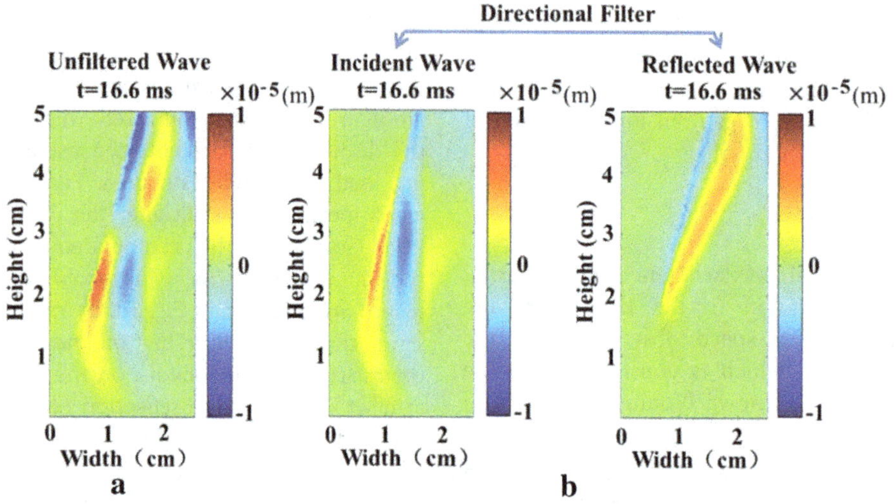

Fig. 4 The use of the directional filtering algorithm for the displacement data obtained from speckle tracking at 16.6 ms. **a** A snapshot of the unfiltered waveform (at 16.6 ms). **b** Snapshots of the incident and reflected waveforms (at 16.6 ms), separated by the directional filter

In Fig. 8, the detected crack locations are compared using speckle tracking and FE simulation, with the given crack location. The contour of the given crack is represented by red lines. The detection results using speckle tracking and FE simulation are represented by blue and green scatter plots. From Fig. 8a, b, it can be seen that for a crack of 1.6 mm thickness, straight or curved, the right edge of the given crack is detected with our method, while the left edge is not detected. The most accurate detection of the right edge is from the FE simulation (the green scatter plot on the left) which is just next to the given right edge and on its left side. The use of speckle tracking moves the detected position further to the left. This is true for Fig. 8c as well, with the only difference that the crack is so slim (0.5 mm thick), that the left edge is also nearby in Fig. 8c. Out of the given crack, sparsely distributed artefacts can be observed in the simulation of the actual USWI by applying speckle tracking. Tissue is less homogeneous in the scattering model, and there is a tradeoff between the resolution and smoothness of the image. Generally a larger filter would reduce such artefacts, but the resolution would also be reduced.

Table 1 presents the quantitative comparison of the transverse positions of the detected and given right edges of different cracks at different depths. In Table 1, USWI represents the simulation result of USWI using speckle tracking. The relative errors of the detected midpoint positions in comparison with the given positions are listed. Except for the depth very near the upper surface, the detected locations are all a bit to the left, in

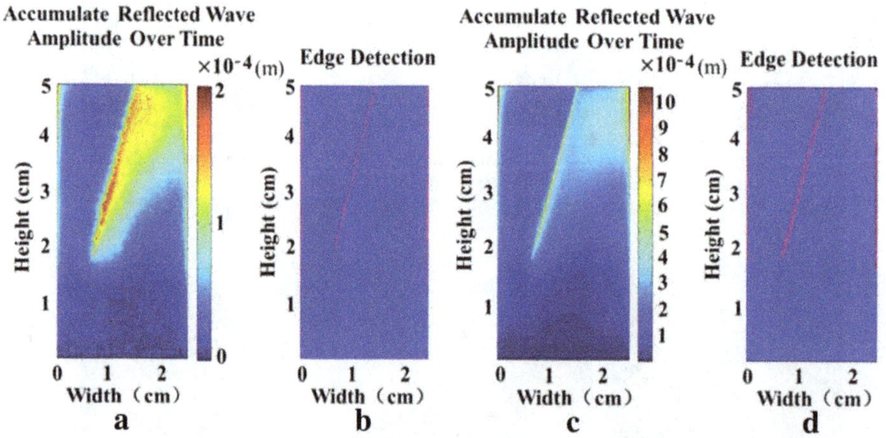

Fig. 5 The crack localization after the use of the directional filter. **a** Accumulated reflected wave amplitude over time for imaging using speckle tracking. **b** Crack localization result for imaging using speckle tracking. **c** Accumulated reflected wave amplitude over time using FE simulation. **d** Crack localization result using FE simulation

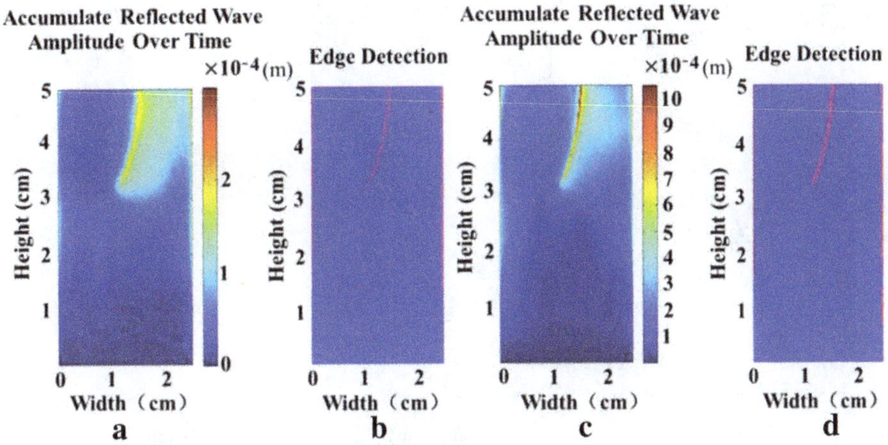

Fig. 6 The crack localization for the curved crack. **a** Accumulated reflected wave amplitude over time for imaging using speckle tracking. **b** Crack localization result for imaging using speckle tracking. **c** Accumulated reflected wave amplitude over time using FE simulation. **d** Crack localization result using FE simulation

comparison with the given locations, but the relative errors are all within 5%. The slimmer crack and the straight crack share the same right edge location, and the detected locations are identical too, except for very near the upper surface where the upper surface has an effect on the detection.

Discussion

Liver trauma, particularly blunt liver trauma, is an important source of morbidity and mortality worldwide. Liver trauma may be induced by road traffic crashes, fall, antisocial, violent behavior, or concussive impacts during military operation. In current emergency medical care, diagnostic peritoneal lavage (DPL) or Focused Assessment with Sonography for Trauma (FAST) is used to diagnose hemoperitoneum in unstable patients with abdominal trauma [26]. The focus of DPL or FAST is to check for free intraperitoneal blood [26–29]. DPL is sensitive, but it is an invasive procedure. FAST is noninvasive and highly specific, but has a relatively limited sensitivity (72 and 46% in detecting blunt and penetrating abdominal trauma, respectively [3]). A negative FAST result does not exclude significant intra-peritoneal bleeding [26] or hepatic injury [3]. Unlike DPL or FAST, computed tomography can determine the source of hemorrhage [4]. CT examination provides superior images of traumatic pathology and is the golden standard for detecting liver injuries. However, it requires patient transport from the emergency department and more time to acquire images which limits its use for unstable patients. There is a critical need to develop

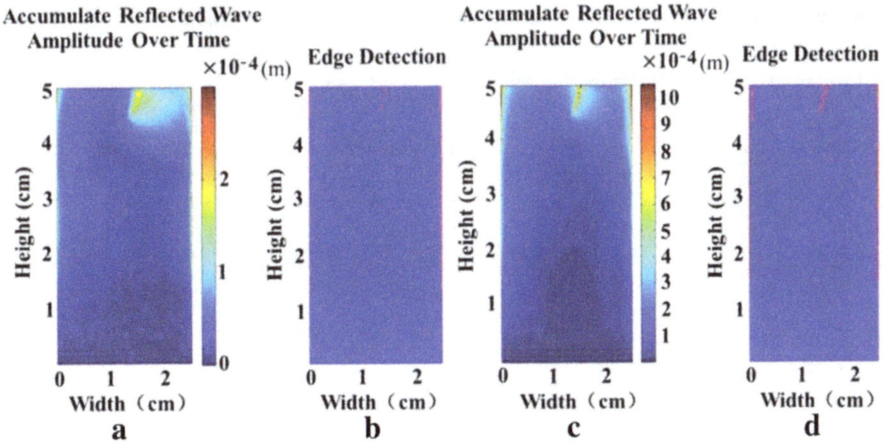

Fig. 7 The crack localization for the slimmer crack. **a** Accumulated reflected wave amplitude over time for imaging using speckle tracking. **b** Crack localization result for imaging using speckle tracking. **c** Accumulated reflected wave amplitude over time using FE simulation. **d** Crack localization result using FE simulation

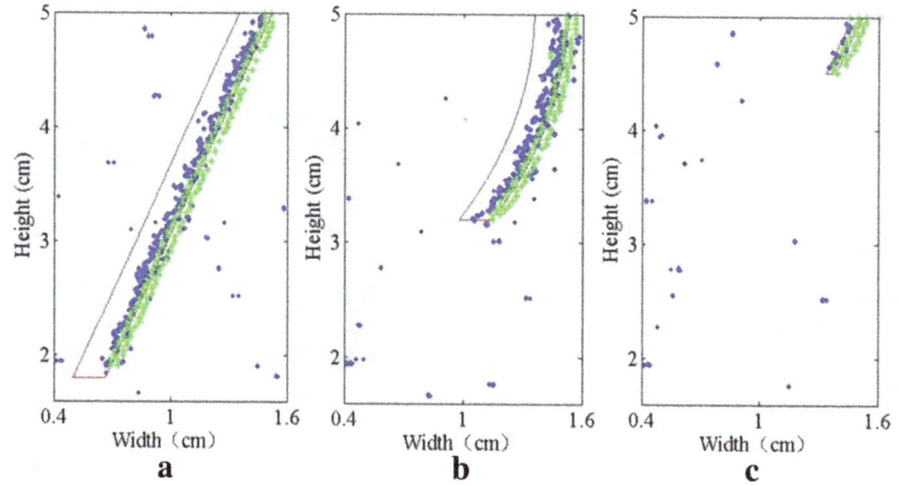

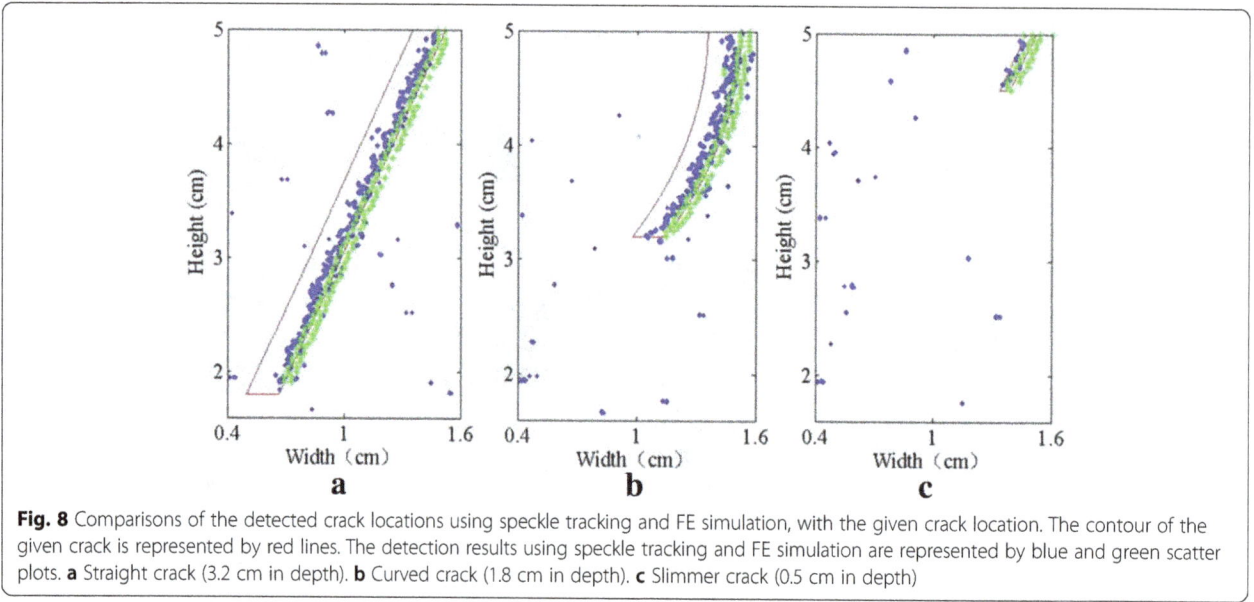

Fig. 8 Comparisons of the detected crack locations using speckle tracking and FE simulation, with the given crack location. The contour of the given crack is represented by red lines. The detection results using speckle tracking and FE simulation are represented by blue and green scatter plots. **a** Straight crack (3.2 cm in depth). **b** Curved crack (1.8 cm in depth). **c** Slimmer crack (0.5 cm in depth)

supplemental diagnostic tool for liver trauma that can rapidly localize and evaluate traumatic liver injuries to be used in clinical situations where CT is not suitable or not easily accessible and FAST is insufficient in characterizing the site of hemorrhage, e.g., pregnant patients and children, patients requiring an emergent bedside procedure, patients under observation or during recovery period requiring serial abdominal examinations, and patients at a community hospital before being transferred to a trauma center, etc.

Since A. P. Sarvazyan, S. Y. Emelianov, et al. [30, 31] proposed the shear wave elasticity imaging method, ultrasound shear wave elasticity imaging has experienced rapid development and has successfully been used in breast lesion detection [32] and liver fibrosis staging [33]. In recent years, with the development of liver trauma research, studies have been carried applying ultrasonic shear wave elastography for liver trauma evaluation [34, 35]. Shear wave elastography was used to diagnose acute liver trauma by measuring the elasticity value of normal liver tissue and traumatic lesions created with a hemostat [35] or to assess the effects of local tissue repair in blunt hepatic trauma after haemostatic injection by measuring the elasticity value of treatment area at different time points [34]. However, to the best of our knowledge, there have been no reports on the application of ultrasound shear wave elasticity imaging (or ultrasonic shear wave elastography) or other USWI based method for the detection and localization of the crack (a.k.a. laceration) in liver, one of the most often ruptured organs in traumatic abdominal injuries.

Ultrasound shear wave elasticity imaging (or ultrasonic shear wave elastography) uses local inversion techniques for measuring tissue elasticity. Typically, these inversion techniques obtain the elasticities by estimating the phase speed from the gradient of the phase or an algebraic

Table 1 The quantitative comparisons of the transverse positions of the detected and given right edges of different cracks at different depths

Depth (cm)	Straight crack (transverse position, cm)			Curved crack (transverse position, cm)			Slimmer crack (transverse position, cm)		
	Given	USWI	Error	Given	USWI	Error	Given	USWI	Error
0.208	1.464	1.431	−2.25%	1.515	1.525	0.66%	1.464	1.422	−2.87%
0.291	1.441	1.431	−0.69%	1.510	1.461	−3.25%	1.441	1.431	−0.69%
0.416	1.408	1.373	−2.49%	1.500	1.476	−1.60%	1.408	1.373	−2.49%
0.917	1.274	1.216	−4.55%	1.425	1.373	−3.65%	–	–	–
1.291	1.173	1.128	−3.84%	1.328	1.265	−4.74%	–	–	–
1.709	1.062	1.039	−2.17%	1.183	1.137	−3.89%	–	–	–
2.083	0.961	0.922	−4.06%	–	–	–	–	–	–
2.500	0.850	0.833	−2.00%	–	–	–	–	–	–
2.917	0.738	0.726	−1.63%	–	–	–	–	–	–

inversion of the elastic wave equation [36]. In estimating phase speed of the shear wave, a very good signal-to-noise ratio (SNR) is required [37]. In the wave equation inversion, the assumption of tissue homogeneity is violated at tissue interfaces, where shear wave reflection at structural interfaces may lead to incorrect speed estimates [38, 39]. Besides, calculation of the spatial-temporal derivatives of the displacements in the inversion algorithm also requires very low noise [40]. The use of USWI combined with a directional filter based technique in this study is motivated by the above perspectives. We expect our method, without elasticity map reconstruction, to be relatively more robust against noise and suitable for delineation of boundary. It is also expected to be computationally faster. Our method, if proved to possess these merits in future studies, even through technical improvements, could potentially be very useful for the in vivo applications. In this paper, we aim to present this method and conduct a preliminary study simulating its use for the detection and delineation of the liver crack.

The generation and propagation of the shear wave in a liver medium with a crack was simulated using a FE method. Numerical simulation suggests that the presence of the crack largely affects the propagation of the shear wave, and reflection of the shear wave at the crack is clearly observed. Despite the crack thickness to be nearly 1/10 of the shear wavelength, little shear wave can pass through the crack and propagate on the other side of the crack. This explains in part why only the near-end edge of the 1.6 mm thick crack is detected in the study. Under such circumstance, in order to detect the far-end boundary, one may move the ultrasound probe to the other side of the crack. As the crack becomes even thinner, a larger proportion of the shear wave will be transmitted through the crack, and the far-end edge of the crack may be detected. However, it may not be necessary to show whether the far-end edge of the crack is detected or not, because, as shown in Fig. 8c for the slimmer crack, as long as the near-end edge is detected, the far-end edge should be just by its left side.

To simulate the USWI method for the detection and localization of the liver crack in silico, the ultrasound RF signal synthesis and 2-D speckle tracking algorithm are used. In this study, the 2-D PSF used to synthesize the 2-D ultrasound RF signal closely mimics a typical commercially available linear probe. The configurations and algorithms for RF signal synthesis and ultrasonic tracking of displaced scatterers are designed to best exploit the shear wave phenomena for better detection and delineation of the crack in liver tissue. 2-D correlation-based speckle tracking is a widely used technique for elasticity imaging studies [20, 41–43]. Different from the techniques based on the signal amplitude which require numerical interpolations, the speckle tracking method used in this study is phase-sensitive. In the literature [44], it was suggested that a small weighted correlation kernel and correlation filter can be used to reduce displacement variance while retaining high spatial resolution. Therefore, for the tissue displacement estimation, we apply correlation kernels that are of the order of the autocorrelation width of the ultrasound signal, along with correlation functions filtering to suppress the errors in the displacement estimation and produce high spatial resolution.

It was observed that the accumulated reflected wave amplitude in Fig. 5a is less than that in Fig. 5c. We surmise that this discrepancy arises from underestimation of the tissue motion caused by correlation-based speckle tracking and resulting shearing under the PSF [45, 46]. The detected crack length using speckle tracking is 96. 6% of the given crack length for the crack that is 3.2 cm in depth. We expect that the detected crack length is slightly shorter than the actual one, because the introduction of the scatterers results in a portion of the sound energy being scattered, which reduces the sensitivity of imaging. Increasing frequency may increase the sensitivity, but the image may become noisier.

Comparing the edge detection results using speckle tracking and FE simulation, the introduction of the speckle limits the accuracy of depicting the near-end boundary location, even for a fully developed speckle field. The detected locations using speckle tracking and FE simulation are on the left side of the given location of the crack's right edge, and we think that it may be because there are still shear waves travelling through this edge into the crack which makes this interface not absolutely "hard" for wave reflection. In this study, the "Sobel" edge detection operator is used; if a more complex edge is to be detected, a more advanced contour extraction algorithm [47, 48] may be needed.

In terms of major findings, the curved crack and the slimmer crack are generally consistent with the straight crack. The contour of the curved crack can also be well delineated with the directional filter method. The slimmer crack that is 0.5 cm in depth and 0.5 mm thick can be detected too. Owing to its size and location that is close to the upper surface, larger errors are yielded in the height estimation. Relative errors of right edge detection for all the cracks are within 5%. Despite that our method proved the capability in capturing small structures like the 0.5 mm thick crack, more studies are needed to further suppress the artefacts in the background.For analyzing convenience, a plane wave model is used for the shear wave in this study. A more realistic simulation would generate a shear wave with a typical Mach cone-shaped acoustic radiation force impulse push. Nevertheless, the results obtained here indicate that although compared with an ideal homogeneous medium, variance in the displacement estimate using USWI in a scattering medium gives a larger error in the crack detection, USWI combined with directional filter based method seems to be a feasible and promising tool for localizing and depicting the liver crack.

As a pilot study, the circumstances considered here are that of the simplest case. Further studies will be necessary to understand the detection of cracks in more complex situations. It is reported that the sensitivity of FAST is higher (88–98%) for injuries of grade III or higher [3, 49]. Therefore, we focus on first studying our method for detecting hepatic lesions that are grade I through III which might be overlooked by FAST. We hope that our method will prove useful in the future, helping emergency clinicians and physicians detect subtle injuries or associated injuries that might be missed in the hepatic trauma setting. According to the American Association for the Surgery of Trauma (AAST), for liver trauma classification, laceration in grade I has capsular tear < 1 cm deep, laceration in grade II has capsular tear 1–3 cm deep, < 10 cm long, and laceration in grade III is > 3 cm deep. The straight crack, the curved crack, and the slimmer crack in this study should be classified as grade III, II, I, respectively. Despite that in clinical scenarios, size and location of the laceration do not have a necessary connection with the severity extent of the liver trauma, we feel that it is necessary to clarify the target of our model.

The three different cracks studied in this paper are all superficial lacerations, which indicate that there is capsular tear occurring for all three cases. As a preliminary study, hematoma is not considered in this paper. In fact, lacerations of liver trauma usually accompany perihepatic or subcapsular or intrahepatic hematoma, especially when the laceration is large. We will incorporate hematoma into our model and further investigate the robustness of our method in future work. Based on studies in Ref. [50], for imaging liver with ultrasound shear wave based method, the operator should verify that the region of interest (ROI) box is free of vascular structures. Properly placing the 2-D ROI box within liver parenchyma is critical for accurate detection of the crack, and it is important to make the size and position of the 2-D ROI box user adjustable. The reflection, the pulsatility, and the increased stiffness of the hepatic vessel wall will lead to measurement bias and variability.

Ref. [51] and Ref. [52] reported that in the clinical applications of shear wave elastography to liver stiffness assessment, ROI located 1–2 cm (or about 1.5–2 cm) below the liver capsule gives the most reliable result. In this paper, we observed the effect of the upper surface on the detection; however, because liver capsule is not modelled in the current study, the influence of the liver capsule on the detection of crack with our method is unknown. It would be interesting to incorporate the liver capsule and other possible interfaces (hepatic veins, two cracks, etc.) into our model and study their effects on the propagation patterns of shear waves and crack detection. It is important to constantly reduce problems that affect quality of imaging and detection, so that a wide exploitation of ultrasound shear wave based techniques will be enabled for new diagnostic applications such as in liver trauma. A multi-directional filter seems to be particularly effective in handling propagation in multiple directions, and different techniques [53, 54] may help improve shear wave motion detection and image processing for better extraction of the crack. It would be also interesting to develop abilities to identify, quantify, and stratify traumatic damage to the liver by area and severity. Technical methods for orientation analysis and damage severity sorting based on automated edge detection [55] are potentially useful for hepatic crack evaluation.

Our future work will also involve in vitro and ex vivo studies for liver crack detection with USWI combined with the directional filter based method. The ultimate goal is to develop USWI based techniques to be a preferred tool in detecting traumatic hepatic injury and delineating the injured site, and use it for additional confirmatory evaluation in an Emergency room or as a supplemental diagnostic tool in the diagnosis of hepatic trauma to be implemented by a bedside ultrasound imaging system. Despite that the clinical feasibility is too early to be known and yet to be proven, the current study should move USWI based technique closer toward the goal for such applications.

Conclusion

In this study, we conduct an in silico simulation of liver crack detection and delineation using ultrasonic shear wave imaging (USWI). The generation and propagation of a shear wave in a liver tissue medium having a crack is simulated using FE model. Ultrasound radio-frequency (RF) signal synthesis and a 2-D speckle tracking algorithm are then applied to simulate the actual USWI in a medium with randomly distributed scatterers. We present a method that applies a directional filter and edge detection algorithm solely without recovering the elasticity map for the detection of the crack, and with our method, the near-end edge of the crack can be well localized. For a crack with a thickness of 1.6 mm (about 1/10 of shear wavelength), we found that little shear wave can pass through it and as a result the far-end edge of the crack cannot be detected. The detected crack length using USWI is slightly shorter than the actual crack length. We test our method for cracks with varied sizes and locations, and the near end edge of the crack can be detected and delineated, with an error within 5%. The robustness of our method for the detection and localization of the crack is demonstrated in a curved crack and a subtle crack of 0.5 mm thickness.

Despite the various limitations in this study, to the authors' knowledge, no other study has yet been reported, which has attempted to detect and delineate a hepatic laceration in traumatic liver injuries by using ultrasound shear wave imaging based techniques. The in silico study presented in this paper provides a basis for more advanced crack detection studies in a tissue phantom or liver.

Abbreviations

2-D: Two-dimensional; AAST: American Association for the Surgery of Trauma; CT: Computed tomography; DPL: Diagnostic peritoneal lavage; FAST: Focused assessment with sonography for trauma; FE: Finite element; PSF: Point spread function; RF: Radio-frequency; ROI: Region of interest; SNR: Signal-to-noise ratio; USWI: Ultrasonic shear wave imaging

Funding

This work was supported by the National Natural Science Foundation of China (Grant No. 11304137) and the Program for Liaoning Excellent Talents in University (Grant No. LJQ2013042).

Authors' contributions

EN performed the in silico study and drafted the manuscript. JY revised the manuscript critically and gave final approval of the version to be published. DD provided support on the forward/reverse directional filter and took part in interpretation of the imaging results. YZ participated in the design of the study and conducted the data analysis. All authors read and approved the final manuscript.

Competing interests

The authors declare that they have no competing interests.

Author details

[1]College of Information and Control Engineering, Liaoning Shihua University, Fushun, People's Republic of China. [2]College of Science, Liaoning Shihua University, Fushun, People's Republic of China. [3]Sensing and Computer Vision, Union Pacific Railroad, Omaha, USA.

References

1. Piper GL, Peitzman AB. Current management of hepatic trauma. Surg Clin N Am. 2010;90:775–85.
2. Chien LC, Lo SS, Yeh SY. Incidence of liver trauma and relative risk factors for mortality: a population-based study. J Chin Med Assoc. 2013;76:576–82.
3. Ali Nawaz Khan. Liver Trauma Imaging. 2017. https://emedicine.medscape.com/article/370508-overview. Accessed 23 Jan 2018.
4. Eric L Legome. Blunt Abdominal Trauma 2017. https://emedicine.medscape.com/article/1980980-overview. Accessed 23 Jan 2018.
5. Ali Nawaz Khan. Ultrasonography. 2017. https://emedicine.medscape.com/article/370508-overview#a5. Accessed 23 Jan 2018.
6. Ophir J, Céspedes I, Ponnekanti H, Yazdi Y, Elastography LX. A quantitative method for imaging the elasticity of biological tissues. Ultrason Imaging. 1991;13:111–34.
7. Sarvazyan AP, Skovoroda AR. The new approaches in ultrasonic visualization of cancers and their qualitative mechanical characterization for the differential diagnostics. In: Abstract of the all-union conference "the actual problems of the cancer ultrasonic diagnostics," Moscow; 1990.
8. Natarajan B, Gupta PK, Cemaj S, Sorensen M, Hatzoudis GI, Forse RAFAST. Scan: is it worth doing in hemodynamically stable blunt trauma patients? Surgery. 2010;148:695–701.
9. He L, Guo Y, Lee WN. Systematic performance evaluation of a cross-correlation-based ultrasound strain imaging method. Ultrasound Med Biol. 2016;42:2436–56.
10. Chen S, Urban MW, Greenleaf JF, Zheng Y, Yao A. Quantification of liver stiffness and viscosity with SDUV: in vivo animal study. In: 2008 IEEE Ultrasonics symposium (IUS); 2008. p. 654–7.
11. Wang MH, Palmeri ML, Rotemberg VM, Rouze NC, Nightingale KR. Improving the robustness of time-of-flight based shear wave speed reconstruction methods using RANSAC in human liver in vivo. Ultrasound Med Biol. 2010;36:802–13.
12. Palmeri ML, Wang MH, Dahl JJ, Frinkley KD, Nightingale KR. Quantifying hepatic shear modulus in vivo using acoustic radiation force. Ultrasound Med Biol. 2008;34:546–58.
13. Fedosov DA, Pan W, Caswell B, Gompper G, Karniadakis GE. Predicting human blood viscosity in silico. Proc Natl Acad Sci. 2011;108:11772–7.
14. Xu J, Tripathy S, Rubin JM, Stidham RW, Johnson LA, Higgins PDR, Kim K. A new nonlinear parameter in the developed strain-to-applied strain of the soft tissues and its application in ultrasound elasticity imaging. Ultrasound Med Biol. 2012;38:511–23.
15. Maurice RL, Bertrand M. Speckle-motion artifact under tissue shearing. IEEE Trans Ultrason Ferroelectr Freq Control. 1999;46:584–94.
16. Shao J, Wang J, Zhang Y, Cui L, Liu K, Bai J. Subtraction elastography for the evaluation of ablation-induced lesions: a feasibility study. IEEE Trans Ultrason Ferroelectr Freq Control. 2009;56:44–54.
17. Wagner RF, Smith SW, Sandrik JM, Lopez H. Statistics of speckle in ultrasound B-scans. IEEE Trans Sonics Ultrason. 1983;30:156–63.
18. Mcaleavey SA, Osapoetra LO, Langdon J. Shear wave arrival time estimates correlate with local speckle pattern. IEEE Trans Ultrason Ferroelectr Freq Control. 2015;62:2054–67.
19. Goodman JW, Narducci LM. Statistical optics. Phys Today. 1986;39:126.
20. Lubinski MA, Emelianov SY, O'Donnell M. Speckle tracking methods for ultrasonic elasticity imaging using short-time correlation. IEEE Trans Ultrason Ferroelectr Freq Control. 1999;46:82–96.
21. Kim K, Johnson LA, Jia C, Joyce JC, Rangwalla S, Higgins PDR, Rubin JM. Noninvasive ultrasound elasticity imaging (UEI) of Crohn's disease: animal model. Ultrasound Med Biol. 2008;34:902–12.
22. Manduca A, Lake DS, Kruse SA, Ehman RL. Spatio-temporal directional filtering for improved inversion of MR elastography images. Med Image Anal. 2002;7:465–73.
23. Deffieux T, Gennisson JL, Bercoff J, Tanter M. On the effects of reflected waves in transient shear wave elastography. IEEE Trans Ultrason Ferroelectr Freq Control. 2011;58:2032–5.
24. Deffieux T, Gennisson JL, Larrat B, Fink M, Tanter M. The variance of quantitative estimates in shear wave imaging: theory and experiments. IEEE Trans Ultrason Ferroelectr Freq Control. 2012;59:2390–410.
25. Mercado KP, Langdon J, Helguera M, McAleavey SA, Hocking DC, Dalecki D. Scholte wave generation during single tracking location shear wave elasticity imaging of engineered tissues. J Acoust Soc Am. 2015;138:138–44.
26. Coccolini F, Montori G, Catena F, Di Saverio S, Biffl W, Moore EE, Peitzman AB, Rizoli S, Tugnoli G, Sartelli M, Manfredi R, Ansaloni L. Liver trauma: WSES position paper. World J Emerg Surg. 2015;10:39.
27. Savatmongkorngul S, Wongwaisayawan S, Kaewlai R. Focused assessment with sonography for trauma: current perspectives. Open Access Emerg Med. 2017;9:57–62.
28. McGahan JP, Wang L, Richards JR. From the RSNA refresher courses: focused abdominal US for trauma. Radiographics. 2001;21(Spec Issue):S191–9.
29. Karim Brohi. Focused Assessment with Sonography for Trauma (FAST). 2006. http://trauma.org/index.php/main/article/214/ Accessed 23 Jan 2018.
30. Rudenko OV, Sarvazyan AP, Emelianov SY. Acoustic radiation force and streaming induced by focused nonlinear ultrasound in a dissipative medium. J Acoust Soc Am. 1996;99:2791–8.
31. Sarvazyan AP, Rudenko OV, Swanson SD, Fowlkes JB, Emelianov SY. Shear wave elasticity imaging: a new ultrasonic technology of medical diagnostics. Ultrasound Med Biol. 1998;24:1419–35.
32. Athanasiou A, Tardivon A, Tanter M, Sigal-Zafrani B, Bercoff J, Deffieux T, Gennisson JL, Fink M, Neuenschwander S. Breast lesions: quantitative elastography with supersonic shear imaging—preliminary results. Radiology. 2010;256:297–303.
33. Bavu E, Gennisson JL, Mallet V. Supersonic shear imaging is a new potent morphological non-invasive technique to assess liver fibrosis. Part 1: technical feasibility. Hepatology. 2010;52(Suppl):S166.
34. Wu R, Luo Y, Lv F, Tang J, Liu Q, Jiao Z. Evaluation of liver trauma after haemostatic injection by shear wave elastography: an experimental study. Chin J Med Ultrasound. 2011;8:1914–21.
35. Wu R, Luo Y, Lv F, Tang J, Liu Q, Jiao Z. An animal experiment of real-time shear wave elastography in diagnosing acute liver trauma. Chin J Med Ultrasound. 2012;20:294–7.
36. Baghani A, Salcudean S, Rohling R. Theoretical limitations of the elastic wave equation inversion for tissue elastography. J Acoust Soc Am. 2009;126:1541–51.

37. Deffieux T, Montaldo G, Tanter M, Fink M. Shear wave spectroscopy for in vivo quantification of human soft tissues visco-elasticity. IEEE Trans Med Imaging. 2009;28:313–22.
38. Sigrist RMS, Liau J, Kaffas AE, Chammas MC, Willmann JK. Ultrasound elastography: review of techniques and clinical applications. Theranostics. 2017;7:1303–29.
39. Shiina T, Nightingale KR, Palmeri ML, Hall TJ, Bamber JC, Barr RG, et al. WFUMB guidelines and recommendations for clinical use of ultrasound elastography: part 1: basic principles and terminology. Ultrasound Med Biol. 2015;41:1126–47.
40. Park E. Finite element formulation for shear modulus reconstruction in transient elastography. Inverse Probl Sci En. 2009;17:605–26.
41. Lubinski MA, Emelianov SY, Raghavan KR, Yagle AE, Skovoroda AR, O'Donnell M. Lateral displacement estimation using tissue incompressibility. IEEE Trans Ultrason Ferroelectr Freq Control. 1996;43:247–56.
42. Konofagou E, Ophir JA. New elastographic method for estimation and imaging of lateral displacements, lateral strains, corrected axial strains and Poisson's ratios in tissues. Ultrasound Med Biol. 1998;24:1183–99.
43. Chaturvedi P, Insana MF, Hall TJ. 2-D companding for noise reduction in strain imaging. IEEE Trans Ultrason Ferroelectr Freq Control. 1998;45:179–91.
44. Nishi T, Funabashi N, Ozawa K, Takahara M, Fujimoto Y, Kamata T, Kobayashi Y. Resting multilayer 2D speckle-tracking transthoracic echocardiography for the detection of clinically stable myocardial ischemic segments confirmed by invasive fractional flow reserve. Part 1: vessel-by-vessel analysis. Int J Cardiol. 2016;218:324–32.
45. Palmeri ML, Sharma AC, Bouchard RR, Nightingale RW, Nightingale KRA. Finite-element method model of soft tissue response to impulsive acoustic radiation force. IEEE Trans Ultrason Ferroelectr Freq Control. 2005;52:1699–712.
46. Mcaleavey SA, Nightingale KR, Trahey GE. Estimates of echo correlation and measurement bias in acoustic radiation force impulse imaging. IEEE Trans Ultrason Ferroelectr Freq Control. 2003;50:631–41.
47. Wang Y, Zhang Q, Luo S. Image tracking method based on fractal-geometry edge extraction. J Appl Optics. 2005;34:S258.
48. Xu P, Li D, Cui X. Qin G. Infrared image edge extraction based on the lateral inhibition network and a new denoising method. In: 2012 international conference on modelling. Identification & Control (ICMIC). 2012:774–8. https://ieeexplore.ieee.org/document/6260200/citations.
49. Adedipe AA, Backlund BH, Basler E, Shah S. Accuracy of the fast exam: a retrospective analysis of blunt abdominal trauma patients. Open Access Emerg Med. 2016;06:1000308.
50. Bruce M, Kolokythas O, Ferraioli G, Filice C, Limitations O'DM. Artifacts in shear-wave elastography of the liver. Biomed Eng Lett. 2017;7:1–9.
51. Wang C, Zheng J, Huang Z, Xiao Y, Song D, Zeng J, Zheng H, Zheng R. Influence of measurement depth on the stiffness assessment of healthy liver with real-time shear wave elastography. Ultrasound Med Biol. 2014;40:461–9.
52. Ferraioli G, Tinelli C, Zicchetti M, Above E, Poma G, Gregorio MD, Filice C. Reproducibility of real-time shear wave elastography in the evaluation of liver elasticity. Eur J Radiol. 2012;81:3102–6.
53. He XN, Diao XF, Lin HM, Zhang XY, Shen YY, Chen SP, Qin ZD, Chen X. Improved shear wave motion detection using coded excitation for transient elastography. Sci Rep. 2017;7:44483.
54. Giachetti A, Zanetti G. Vascular modeling from volumetric diagnostic data: a review. Curr Med Imaging Rev. 2006;2:415–23.
55. Ros SJ, Andarawis-Puri N, Flatow EL. Tendon extracellular matrix damage detection and quantification using automated edge detection analysis. J Biomech. 2013;46:2844–7.

17

Value of flaccid penile ultrasound in screening for arteriogenic impotence

Li-Da Chen[1], Fu-Shun Pan[1], Lu-Yao Zhou[1], Yu-Bo Liu[2], Jian-Yao Lv[1], Ming Xu[1], Xiao-Yan Xie[1], Ming-De Lu[1,3], Zhu Wang[1*] and Wei Wang[1*]

Abstract

Background: This prospective study is to evaluate the potential value of sonographic measurements in the flaccid penis for the screening of arteriogenic impotence.

Methods: A consecutive series of 260 Chinese males consulting for sexual dysfunction and 54 controls underwent sonographic examination. The sonographic parameters were correlated with the clinical gold standards, including the international index of erectile function (IIEF) and penile erectile hardness grading scale (EHGS). The sensitivity, specificity, positive predictive value (PPV), negative predictive value (NPV) and area under the receiver operating characteristic curve (AUROC) of flaccid peak systolic velocity (PSV) in predicting patients with normal function were analyzed.

Results: The mean cavernous PSV of both sides in the patients with sexual dysfunction ranged from 7.76 to 11.12 cm/sec with a stepwise increase in IIEF and EHGS grading scale ($P < .05$). The cutoff value of flaccid PSV for the differential diagnosis of grade 4 of IIEF-5 or EHGS was 8.20–8.90 cm/sec, with an AUROC of 0.657–0.724, specificity of 82.96–86.84% and PPV of 95.20–96.60%, respectively.

Conclusions: This simple flaccid PSV measurement is a specific tool for screening arteriogenic impotence.

Keywords: Erectile dysfunction, Ultrasound, Peak systolic velocity, Receiver operating characteristic, International index of erectile function, Erectile hardness grading scale

Background

Erectile dysfunction (ED) is a common worldwide and potentially treatable problem with an incidence of 50% in the general male population aged between 40 and 70 years [1]. In addition to psychological and metabolic factors and relational problems, arteriogenic causes play important roles in erectile dysfunction [2–4]. Changes in any one of these factors may result in ED.

For diagnosis of arteriogenic causes, color Doppler ultrasound is one of the most noninvasive, simple and promising tools [1–3, 5–8]. The peak systolic velocity (PSV) of the cavernous artery measured after the intra-cavernous injection (ICI) of vasoactive agents is a widely accepted criterion for evaluating penile circulation [2, 6]. A post-ICI PSV value less than 25 cm/sec is recognized as a severely insufficient arterial supply [2, 5]. However, the clinical adaptability of this method is relatively limited because of the time consuming, lack of standardization, and side effects due to vasoactive agents [2]. Currently, a growing number of male are anxious about their sexual lives. A simple parameter for evaluating penile arteriogenic health, with limited costs in terms of time and money and without the inconvenience of priapism, is an ideal goal. Therefore, post-ICI PSV is not an optimal method of screening for arteriogenic impotence.

Doppler investigation in the flaccid state would avoid these disadvantages. It has been reported that PSV values that were measured in the flaccid state show a significant correlation with post-ICI PSV and might be

* Correspondence: wangzhu@mail.sysu.edu.cn; wangw73@mail.sysu.edu.cn
[1]Department of Medical Ultrasonics, Institute of Diagnostic and Interventional Ultrasound, The First Affiliated Hospital of Sun Yat-Sen University, 58 Zhongshan Road 2, Guangzhou 510080, People's Republic of China
Full list of author information is available at the end of the article

predictive in the determination of arterial insufficiency [2, 7, 9]. However, these studies all used the PSV measured in the flaccid state as an additional tool to evaluate penile circulation. In our opinion, the evaluation of PSV in the flaccid penis alone for screening arteriogenic impotence remains underestimated. It has been reported that flaccid PSV in the general population is above 13 cm/sec for Europeans [2], but no data about Chinese population has been reported.

In this prospective study, we tried to evaluate the potential value of ultrasound (US) parameters measured in the flaccid state for the diagnosis of arteriogenic impotence, correlated with the international index of erectile function (IIEF) and penile erectile hardness grading scale (EHGS) [10–12].

Methods

Patients population

This prospective study was approved by the research ethics board of our institution, and informed consent was obtained. Participants recruited from our hospital consented to receive this noninvasive US examination, and this aspect of the study was approved by the Ethical Committee of the First Affiliated Hospital of Sun Yat-Sen University as IRB_2011 [168] entitled "Assessment of cavernous endothelial dysfunction in patients consulting for sexual dysfunction". From October 2014 to October 2016, a consecutive series of 310 Chinese male patients consulting for sexual dysfunction were referred. Among them, 6 patients declined the US examination. Another 44 patients were excluded if (a) US data were not collected according to the standard protocol ($n = 25$), (b) no reference standard was obtained ($n = 13$), or (c) clinical or US data were missing ($n = 6$).The remaining 260 eligible patients underwent color Doppler sonographic examination. Fifty-four healthy adult volunteers who did not have a history of sexual dysfunction were examined by US and served as a control group for which the same US parameters were obtained. No volunteers had taken any medication or drugs at the time of the US examination. The mean ages of the two groups were 32.9 ± 8.3 years (range 19–72 years) and 29.9 ± 8.9 years (range 19–40 years), respectively ($P = 0.200$). All patients were in a stable monogamous relationship with a female partner and had made at least one attempt at sexual intercourse over the last 8 weeks. All patients underwent an erectile dysfunction evaluation that included IIEF-5 and EHGS.

US examination

All patients in each group were examined using an Aplio XV or 500 (Toshiba Medical Systems, Tokyo, Japan) or Mylab Twice (Esaote Medical Systems, Genoa, Italy) by three operators (W.W., Z. W., L.Y Z.). To ensure patient privacy, all exams were performed in a quiet, comfortable room. Excessive compression with the transducer was avoided. First, in grayscale US, the penis was evaluated in both the longitudinal and transverse planes in the flaccid state. Then, color Doppler sonography was optimized to obtain the best longitudinal plane of the cavernosal arteries. In this longitudinal plane, spectral analysis of the cavernosal arteries was performed in the proximal part of the penis. The optimal site for spectral analysis was the proximal part of the cavernosal arteries where the vessels curved. This location allowed an angle of insonation as low as < 30° for accurate angle-corrected velocity calculations. The PSV, resistance index (RI) and diameters of both cavernosal arteries were recorded. When analyzing the spectral Doppler, the optimized pulse repetition frequency and wall filter were selected, and the width of the Doppler sample size was set at 0.5 mm - 1 mm. Three consecutive similar waveforms were considered to constitute a satisfactory test.

IIEF-5 and EHGS

The IIEF-5, a 5-item questionnaire, is used for clinical diagnosis of the severity of ED, including scores on the 5-item form (that is, Erection confidence, Penetration ability, Maintenance frequency, Maintenance ability, Intercourse satisfaction) [12]. These items focus on erectile function and intercourse satisfaction. This tool has become the 'gold standard' for the clinical evaluation of therapy efficacy. The degree of ED is classified as follows: grade1 = severe ED (scores between 5 and 7), grade2 = mild ED (scores between 8 and 11), grade 3 = moderate ED (scores between 12 and 21), grade 4 = no ED (scores between 22 and 25).

The erection hardness grading scale (EHGS) was developed in 1998 by Goldstein et al. [11]. It is a convenient, four-grade scale for ED that provides a reliable measure of the degree and duration of penile rigidity, according to data reported at the European Association of Urology. The erection hardness of the penis is graded according to the EHGS as follows: grade 1 = increased in size without hardness, grade 2 = hard but not hard enough for penetration, grade 3 = hard enough for penetration but not completely hard, and grade 4 = completely hard and fully rigid.

Statistical analysis

The data were expressed as the mean ± SD or median and inter-quartile range (IQR), as appropriate. The chi-square test or Fisher's exact test was used to evaluate the difference between the IIEF-5 and EHGS groups in PSV, diameter and RI. Receiver operating characteristic (ROC) curves were compared to evaluate the diagnostic performance of PSV using the MedCalc version 9.0 software (MedCalc Software, Mariakerke, Belgium). The

Table 1 IIEF-5 and EHGS findings, Cavernous PSV, Diameter and RI Measurements in Patients with ED

Parameters	No. of Patients	Left Cavernous Artery							Right Cavernous Artery						
		PSV(cm/s)		Diameter(mm)		RI			PSV(cm/s)		Diameter(mm)		RI		
		Mean ± SD	*P** Value	Mean ± SD	*P** Value	Median(Mean ± SD)		*P** Value	Mean ± SD	*P** Value	Mean ± SD	*P** Value	Median(Mean ± SD)		*P** Value
IIEF-5			0.025		0.142			0.528		0.012		0.307			0.174
1	57	7.87 ± 3.44		0.50 ± 0.16		1.00	0.93 ± 0.20		7.76 ± 3.18		0.49 ± 0.17		1.00	0.93 ± 0.20	
2	48	8.56 ± 4.14		0.49 ± 0.16		1.00	0.92 ± 0.22		7.81 ± 4.01		0.46 ± 0.18		1.00	0.92 ± 0.22	
3	135	8.86 ± 3.75		0.53 ± 0.16		1.00	0.97 ± 0.13		8.46 ± 3.97		0.50 ± 0.16		1.00	0.96 ± 0.16	
4	20	10.82 ± 3.29		0.58 ± 0.18		1.00	0.97 ± 0.08		10.82 ± 2.79		0.54 ± 0.15		1.00	0.99 ± 0.03	
EHGS			0.004		0.172			0.073		0.001		0.093			0.197
1	11	8.68 ± 3.53		0.58 ± 0.13		1.00	0.99 ± 0.04		8.85 ± 2.75		0.59 ± 0.19		1.00	1.00 ± 0.00	
2	79	7.70 ± 3.58		0.49 ± 0.16		1.00	0.91 ± 0.23		7.43 ± 3.54		0.48 ± 0.17		1.00	0.92 ± 0.23	
3	148	9.00 ± 3.88		0.52 ± 0.16		1.00	0.97 ± 0.13		8.42 ± 3.90		0.49 ± 0.16		1.00	0.96 ± 0.16	
4	22	10.79 ± 2.84		0.56 ± 0.18		1.00	0.96 ± 0.08		11.12 ± 3.20		0.54 ± 0.13		1.00	0.99 ± 0.04	

*Comparisons among IIEF-5 subgroups or EHGS subgroups were made by using the variance analysis

diagnostic performance was expressed as the area under the ROC curve (AUROC). The sensitivity, specificity, accuracy, positive predictive value (PPV) and negative predictive value (NPV) were calculated. Figures were drawn using the Origin 8.5 software (OriginLab, Northampton, MA, USA). $P < 0.05$ was considered to indicate statistical significance.

Results

Relationships between US parameters and IIEF-5 and EHGS

The IIEF-5 and EHGS of ED patients are shown in Table 1. The mean PSVs of both sides in the patients consulting for sexual dysfunction ranged from 7.76 to 11.12 cm/sec with a stepwise increase in IIEF and EHGS grading ($P < .05$) (Table 1, Fig. 1).Moreover, the differences between grade 4 of IIEF-5 or EHGS and other grades were significant (grade 1 vs. 4 in the left cavernous PSV, grade1 or 2 vs. 4 in the right cavernous PSV for IIEF-5; grade 2 vs. 4 in the left cavernous PSV, grade 2 or 3 vs. 4 in the right cavernous PSV for EHGS, all $P < .05$) (Fig. 1).

Diameter and RI in both sides of the cavernous artery showed no significant difference among different grades of IIEF-5 or EHGS (all $P > .05$), with a mean value of 0.48–0.58 mm for diameter and a median value of 1.00 for RI.

The flaccid PSV on both sides in the patients consulting for sexual dysfunctions with grade 4 of IIEF-5 or EHGS showed no statistically significant difference from the control group ($P > .05$) (Fig. 2).In the control group, 45/54 (83.3%) volunteers were classified as grade 4 of IIEF-5, and 48/54 (88.9%) were classified as grade 4 of EHGS.

Receiver operating characteristic curves

The AUROC for estimating the performance of flaccid PSV in the patients with no ED (grade 4 of IIEF-5, scores between 22 and 25) was 0.657 (cutoff value, 8.20 m/sec; sensitivity, 49.38%; specificity, 82.86%; PPV, 95.20%; NPV, 19.10%) for the left cavernous artery and 0.706 (cutoff value, 8.90 m/sec; sensitivity, 59.26%; specificity, 85.71%; PPV, 96.60%; NPV, 23.30%) for the right cavernous artery (Fig. 3, Table 2).

The AUROC for estimating the performance of flaccid PSV in the patients with grade 4 of EHGS (completely hard and fully rigid) was 0.679 (cutoff value, 8.20 m/sec; sensitivity, 50.42%; specificity, 86.84%; PPV, 96.00%; NPV, 21.70%) for the left cavernous artery and 0.724 (cutoff value, 8.70 m/sec; sensitivity, 58.33%; specificity, 86.84%; PPV, 96.60%; NPV, 24.80%) for the left cavernous artery (Fig. 3, Table 2).

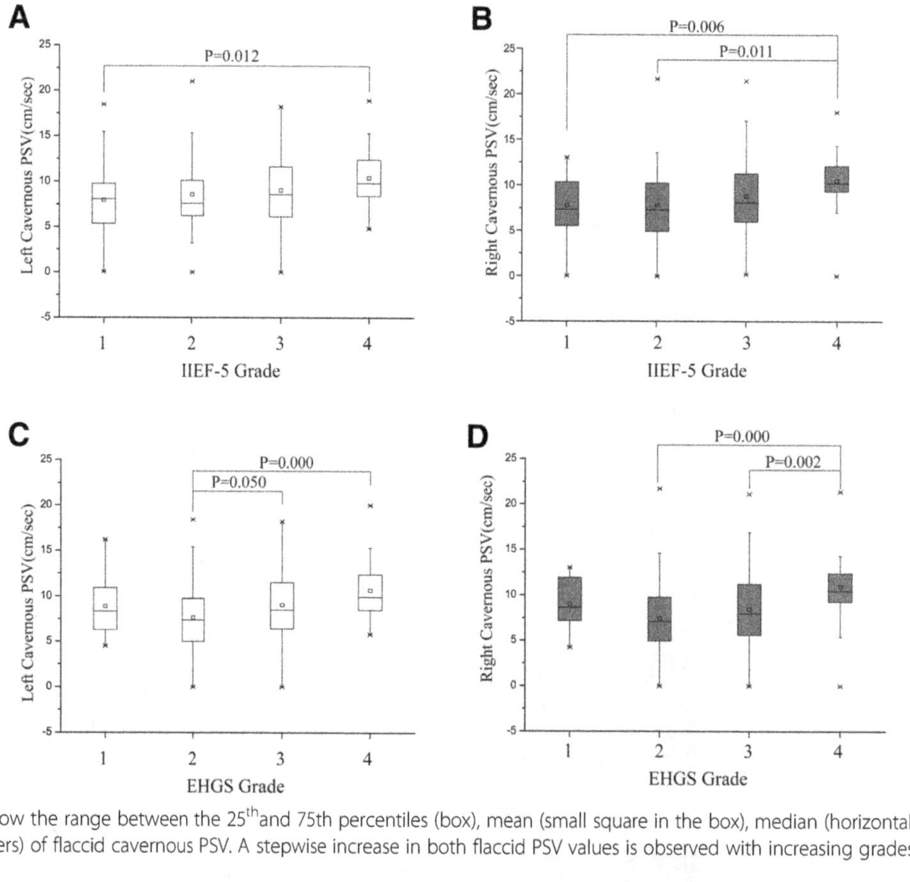

Fig. 1 Box plots show the range between the 25th and 75th percentiles (box), mean (small square in the box), median (horizontal line in the box), and outliers (whiskers) of flaccid cavernous PSV. A stepwise increase in both flaccid PSV values is observed with increasing grades of IIEF-5 or EHGS ($P < 0.05$)

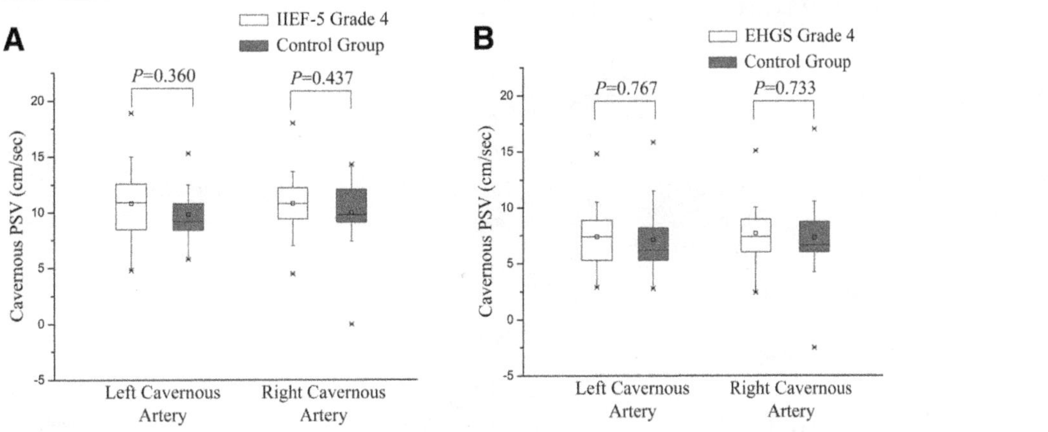

Fig. 2 Box plots show the range between the 25th and 75th percentiles (box), mean (small square in the box), median (horizontal line in the box), and outliers (whiskers) of flaccid cavernous PSV. PSV in the flaccid state in patients consulting for sexual dysfunctions with grade 4 of IIEF-5 or EHGS show no statistically significant difference from the control group ($P > .05$)

Discussion

This study was performed to determine the potential value of sonographic measurements in the flaccid penis for diagnosing arteriogenic impotence. Our prospective study demonstrated that flaccid PSV values were correlated with IIEF-5 and EHGS grading. The optimal cutoff for PSV is 8.2–8.9 cm/sec, which yielded a specificity and PPV of approximately 82–87 and 95%–97%, respectively.

The incidence of ED in adults is rapidly increasing [13]. Although there are complicating factors, arteriogenic impotence is among the most important cause of erectile dysfunction [14–16]. Color Doppler sonographic examination is a noteworthy diagnostic tool for detecting failure of the penile arterial supply [2, 5]. For patients consulting for sexual dysfunction, the most commonly used evaluation is Doppler investigation in conjunction with ICI of vasoactive substances. The proposed cutoff values of post-ICI PSV for arterial insufficiency range widely, from 25 to 40 cm/sec [2]. Meanwhile, Doppler investigation after ICI is a time-consuming technique. Psychological inhibition and anxiety during ICI may disturb the assessment of arterial supply [1].

Kahvecioglu et al. [7] had demonstrated that flow in the cavernosal arteries in the flaccid state could determine nondiabetic patients with vasculogenic impotence with a high accuracy rate. Furthermore, Corona et al. [2] found that flaccid PSV showed a significant ($r = 0.513$, $P < 0.0001$) correlation with post-ICI PSV, similar to that ($r = 0.477$) proposed by Mancini et al. [17]. They also concluded that flaccid PSV < 13 cm/s predicted reduced dynamic PSV with an accuracy greater than 80%, the cut off of which was higher than that previously reported by Sen et al. and Roy et al. [5, 6]. Those European reports had documented normal flaccid PSV values varied from 10 cm/s to 25 cm/s, but these results were not applicable for Asians. Furthermore, the utility of flaccid PSV alone had not been sufficiently studied. In our study, we aimed to test this easier method's correlation with the clinical

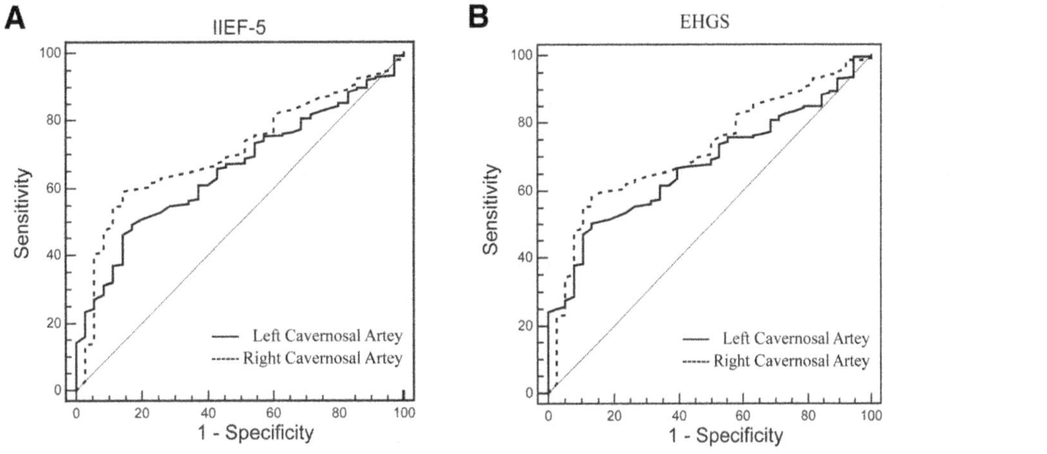

Fig. 3 Receiver operating characteristic curves for estimation of the performance of flaccid PSV in patients with grade 4 of IIEF-5 or EHGS

Table 2 Cavernous PSV Measurements for Determination of ED

Parameter	IIEF-5 Grade 1–3 vs. 4		EHGS Grade 1–3 vs. 4	
	Left Cavernous Artery	Right Cavernous Artery	Left Cavernous Artery	Right Cavernous Artery
Cutoff Value (cm/sec)	8.20	8.90	8.20	8.70
AUC	0.657	0.706	0.679	0.724
95% Confidence Interval	0.598 to 0.713	0.649 to 0.759	0.620 to 0.733	0.668 to 0.776
Sensitivity (%)	49.38	59.26	50.42	58.33
Specificity (%)	82.86	85.71	86.84	86.84
Positive Predictive Value (%)	95.20	96.60	96.00	96.60
Negative Predictive Value (%)	19.10	23.30	21.70	24.80

gold standard. The correlations between flow parameters and IIEF-5 or EHGS were evaluated. Only the PSV in both sides showed significant differences among the different IIEF-5 or EHGS groups. Furthermore, there was no difference between grade 4 of IIEF-5 or EHGS and the control group (all $P > 0.05$), which may indicate that for most patients consulting for sexual dysfunction in grade 4, arteriogenic impotence is a minimal factor.

Considering the patients consulting for sexual dysfunction and the controls as a whole, the ROC curve indicated that a threshold of 8.2–8.9 cm/sec should be chosen. The AUROC of PSV diagnosis was 0.657–0.724, the sensitivity was as low as 49.38%, the specificity was high at 82.96–86.84%, and the PPV values were 95.2–96.6%. The findings of the current study indicated that when the PSV cutoff was set at 8.2–8.9 cm/sec, it was possible to distinguish arteriogenic causes from psychological factors. We believe that this finding is of interest because a PSV of 8.2 cm/sec or lower could be recognized as associated with a higher risk of arteriogenic incompetence in the Chinese population. In this study, our data showed that the flaccid penile US evaluation has the potential to become a specific tool to diagnose arteriogenic impotence. Nonetheless, many other factors regulate sexual function in ED patients, which may explain the low sensitivity and NPV in this study.

One limitation of our study is that we did not include post-ICI PSV as a reference standard because of the complexity and invasiveness. We intended to explore the clinical importance of flaccid PSV for screening for arteriogenic impotence. It was suggested for high-risk patients as the first-line exam at the high PPV of 96%. However, flaccid penile Doppler is not sufficient for management decision making at a low sensitivity of 50 to 60%. Moreover, It has been reported that up to 47% of patients with a diagnosis of venous leakage by dynamic infusion cavernosometry showed completely normal hemodynamics [18, 19]. Repeated US exam with ICI was mandatory to exclude venous leakage [20]. Second, the mean age of the patients in our study was lower than the general mean age of patients with ED, which might be due to selection bias. The percentage of patients between 20 years and 39 years in our study is 80.8% (210/260). We infer that those men are in an active stage of their sexual life with higher expectations. Thus, they were more likely to seek help from doctors when they were included in our study.

Conclusion

In conclusion, our results show that flaccid PSV values correlate with IIEF-5 or EHGS grading in the Chinese population. The best flaccid PSV cutoff value was 8.2–8.9 cm/sec, with a specificity of 82.96–86.84% and PPV of 95.2–96.6%. This easily performed method has the potential to become a specific tool in screening for arteriogenic impotence.

Abbreviations

AUROC: Area under the receiver operating characteristic curve; ED: Erectile dysfunction; EHGS: Penile erectile hardness grading scale; ICI: Intra-cavernous injection; IIEF: International index of erectile function; IQR: Inter-quartile range; NPV: Negative predictive value; PPV: Positive predictive value; PSV: Peak systolic velocity; RI: Resistance index; ROC: Receiver operating characteristic; US: Ultrasound

Acknowledgements

Not applicable.

Funding

This study was funded by the National Nature Science Foundation of China (No: 81701719), the Guangdong Science and Technology Foundation (No: 2016A020215042 and 2016A030310143), and the Guangdong Medical Scientific Research Foundation (No: 201611610484333).

Authors' contributions

Conception and design: WW, WZ; Development of methodology: WW, CLD, WZ; Acquisition of data (e.g., collected patients, imaging performed): WW, WZ, PFS, ZLY, LYB, LJY, XM; Analysis and interpretation of data (e.g., computational analysis, statistical analysis): CLD, WZ, PFS; Editing and review of the manuscript: CLD, WW, LMD, XXY; Study supervision: WW, LMD. All authors read and approved the final manuscript.

Consent for publication
Not applicable.

Competing interests
The authors declare that they have no competing interests.

Author details
[1]Department of Medical Ultrasonics, Institute of Diagnostic and Interventional Ultrasound, The First Affiliated Hospital of Sun Yat-Sen University, 58 Zhongshan Road 2, Guangzhou 510080, People's Republic of China. [2]Department of Ultrasound, State Key Laboratory of Oncology in South China, Sun Yat-Sen University Cancer Center, Guangzhou, China. [3]Department of Hepatobiliary Surgery, The First Affiliated Hospital of Sun Yat-Sen University, Guangzhou, China.

References

1. Celermajer DS, Sorensen KE, Gooch VM, Spiegelhalter DJ, Miller OI, Sullivan ID, et al. Non-invasive detection of endothelial dysfunction in children and adults at risk of atherosclerosis. Lancet. 1992;340:1111–5.
2. Corona G, Fagioli G, Mannucci E, Romeo A, Rossi M, Lotti F, et al. Penile doppler ultrasound in patients with erectile dysfunction (ED): role of peak systolic velocity measured in the flaccid state in predicting arteriogenic ED and silent coronary artery disease. J Sex Med. 2008;5:2623–34.
3. Caretta N, Palego P, Schipilliti M, Ferlin A, Di Mambro A, Foresta C. Cavernous artery intima-media thickness: a new parameter in the diagnosis of vascular erectile dysfunction. J Sex Med. 2009;6:1117–26.
4. Corona G, Petrone L, Mannucci E, Magini A, Lotti F, Ricca V, et al. Assessment of the relational factor in male patients consulting for sexual dysfunction: the concept of couple sexual dysfunction. J Androl. 2006;27:795–801.
5. Roy C, Saussine C, Tuchmann C, Castel E, Lang H, Jacqmin D. Duplex Doppler sonography of the flaccid penis: potential role in the evaluation of impotence. J Clin Ultrasound. 2000;28:290–4.
6. Sen J, Godara R, Singh R, Airon RK. Colour Doppler sonography of flaccid penis in evaluation of erectile dysfunction. Asian J Surg. 2007;30:122–5.
7. Kahvecioglu N, Kurt A, Ipek A, Yazicioglu KR, Akbulut Z. Predictive value of cavernosal peak systolic velocity in the flaccid penis. Adv Med Sci. 2009;54: 233–8.
8. Grenier N. Color Doppler imaging of erectile dysfunction: a new place in strategy? Eur Radiol. 2002;12:2133–5.
9. Debora M, Daniele A, Alessandro B, Ferri C, Giuseppe M. The role of Doppler ultrasound in the diagnosis of vasculogenic impotence. Arch Ital Urol Androl. 2010;82:159–63.
10. Rosen RC, Riley A, Wagner G, Osterloh IH, Kirkpatrick J, Mishra A. The international index of erectile function (IIEF): a multidimensional scale for assessment of erectile dysfunction. Urology. 1997;49:822–30.
11. Goldstein I, Lue TF, Padma-Nathan H, Rosen RC, Steers WD, Wicker PA. Oral sildenafil in the treatment of erectile dysfunction. Sildenafil Study Group. N Engl J Med. 1998;338:1397–404.
12. Rosen RC, Cappelleri JC, Smith MD, Lipsky J, Pena BM. Development and evaluation of an abridged, 5-item version of the international index of erectile function (IIEF-5) as a diagnostic tool for erectile dysfunction. Int J Impot Res. 1999;11:319–26.
13. Uslu N, Gorgulu S, Alper AT, Eren M, Nurkalem Z, Yildirim A, et al. Erectile dysfunction as a generalized vascular dysfunction. J Am Soc Echocardiogr. 2006;19:341–6.
14. Kaya C, Uslu Z, Karaman I. Is endothelial function impaired in erectile dysfunction patients? Int J Impot Res. 2006;18:55–60.
15. Mazo E, Gamidov S, Anranovich S, Iremashvili V. Testing endothelial function of brachial and cavernous arteries in patients with erectile dysfunction. J Sex Med. 2006;3:323–30 discussion 30, author reply 30.
16. Schwartz BG, Economides C, Mayeda GS, Burstein S, Kloner RA. The endothelial cell in health and disease: its function, dysfunction, measurement and therapy. Int J Impot Res. 2010;22:77–90.
17. Mancini M, Bartolini M, Maggi M, Innocenti P, Villari N, Forti G. Duplex ultrasound evaluation of cavernosal peak systolic velocity and waveform acceleration in the penile flaccid state: clinical significance in the assessment of the arterial supply in patients with erectile dysfunction. Int J Androl. 2000;23:199–204.
18. Teloken PE, Park K, Parker M, Guhring P, Narus J, Mulhall JP. The false diagnosis of venous leak: prevalence and predictors. J Sex Med. 2011;8:2344–9.
19. Li L, Fan W, Li J, Li Q, Wang J, Fan Y, et al. Abnormal brain structure as a potential biomarker for venous erectile dysfunction: evidence from multimodal MRI and machine learning. Eur Radiol. 2018;28:3789–800.
20. Cavallini G, Maretti C. Unreliability of the duplex scan in diagnosing corporeal venous occlusive disease in young healthy men with erectile deficiency. Urology. 2018;113:91–8.

18

Microbubbles in macrocysts – Contrast-enhanced ultrasound assisted sclerosant therapy of a congenital macrocystic lymphangioma

Carlos Menendez-Castro*, Maren Zapke, Fabian Fahlbusch, Heiko von Goessel, Wolfgang Rascher and Jörg Jüngert

Abstract

Background: Congenital cystic lymphangiomas are benign malformations due to a developmental disorder of lymphatic vessels. Besides surgical excision, sclerosant therapy of these lesions by intracavitary injection of OK-432 (Picibanil®), a lyophilized mixture of group A Streptococcus pyogenes, is a common therapeutical option. For an appropriate application of OK-432, a detailed knowledge about the structure and composition of the congenital cystic lymphangioma is essential. SonoVue® is a commercially available contrast agent commonly used in sonography by intravenous and intracavitary application.

Case presentation: Here we report the case of 2 month old male patient with a large thoracic congenital cystic lymphangioma. Preinterventional imaging of the malformation was performed by contrast-enhanced ultrasound after intracavitary application of SonoVue® immediately followed by a successful sclerotherapy with OK-432.

Conclusions: Contrast agent-enhanced ultrasound imaging offers a valuable option to preinterventionally clarify the anatomic specifications of a congenital cystic lymphangioma in more detail than by single conventional sonography. By the exact knowledge about the composition and especially about the intercystic communications of the lymphangioma sclerosant therapy becomes safer and more efficient.

Keywords: Contrast agent-enhanced ultrasound, CEUS, Congenital cystic lymphangioma, SonoVue®, Sclerosant therapy, OK-432, Picibanil

Background

Congenital cystic lymphangioma (CCL) is defined as a congenital tumorous formation of lymphatic vessels. About 60% of all lymphangiomas occur at birth, 80–90% before the age of two years. The most frequent localization of CCL is the neck and head region [1]. The fact that the lesions usually have no spontaneous regression, tend to augment in size and can cause life-threatening complications such as occlusion or infiltration of neighbouring organs and structures, underlines the need of an early adequate therapy of lymphangiomas. Surgical excision used to be the first-line treatment of macrocystic lymphangiomas. However, complete excision often is not possible. If the tumor is excised only partially, the recurrence rate is significantly increased [2].

Sclerosant therapy is an alternative to surgical excision, especially in the case of macrocystic lymphangiomas with communicating cysts. Among the different sclerosant agents, OK-432 (Picibanil®) has become the favorite preparation since no perilesional fibrosis occurs after treatment [3]. It is a lyophilized mixture of group A Streptococcus pyogenes cells, which were preincubated with Penicillin G. The efficacy of lymphangioma sclerosant therapy with OK-432 in children has been proven by several clinical studies [3].

Before the injection of OK-432, conventional sonography is required to depict localization, size and structure of the tumor. But one crucial characteristic of CCL, the communication between the cysts, cannot be

* Correspondence: carlos.menendez-castro@uk-erlangen.de
Department of Pediatrics and Adolescent Medicine, University Hospital of Erlangen, Loschgestrasse 15, D-91054 Erlangen, Germany

evaluated sufficiently by regular B-scan ultrasound or by native CT and MRI. Radioscopy with injection of contrast agent, a diagnostic option to test intercystic communication, does not seem appropriate in children because of the radiation exposure.

To our knowledge we report here for the first time a case of preinterventional contrast-enhanced ultrasound (CEUS) of a macrocystic congenital lymphangioma as an alternative method to examine the communication between lesional cysts. Standardized preinterventional usage of CEUS would help to improve the sclerosant therapy of CCL by avoiding unnecessary multiple punctions, and would offer the possibility to reduce the amount of administered OK-432.

Case presentation

A male Caucasian term newborn (Table 1) presented with a soft tumor of the left axilla with a size of 6.5 × 6.0 cm (Fig. 1a). Sonographically the tumor showed the typical signs of a macrocystic lymphangioma with multiple cysts of a diameter up to 3 cm (Fig. 1b). Color doppler imaging did not reveal perfusion as a sign of combined hemangioma. A spontaneous augmentation in size occurred at the age of 4 weeks. MRI confirmed the diagnosis of a CCL without intrathoracic expansion. Since the axillary swelling persisted until the age of 2 months, sclerotherapy was indicated. Treatment was performed under mild anesthesia with ketamine and propofol in an aseptic environment. SonoVue®-supported CEUS was performed using the linear probe 9 L4 on a Siemens S2000 system equipped with the "Cadence Pulse Sequencing" (CPS) technology at low mechanical index (MI). After aspiration of the cystic fluid, 0.1 ml of SonoVue®, a dispersion of phospholipid-stabilized microbubbles containing sulfurhexafluorid, and 4 ml of sodium chloride 0.9% were injected into the lymphangioma via an intralesional 18 Charrière catheter. (Fig. 2a). The connection between the cysts was proved by depiction of a homogenous diffusion of SonoVue® in the whole tumor (Fig. 2b, c). Before sclerotherapy the injected contrast agent and liquid content of the cysts were aspirated. Then a single injection of OK-432 (0.01 mg/ml sodium chloride 0.9%) was performed via the same catheter. Expectedly one day after intervention fever and a local swelling occurred. C-reactive protein (CRP) increased up to 104 g/dl, normalizing five days after injection. An antibiotic therapy with piperacilline and tobramycin was applied for seven days. Sonographic follow-up examinations showed that the cysts became more solid, accompanied by a subcutaneous edema. Three weeks after intervention we saw a significant involution of the lymphangioma (Fig. 3a). After eight weeks only few singular cysts up to 3 mm (Fig. 3b) could be depicted by sonography.

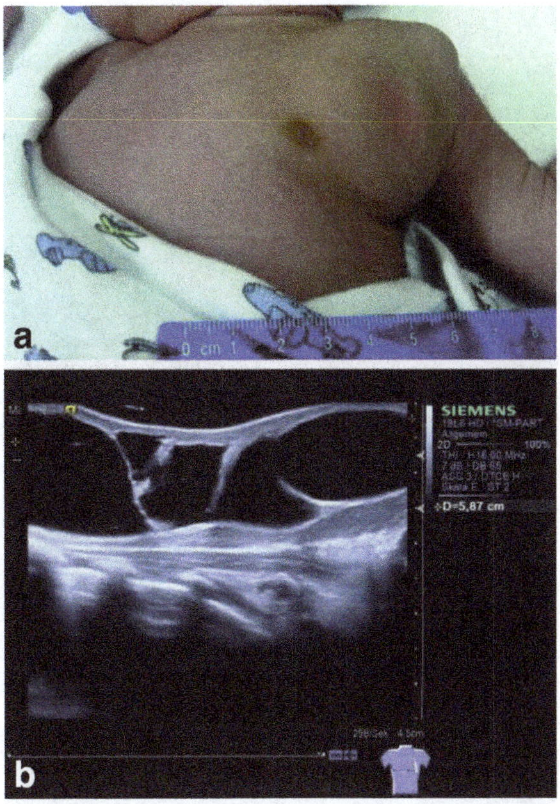

Fig. 1 Large congenital macrocystic lymphangioma in the area of the left axilla. **a** Clinical, macroscopic aspect. **b** B-mode ultrasound showing the typical finding of a subcutaneous tumor with multiple homogenous anechoic cysts

Table 1 Timeline

08/2013	Male term newborn with a congenital soft tumor of the left axilla, postnatal sonography: see Fig. 1a, b
09/2013	Spontaneous augmentation of the tumor, MRI: diagnosis of a CCL without intrathoracic expansion
10/2013	SonoVue® supported CEUS and sclerotherapy of CCL with OK-432
11/2013	Follow up examination by sonography: see Fig. 3a
12/2013	Follow up examination by sonography: see Fig. 3b

Discussion

We report the successful intracavitary use of CEUS to elucidate intercystic communications in a macrocystic congenital lymphangioma prior to sclerosant therapy with OK-432.

Among the cavernous and capillary lymphangiomas, the cystic lymphangioma is the leading lymphangioma subtype. It is characterized by dilated lymphatic ducts coated by an endothelial layer [1]. Besides surgical resection, sclerosant therapy with OK-432 is a well described and validated therapeutic option for macrocystic

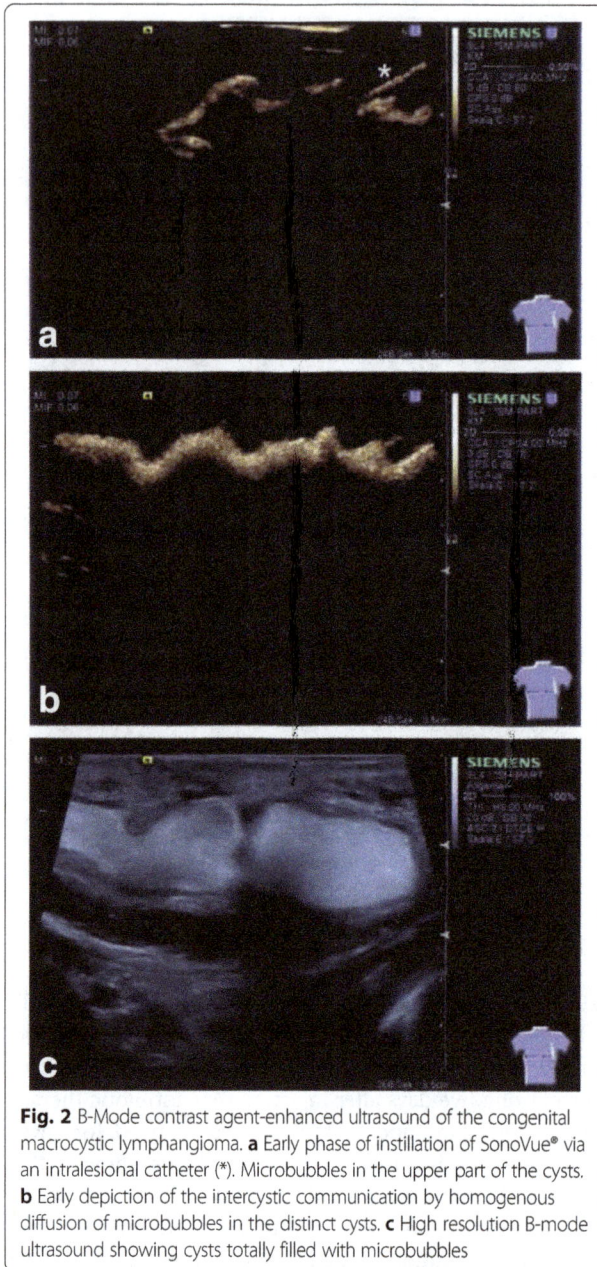

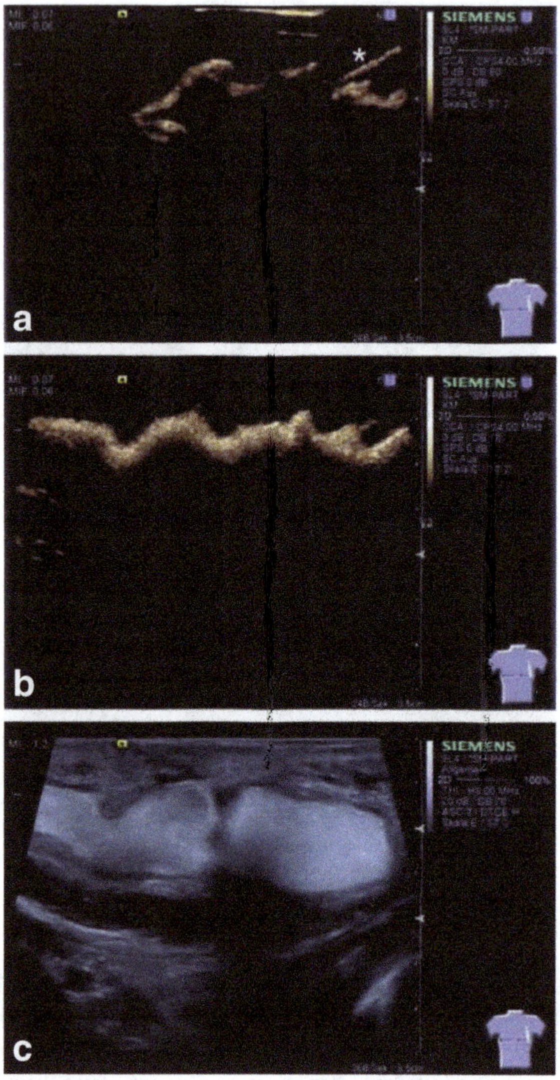

Fig. 2 B-Mode contrast agent-enhanced ultrasound of the congenital macrocystic lymphangioma. **a** Early phase of instillation of SonoVue® via an intralesional catheter (*). Microbubbles in the upper part of the cysts. **b** Early depiction of the intercystic communication by homogenous diffusion of microbubbles in the distinct cysts. **c** High resolution B-mode ultrasound showing cysts totally filled with microbubbles

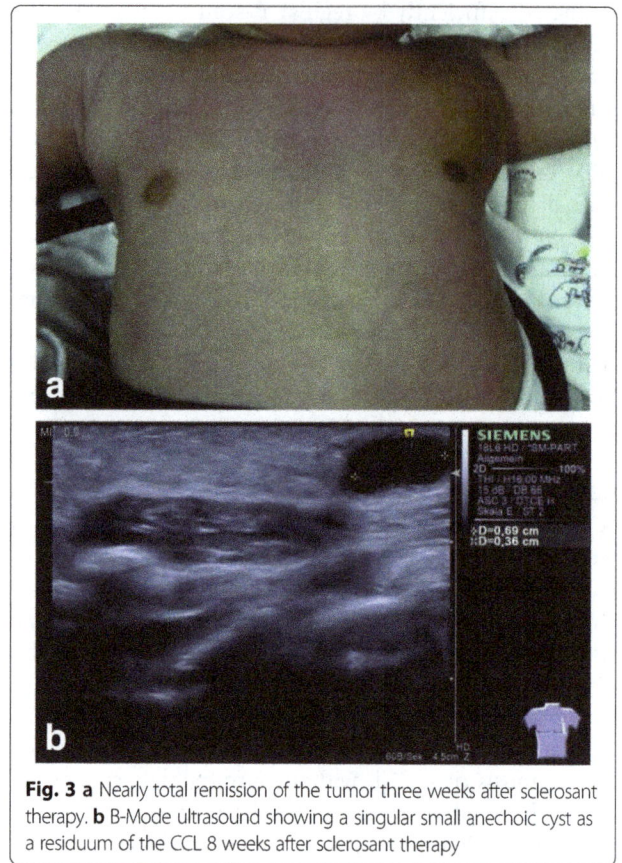

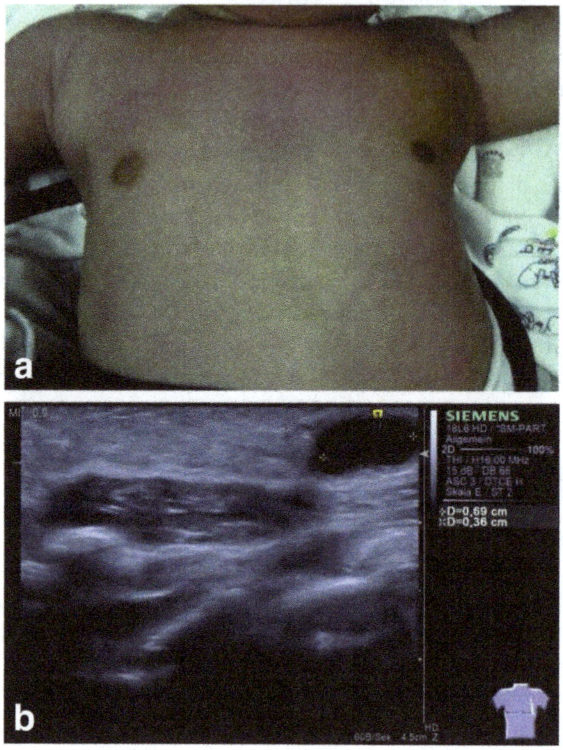

Fig. 3 **a** Nearly total remission of the tumor three weeks after sclerosant therapy. **b** B-Mode ultrasound showing a singular small anechoic cyst as a residuum of the CCL 8 weeks after sclerosant therapy

congenital lymphangiomas. The lyophilized mixture of group A streptococcus pyogenes induces a local inflammatory reaction, thus reducing the production of the lymphatic fluid and improving its drainage. Complete aspiration of cystic contents seems to be crucial for the success of OK-432 sclerotherapy of macrocystic lymphangiomas [4].

Conventional sonography is a radiation-free diagnostic tool to describe location, size and structure of the lymphangioma. It combines the main advantages of sonographic imaging like mobility, realtime assessment and high spatial resolution. Yet, for sclerosant therapy it is necessary to gain knowledge about the intercystic communication of the tumor. In this context CEUS provides a valuable diagnostic tool.

By preinterventional CEUS we were able to prove extensive intercystic communication in the lymphangioma and thereby to avoid multiple punctions. Thus, not only the risk of periinterventional infection can be reduced, but also the amount of administered OK-432 can be individually case-adapted. Furthermore by utilizing CEUS we were able to verify the proper intracystic positioning of the catheter prior to the injection of the sclerosant agent, which significantly reduces the risk of paratumorous application of OK-432.

While the utilization of CEUS with SonoVue® was approved for diagnostic liver imaging in children in 2016 in the USA, the utilization of CEUS with SonoVue® in children is still off-label in Europe. There is a long history of safe use of SonoVue® in echocardiography [5] and recent clinical studies document the drug safety of SonoVue® in children [6, 7]. Thus, in our opinion, the advantages of preinterventional CEUS in CCL, including improved application guidance of the sclerosant agent and reduced risk of periinterventional infection due to unnecessary punctions, justify off-label use of SonoVue® in CCL in children. The use of SonoVue® is still quite expensive but this might be compensated by the advantage of a case-adapted and therefore dosage-reduced application of OK-432.

Conclusions

In summary, this case report shows that contrast-enhanced ultrasound with intracavitary application of SonoVue® might be a helpfull diagnostic technique to depict the communications of cysts in CCL and to optimize sclerotherapy with OK-432 in children. Further clinical studies are needed to analyze the benefits and limits of this procedure.

Abbreviations

CCL: Congenital cystic lymphangioma; CEUS: Contrast-enhanced ultrasound; CPS: Cadence pulse sequencing; CRP: C-reactive protein

Acknowledgments

Not applicable.

Funding

Not applicable.

Authors' contribution

CM-C and JJ participated in the design of the reported diagnostic procedure and in the acquisition and interpretation of images and wrote the manuscript. MZ, FF and HvG participated in the acquisition and interpretation of sonographic images. WR participated in the design of the reported diagnostic procedure and in the interpretation of sonographic images. All authors read and approved the final manuscript.

Consent for publication

Written informed consent for publication of the case report was given by the parents of the patient. A copy of the written consent is available for review by the Editor-in-Chief of this journal.

Competing interests

The authors declare that they have no competing interests.

References

1. Zadvinskis DP, Benson MT, Kerr HH, Mancuso AA, Cacciarelli AA, Madrazo BL, Mafee MF, Dalen K. Congenital malformations of the cervicothoracic lymphatic system: embryology and pathogenesis. Radiographics. 1992;12(6): 1175–89.
2. Riechelmann H, Muehlfay G, Keck T, Mattfeldt T, Rettinger G. Total, subtotal, and partial surgical removal of cervicofacial lymphangiomas. Arch Otolaryngol Head Neck Surg. 1999;125(6):643–8.
3. Poldervaart MT, Breugem CC, Speleman L, Pasmans S. Treatment of lymphatic malformations with OK-432 (Picibanil): review of the literature. J Craniofac Surg. 2009;20(4):1159–62.
4. Kim DW. OK-432 sclerotherapy of lymphatic malformation in the head and neck: factors related to outcome. Pediatr Radiol. 2014;44(7):857–62.
5. Broillet A, Puginier J, Ventrone R, Schneider M. Assessment of myocardial perfusion by intermittent harmonic power Doppler using SonoVue, a new ultrasound contrast agent. Investig Radiol. 1998;33(4):209–15.
6. Rosado E, Riccabona M. Off-Label Use of Ultrasound Contrast Agents for Intravenous Applications in Children: Analysis of the Existing Literature. J Ultrasound Med. 2016;35(3):487–96.
7. Knieling F, Strobel D, Rompel O, Zapke M, Menendez-Castro C, Wolfel M, Schulz J, Rascher W, Jungert J: Spectrum, Applicability and Diagnostic Capacity of Contrast-Enhanced Ultrasound in Pediatric Patients and Young Adults after Intravenous Application - A Retrospective Trial. Ultraschall in der Medizin 2016; doi:10.1055/s-0042-108429.

19

Comparison of contrast in brightness mode and strain ultrasonography of glial brain tumours

Tormod Selbekk[1,2*], Reidar Brekken[1,2], Marit Indergaard[2], Ole Solheim[2,3] and Geirmund Unsgård[2,3]

Abstract

Background: Image contrast between normal tissue and brain tumours may sometimes appear to be low in intraoperative ultrasound. Ultrasound imaging of strain is an image modality that has been recently explored for intraoperative imaging of the brain. This study aims to investigate differences in image contrast between ultrasound brightness mode (B-mode) images and ultrasound strain magnitude images of brain tumours.

Methods: Ultrasound radiofrequency (RF) data was acquired during surgery in 15 patients with glial tumours. The data were subsequently processed to provide strain magnitude images. The contrast in the B-mode images and the strain images was determined in assumed normal brain tissue and tumour tissue at selected regions of interest (ROI). Three measurements of contrast were done in the ultrasound data for each patient. The B-mode and strain contrasts measurements were compared using the paired samples t- test.

Results: The statistical analysis of a total of 45 measurements shows that the contrasts in the strain magnitude images are significantly higher than in the conventional ultrasound B-mode images (P < 0.0001).

Conclusions: The results indicate that ultrasound strain imaging provides better discrimination between normal brain tissue and glial tumour tissue than conventional ultrasound B-mode imaging. Ultrasound imaging of tissue strain therefore holds the potential of becoming a valuable adjunct to conventional intraoperative ultrasound imaging in brain tumour surgery.

Keywords: Ultrasound, Elastography, Elastogram, Strain, Brain, Neurosurgery, Brain tumours, Image contrast

Background

Prior to modern neuroimaging, the neurosurgeon could detect pathological tissue by palpating the suspected areas of the brain during surgery. The tumour would be felt as a region with different elasticity compared to the surrounding normal brain, as such tumours most often have a firmer consistency than normal tissue. Even today when an operating microscope is used, the surgeon may palpate the tissue using the surgical instruments in order to find areas of the brain with differences in tissue hardness. This manual inspection of tissue hardness may aid to identify remaining tumour tissue that may be difficult to detect with direct visualisation using the operating microscope. Ultrasound imaging can also be used for the assessment of tissue hardness through imaging of *strain* in the tissue. Assuming that the stress applied to the tissue is uniform, the calculated and displayed strain values should in ideal circumstances be proportional to the modulus of elasticity (Young's modulus) of the tissues. The imaging technique is therefore often also referred to as *ultrasound elastography* and the corresponding images are often called *elastograms.*

Several research groups have investigated the use of ultrasound elastography in imaging brain tumours [1-3]. However, the clinical benefit of ultrasound strain imaging compared to conventional ultrasound imaging is still to be determined. The publications so far have shown only a few example images of brain tumours and have mainly demonstrated that it is feasible to generate elastograms of brain tumours. The measurements and display of strain require some form of displacement of the tissue, which means that internal or external forces need to act on the organ. Previous studies have demonstrated strain images (elastograms) generated by the internal displacements in

* Correspondence: tormod.selbekk@sintef.no
[1]Department of Medical Technology, SINTEF, Olav Kyrres gate 9, Trondheim, Norway
[2]Faculty of Medicine, Norwegian University of Science and Technology, Olav Kyrres gate 9, Trondheim, Norway
Full list of author information is available at the end of the article

the brain parenchyma caused by arterial pulsation, or generated by the use of either a mechanical shaker device or manual palpation to induce tissue displacements [1-3]. Quantitative assessments of ultrasound strain images of brain tumours have been performed in one study, which used the natural pulsation of the brain parenchyma to generate strain images. The study concluded that strain magnitudes of brain tumours are significantly lower than the strain magnitudes of normal brain tissue [4]. However, quantitative comparisons between ultrasound *strain images* and conventional *brightness mode images* have not been published so far.

The clinical performance of ultrasound strain imaging has been evaluated more thoroughly in breast tumours. In a study by Burnside *et al.*, the use of ultrasound strain imaging in combination with ultrasound B-mode imaging led to a higher area under the receiver operating characteristics (ROC) curve then by using ultrasound B-mode images alone [5].

A few ultrasound machines have implemented the option of calculating the *strain ratio* between strain levels in assumed tumour and in assumed normal tissue. This has resulted in several recent papers on the use of strain ratio (also referred to as *strain index*) for diagnostic purposes. One study compared the performance of B-mode images, strain images and strain ratio in differentiating benign and malignant tumours in a group of 227 women with focal breast lesions [6]. The authors concluded that B-mode images provided the highest sensitivity, but the strain images and strain ratio provided higher specificity. In another study Cho *et al.* compared the diagnostic performance of ultrasound B-mode sonography and strain rate in differentiation of malignant and benign breast masses and found no significant difference in the area under the ROC curve [7].

These and other studies indicate that ultrasound strain imaging may to some extent provide an improvement in diagnostics of some tumours compared to using conventional ultrasound alone. It might be asked what features of strain imaging do account for an increase in diagnostic performance compared to conventional B-mode imaging. Ultrasound is able to produce B-mode images with high spatial and temporal resolution, but the contrast resolution may be limited compared to other imaging techniques like Magnetic Resonance Imaging (MRI) or Computed Tomography (CT). The difference in brightness intensity between the lesion to diagnose and the normal tissue may in some cases appear to be low, thus having a poor contrast resolution. An improved image contrast would probably lead to improved diagnostics of these low-contrast lesions. It could be speculated that the ultrasound strain images might possess a higher image contrast than conventional ultrasound. The imaging of strain is related to other properties of tissue than the generation of ultrasound B-mode images, and therefore holds the potential to provide unique information about tissue pathology [8].

It is therefore of clinical interest to make comparisons of attributes like image contrast between the two modalities, to assess potential differences in imaging of lesions.

In this study we have processed and analysed ultrasound data acquired during surgery of glial tumours in order to compare the image contrast in conventional ultrasound images (B-mode) versus the image contrast in ultrasound strain images. We have performed a quantitative comparison of image contrast between ultrasound strain images generated by the natural pulsation of the brain parenchyma and the corresponding B-mode images. The measurements of image contrast have been performed in the peripheral parts of the tumour, covering the transition from cancerous tissue towards more normal brain tissue. The hypothesis of the study was that the contrast between tumour and normal tissue is higher in the ultrasound strain images than in the ultrasound B-mode images.

Methods

Regional Research Ethics Committee of Central Norway approved the study protocol and the use of previously acquired ultrasound data in this retrospective study. The anonymous ultrasound data used in this study has been acquired with the patient's informed consent as a part of a prior study.

Data acquisition

Ultrasound radiofrequency (RF) data was acquired during surgery of 15 glial tumours. The patients were diagnosed by histopathology. Eight patients had low-grade glioma (WHO-grade I and II) and 7 patients had high-grade astrocytoma (WHO grade III & IV). The data were acquired after craniotomy with the 10 MHz flat linear probe (System FiVE, GE Vingmed, Horten, Norway) kept motionless on intact dura. An engineer (TS) adjusted the settings of the ultrasound scanner (power, gain, time gain control-TGC) prior to acquisition, aiming to provide ultrasound B-mode images with a homogenous appearance but avoiding brightness saturation. The acquired data covered at least one cardiac cycle in time.

Strain processing

The axial strain was calculated by differentiation of time delays that were estimated by processing of the ultrasound RF-data. The time delays were calculated by implementing in Matlab (MathWorks, Natic, MA, USA) a method initially suggested by Cabot [9], which has been further refined for time delay estimation in later publications [10,11]. The strain processing of the RF-data is described in details in an earlier publication from our research group [1].

Performing the measurements

The B-mode and strain magnitude images were analysed with measuring methods implemented in Matlab. For each dataset a total of three measurements of contrast for both strain and B-mode were done at three different locations in the images. That is, a different location in the image was selected for each measurement. All three measurements for a given tumour were done at the same image frame, i.e. at the same point in time. With reference to the B-mode images, the measurements were performed in the hyperechoic tumour and the surrounding isoechoic regions presumably representing normal brain tissue.

The procedure for obtaining the contrast measurements is illustrated in Figure 1. After import and strain processing of the ultrasound data, the B-mode image was displayed. As a first step, the operator (MI) identified the tumour border as seen in the ultrasound B-mode images, and selected one position (using the mouse) on the border for contrast measurement. The B-mode intensity and strain magnitude were subsequently plotted along the lateral direction for the given depth, with a cross mark (X) indicating the lateral position of the point selected by the operator (Figure 1C-D). The plotted strain magnitudes and B-mode intensity were calculated by averaging the values over an area of approx. 1 mm^2 in the images.

The second step of the measurements was to calculate the contrast between expected cancerous tissue and normal tissue for both image modalities. The calculation was based on the local minimum and maximum values found closest to the cross mark (X) in the respective plotted curves, i.e. the local extrema close to the tumour border as identified by the operator.

The maximum allowable lateral range for the amplitude picking was defined with the aid of a low-pass (LP) filtered version of the curves (shown as a light grey stepwise curve in Figure 1C-D), in order to increase the

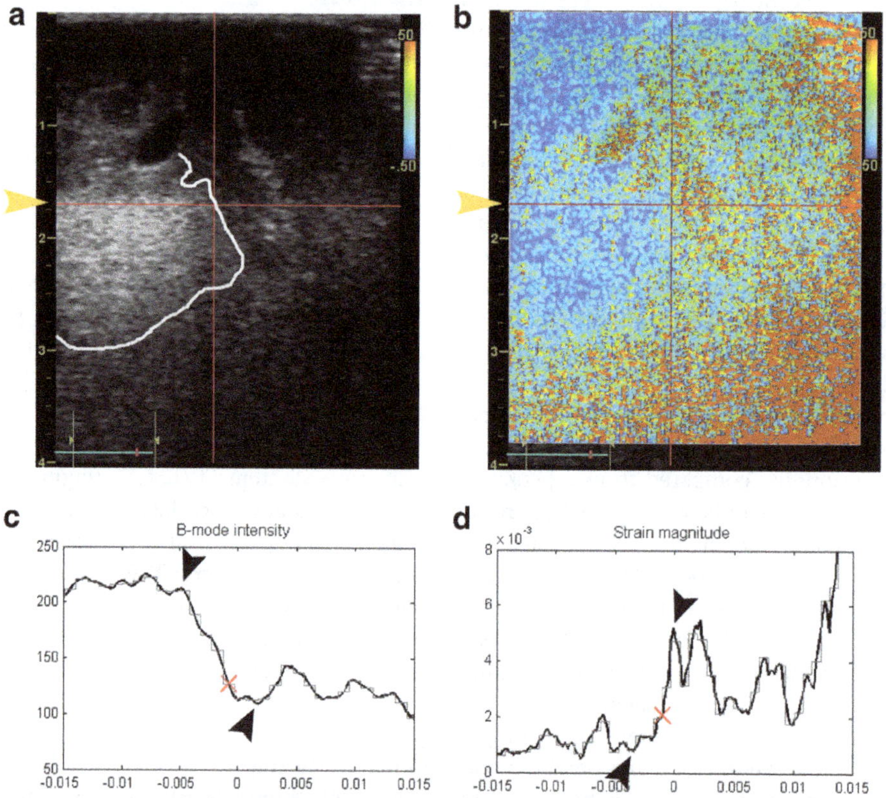

Figure 1 Ultrasound B-mode and strain images. The ultrasound B-mode image of a glioblastoma (grade IV) in **(a)** and the corresponding strain magnitude image **(b)**. For display purposes the delineation of the solid tumour close to the location of the measurements is marked with a bright line in the B-mode image. The B-mode intensity plotted along the lateral direction at a user- selected depth is shown in **(c)**, with the numbers of the x-axis referring to the distance [m] from the lateral midpoint of the image. The strain magnitudes are plotted in similar way and displayed in **(d)**, with the Y-axis showing strain magnitude values from 0–8 ‰. The depth of the plotted magnitudes is for display purposes indicated with a bright arrow in **(a)** and **(b)**. The values picked for estimation of contrast between tumour tissue and assumed normal tissue are indicated by black arrowheads in **(c)** and **(d)**.

Table 1 Strain and B-mode contrast

Glioma grading	Dataset No.	Average strain magnitude contrast (σ)	Average B-mode contrast (σ)
low-grade glioma	1	0.55 (0.11)	0.43 (0.20)
	2	0.56 (0.27)	0.61 (0.20)
	3	0.57 (0.08)	0.27 (0.04)
	4	0.58 (0.19)	0.46 (0.13)
	5	0.51 (0.04)	0.32 (0.06)
	6	0.64 (0.12)	0.36 (0.07)
	7	0.66 (0.25)	0.35 (0.12)
	8	0.84 (0.04)	0.56 (0.11)
high-grade glioma	9	0.58 (0.22)	0.31 (0.06)
	10	0.48 (0.21)	0.24 (0.09)
	11	0.58 (0.11)	0.25 (0.19)
	12	0.50 (0.07)	0.29 (0.06)
	13	0.69 (0.17)	0.42 (0.08)
	14	0.65 (0.17)	0.60 (0.12)
	15	0.60 (0.03)	0.44 (0.24)
	All data	0.60 (0.16)	0.39 (0.16)

The average and standard deviation (σ) of the three contrast measurements obtained for each patient.

robustness towards minor amplitude deviations. The valid lateral range was between the first minimum and first maximum values for the LP-curve found locally around the user-selected position (marked X) of the tumour border as seen in the ultrasound images. The local extrema of the original and unfiltered curves within this lateral range were found by manual inspection, and used for the calculation of contrast. Thus, the contrast was calculated by selecting one extremum value in the tumour and a second extremum value in the supposedly normal brain tissue. The contrast between the assumed normal tissue and the tumour tissue for the two image modalities was calculated as

$$C = \frac{|A_1 - A_2|}{A_1 + A_2} \quad (1)$$

where A_1 and A_2 are the respective local minimum and maximum values for strain magnitude or brightness intensity observed across the tumour border as depicted by ultrasound. A value of $C = 0$ means no difference in contrast between areas of tumour and areas of assumed normal brain tissue.

Statistics

The differences in contrast between ultrasound strain and B-mode were statistically analysed using the paired samples t-test (SPSS Statistics, v 19.0, IBM corporation, NY, USA), using a significance level $\alpha = 0.05$. Normal quantile plots (Q-Q plots) were used for assessment of the sample populations' probability distribution. The independent samples t-test was used to investigate differences in contrast between the subgroups of low-grade and high-grade gliomas for a given image modality.

Results

For each glial tumour (15 cases) three analyses of contrast were done on ultrasound strain magnitude and B-mode images, giving a total of 45 measurements for each modality. The measurements were performed at depths between 0.7 and 3.0 cm, with the average measurement depth being 1.9 cm for the 45 samples. Table 1 shows the average contrast and standard deviation of the three measurements performed for each patient. The average contrast is higher for the strain magnitude than for the B-mode intensity in all cases except one with a low-grade glioma. Box plot of the strain and B-mode contrast measurements is shown for the subgroups of low-grade and high-grade gliomas (Figure 2).

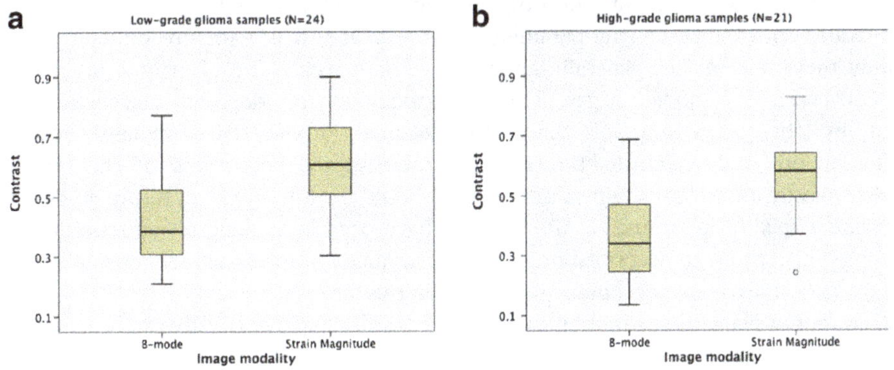

Figure 2 Box plot of B-mode and strain contrast. Box plot of brightness mode and strain magnitude contrast for the low-grade glioma samples **(a)** and the high-grade glioma samples **(b)**. The lower and upper edges of the box represent the first and third quartile respectively, while a horizontal line within the box indicates the median. The vertical length of the box represents the interquartile range (IQR). The most extreme sample values (within a distance of 1.5 IQR from the median) are the endpoints of the lines extending from the box. Possible outliers are shown as circles.

The difference in contrast between the two image modalities was statistically investigated for all contrast measurements of the tumours ($N = 45$), and for the measurements in the subgroups low-grade gliomas ($N_l = 24$) and high-grade gliomas ($N_h = 21$). The normal probability distributions of the sample populations were confirmed by inspection of Q-Q-plots. For the glial tumours as a whole the contrasts between tumour and presumably normal tissue in the strain images were significantly higher than the corresponding contrast in the B-mode images ($P < 0.0001$). For the subgroup of patients with high-grade gliomas the contrast in the strain images were significantly higher than the contrast in the B-mode images ($P < 0.0001$), and the same was observed for the subgroup with low-grade gliomas ($P < 0.0001$).

There was not a significant difference in contrast between the two subgroups' low-grade and high-grade gliomas, neither for the strain images ($P = 0.49$) nor the B-mode images ($P = 0.25$).

Discussion

In this study we have performed measurements of strain magnitude and brightness intensity across the ultrasound depicted border of glial tumours, with subsequent analysis of differences in contrast between the image modalities. The results of the analyses show a significantly higher contrast between tumour tissue and presumed normal tissue in the strain images, as compared to the B-mode images. From Table 1 we observe that the mean contrast for all B-mode measurements is 0.39 while it is 0.60 for the strain magnitude measurements, which is 54 % higher. One interpretation of the results could be that ultrasound strain imaging should be the preferred image modality to use during surgery of brain tumours, since the strain images provide better discrimination (higher contrast) between the tumour tissue and the normal brain tissue. However, in a clinical setting there are still several key issues to solve before the surgeons can use ultrasound strain imaging as a practical tool for identification of the resectable tumour tissue. With the processing parameters applied in this study the strain images generally appear noisier than the conventional B-mode images. This is partly introduced by the processing of the data where e.g. the differentiation of the calculated time delays in the axial direction typically introduces strain values with alternating polarity and a spiking appearance in the strain image. The processing is also prone to decorrelation of the echo signal due to low signal levels (hypoechoic regions in the B-mode image) or "out of plane" tissue motion causing loss of temporally coherent signals. This may cause the processing to produce false results with abnormally high strain values. Also, our method for estimation of time delays assumes that the delay is smaller than the sampling time Ts, i.e. that the tissue velocity is low compared to the number of frames acquired per second. If this assumption is not met the processing may produce incorrectly high strain values.

In our processed strain images we have indeed seen that noise can be present in parts of the image. This is typically seen in regions with low intensity in the B-mode image, for example when imaging homogenous tissue like the brain stem and deeper white brain matter that appear hypoechoic compared to other brain tissue. However, our measurements are intentionally performed in the transition zone from tumour to presumed normal brain tissue. In this short distal range we expect the data to be least influenced by noise, with the B-mode intensity ranging from the hyperechoic tumour to the isoechoic areas with presumed normal tissue. The inspection of the strain magnitude curves did not indicate any abrupt change of signal level within the spatial distance analysed, as could be expected if the strain processing produced invalid results.

It can be argued that the measurements performed in the transition zone from tumour to normal tissue impose a selection bias for the contrast analysis. This is the region that is of interest to the surgeon, but it is also the region where we should expect the strain images to be least affected by noise. The contrast measurements are only valid for analysis of image contrast between glial tumour tissue and adjacent normal tissue. It should not be interpreted to represent differences in contrast resolution between the image modalities in general.

The methodology for the analysis of image contrast in the peripheral parts of tumour involves a subjective assessment of the approximate position of the depicted tumour border and manual reading of the displayed strain magnitude and brightness curves. Even if the implemented method of analysis is not fully automatic, the measurements were obtained by following a standardized procedure, as outlined in the Methods section. Quantitative image quality measures will usually imply some subjective decisions about where to perform the analysis in the image. It is therefore difficult to establish a method without some kind of manual intervention. However, the calculation of additional measures like e.g. the contrast-to-noise ratio (CNR), or signal-to-noise ratio (SNR) would increase the robustness of the image assessment and should be considered in future studies [12]. It would also have been interesting to address intra- and interobserver variability of the measurements, which was not performed in this study.

As discussed above there are different factors that may have affected the measurements. However, we have found the obtained measurements to be quite robust and we believe that the differences in contrast found between ultrasound strain magnitude and B-mode intensity should represent actual differences between the image modalities.

Ultrasound strain imaging in brain surgery is a quite novel approach and we have not found other studies performing a similar comparison between strain images and conventional B-mode images. It is therefore difficult to compare our results with previous findings. Some studies have however explored the use of strain ratio for diagnostic purposes, but the similar ratio for B-mode intensity has not been reported. The strain ratio is a quantitative index but should not be considered as an objective *diagnostic* parameter as its value may be heavily dependent on which regions are selected for comparison and is therefore prone to variations between observers and within the patient population, which has also been pointed out by others [13]. It should be noted that the contrasts calculated in our study are not intended to serve a diagnostic purpose; the sole purpose is the pairwise comparison between the ultrasound modalities.

The *diagnostic value* of ultrasound strain imaging of brain tumours has not been assessed in this study. This would require a comparison between image findings and histology, which was not available for the current study. Glial tumours are diffuse infiltrating and tumour cells are likely to be present also beyond the border zone seen in the ultrasound B-mode image [14]. Scattered tumour cells are likely to be present in the isoechoic regions interpreted to be mainly normal brain tissue, but to a substantially less extent than in the hyperechoic regions. The calculated contrasts should therefore represent differences in magnitude (strain/brightness) between areas in the brain predominated by glial tumour cells and areas predominated by normal brain cells, respectively.

The results obtained should provide a rationale for further technical developments and investigations of methods for real-time intraoperative ultrasound strain imaging of brain tumours. The ultrasound strain magnitude images possess a higher contrast between tumour and normal brain tissue in the peripheral parts of the tumour than the conventional B-mode images. This suggest that the surgeon may use imaging of strain to improve detection of remaining tumour towards the end of surgery, compared to using conventional ultrasound imaging alone.

Conclusions

Off-line processing of ultrasound RF-data to yield strain magnitude images has been performed on *in vivo* data acquired during brain tumour surgery. The strain magnitude images have a significantly higher contrast between normal tissue and tumour tissue than conventional B-mode images. We conclude that for glial brain tumours, ultrasound imaging of strain holds the potential to become a valuable adjunct to conventional brightness mode imaging. However, the practical aspects of acquisition and display of strain images in real time as well as evaluation of diagnostic value must be addressed in future studies.

Competing interests

The authors declare that they have no competing interests.

Authors' contributions

TS contributed to the study design, acquisition of data, data analyses and drafting of manuscript, RB contributed to the study design and implementation of the strain processing methods and measurements method in Matlab, MI performed the measurements and contributed to the statistical analyses and drafting of manuscript, OS contributed to data acquisition and drafting of manuscript and GU contributed to the study design, acquisition of data and drafting of manuscript. All authors read and approved the final manuscript.

Acknowledgements

The study has been financed by the regional health authorities in central Norway through the financing of the National Centre for 3D ultrasound in Neurosurgery, the independent research institute SINTEF and the MI Lab and Department of Circulation and Medical Imaging, Norwegian University of Science and Technology, Trondheim, Norway. We acknowledge our former colleague Dr Jon Bang for implementation in Matlab some of the algorithms used in the strain processing.

Author details

[1]Department of Medical Technology, SINTEF, Olav Kyrres gate 9, Trondheim, Norway. [2]Faculty of Medicine, Norwegian University of Science and Technology, Olav Kyrres gate 9, Trondheim, Norway. [3]Department of Neurosurgery, St. Olav University Hospital, Olav Kyrres gate 9, Trondheim, Norway.

References

1. Selbekk T, Bang J, Unsgaard G: **Strain processing of intraoperative ultrasound images of brain tumours: initial results.** *Ultrasound Med Biol* 2005, **31**(1):45–51.
2. Scholz M, Noack V, Pechlivanis I, Engelhardt M, Fricke B, Linstedt U, Brendel B, Ing D, Schmieder K, Ermert H, Harders A: **Vibrography during tumor neurosurgery.** *J Ultrasound Med* 2005, **24**(7):985–992.
3. Uff CE, Garcia L, Fromageau J, Dorward N, Bamber JC: **Real time ultrasound elastography in neurosurgery.** *Proceedings of the IEEE International Ultrasonics Symposium* 2009, 467–470.
4. Selbekk T, Brekken R, Solheim O, Lydersen S, Hernes TAN, Unsgard G: **Tissue motion and strain in the human brain assessed by intraoperative ultrasound in glioma patients.** *Ultrasound Med Biol* 2010, **36**(1):2–10.
5. Burnside ES, Hall TJ, Sommer AM, Hesley GK, Sisney GA, Svensson WE, Fine JP, Jiang J, Hangiandreou NJ: **Differentiating benign from malignant solid breast masses with US strain imaging.** *Radiology* 2007, **245**(2):401.
6. Thomas A, Degenhardt F, Farrokh A, Wojcinski S, Slowinski T, Fischer T: **Significant differentiation of focal breast lesions: calculation of strain ratio in breast sonoelastography.** *Acad Radiol* 2010, **17**(5):558–563.
7. Cho N, Moon WK, Kim HY, Chang JM, Park SH, Lyou CY: **Sonoelastographic strain index for differentiation of benign and malignant nonpalpable breast masses.** *J Ultrasound Med* 2010, **29**(1):1–7.
8. Wells PNT, Liang HD: **Medical Ultrasound: imaging of soft tissue strain and elasticity.** *J R Soc Interface* 2011, **8**(64):1521–1549.
9. Cabot RC: **A note on the application of Hilbert transform to time delay estimation.** *IEEE Trans. Acoust. Speech Signal Processing* 1981, **29:**607–609. ASSP.
10. Loupas T, Powers JT, Gill RW: **An axial velocity estimator for ultrasound blood flow imaging, based on a full evaluation of the Doppler equation by means of a two-dimensional autocorrelation approach.** *IEEE Trans Ultrason Ferroelect Freq Control.* 1995, **42:**672–688.

11. Simon C, VanBaren P, Ebbini ES: **Two-dimensional temperature estimation using diagnostic ultrasound.** *IEEE Trans Ultrason Ferroelect Freq Control* 1998, **45**:1088–1099.
12. Varghese T, Ophir J: **An analysis of elastographic contrast-to-noise ratio.** *Ultrasound Med Biol* 1998, **24**:915–924.
13. Kagoya R, Monobe H, Tojima H: **Utility of elastography for differential diagnosis of benign and malignant thyroid nodules.** *Otolaryngol Head Neck Surg* 2010, **143**(2):230–234.
14. Unsgaard G, Selbekk T, Müller TB, Ommedal S, Torp SH, Myhr G, Bang J, Hernes TAN: **Ability of navigated 3D ultrasound to delineate gliomas and metastases - comparison of image interpretations with histopathology.** *Acta Neurochir* 2005, **147**(12):1259–1269.

Reliability and validity of the ultrasound technique to measure the rectus femoris muscle diameter in older CAD-patients

Tom Thomaes[1], Martine Thomis[2], Steven Onkelinx[1], Walter Coudyzer[3], Véronique Cornelissen[1] and Luc Vanhees[1*]

Abstract

Background: The increasing age of coronary artery disease (CAD) patients and the occurrence of sarcopenia in the elderly population accompanied by 'fear of moving' and hospitalization in these patients often results in a substantial loss of skeletal muscle mass and muscle strength. Cardiac rehabilitation can improve exercise tolerance and muscle strength in CAD patients but less data describe eventual morphological muscular changes possibly by more difficult access to imaging techniques. Therefore the aim of this study is to assess and quantify the reliability and validity of an easy applicable method, the ultrasound (US) technique, to measure the diameter of rectus femoris muscle in comparison to the muscle dimensions measured with CT scans.

Methods: 45 older CAD patients without cardiac event during the last 9 months were included in this study. 25 patients were tested twice with ultrasound with a two day interval to assess test-retest reliability and 20 patients were tested twice (once with US and once with CT) on the same day to assess the validity of the US technique compared to CT as the gold standard. Isometric and isokinetic muscle testing was performed to test potential zero-order correlations between muscle diameter, muscle volume and muscle force.

Results: An intraclass correlation coefficient (ICC) of 0.97 ((95%CL: 0.92 - 0.99) was found for the test-retest reliability of US and the ICC computed between US and CT was 0.92 (95%CL: 0.81 - 0.97). The absolute difference between both techniques was 0.01 ± 0.12 cm ($p = 0.66$) resulting in a typical percentage error of 4.4%. Significant zero-order correlations were found between local muscle volume and muscle diameter assessed with CT ($r = 0.67$, $p = 0.001$) and assessed with US ($r = 0.49$, $p < 0.05$). Muscle strength parameters were also significantly correlated with muscle diameter assessed with both techniques (range r = 0.45-r = 0.61, $p < 0.05$).

Conclusions: Ultrasound imaging can be used as a valid and reliable measurement tool to assess the rectus femoris muscle diameter in older CAD patients.

Keywords: Cardiac Rehabilitation, Coronary Artery Disease, Ultrasound Imaging, CT scan

Background

According to the World Health Association, coronary heart disease (CHD) is the leading cause of death worldwide with age as the most powerful independent risk factor [1]. Ageing is characterized by a decline in functionality due to progressive loss of muscle tissue coupled with a decrease in strength and force output. Low skeletal muscle strength has been shown to be an important predictor of all-cause mortality in healthy as well as diseased individuals [2-4]. The increasing age of coronary artery disease (CAD) patients and the occurrence of sarcopenia in the elderly population accompanied by 'fear of moving' and hospitalization in these patients often results in a substantial loss of skeletal muscle mass and muscle strength.

That is, compared to healthy subjects, CAD patients have an impaired peak VO_2 and show accompanying increased muscle fatigability [5]. Previous studies have demonstrated that cardiac rehabilitation improves exercise tolerance and muscle strength in patients with

* Correspondence: luc.vanhees@faber.kuleuven.be
[1]Cardiovascular Rehabilitation Unit, Department of Rehabilitation Sciences, Katholieke Universiteit Leuven, Tervuursevest 101, 3001 Heverlee, Belgium
Full list of author information is available at the end of the article

myocardial infarction and in patients after cardiac surgery. In addition, Sumide et al. [6] reported that the improvement in exercise tolerance was significantly correlated with the changes in lower limb leg strength in post-cardiac valve surgery patients ($r = 0.51$, $P < 0.01$). A positive and significant correlation between the change in peak VO_2 and the change in peak torque of knee extension ($r = 0.50$, $P < 0.005$) was also observed in the acute phase after a myocardial infarction (MI) in patients with a lower limb muscle volume of less than 22 kg at baseline [7].

Repeated ionisation radiation exposure and high costs, accessibility and long scanning times when using CT or MRI, limits the use of both techniques to measure muscle cross sectional area (CSA) and muscle diameter on a broad scale in the clinical and research setting. By contrast ultrasound systems (US) are more easily available and may offer a useful alternative. In asthmatic (mean age 56 ± 8) and chronic obstructive pulmonary disease (COPD) (mean age 67 ± 9) patients it was shown that US can be used as a valid and reliable alternative to CT for measuring mm. rectus femoris (RF) CSA [8,9]. To the best of our knowledge, the validity and reliability of the US technique to measure muscle diameter has not been investigated in an elderly CAD population. Therefore, the aim of this study is to assess and quantify the reliability and validity of the US technique to measure the diameter of RF compared to the muscle dimensions measured with CT scans. In addition, muscle testing was performed to test potential zero-order correlations between muscle diameter, muscle volume and muscle force and to investigate whether correlations found with CT are similar to those with US. Peripheral skeletal muscle strength of the lower limb may be assessed by isokinetic dynamometry and provides a reliable and safe assessment of dynamic muscle function [5,6].

Methods

Study sample

Forty five CAD patients (age: 68.4 ± 6.2 years; BMI: 26.6 ± 2.9 kg/m^2; mean ± SD) without cardiovascular incident during the last year, participating in sporting activities of a maintenance program for patients with cardiovascular disease, volunteered for this study. The first 20 patients (hence forward called 'group 1') (age: 68.3 ± 7.3 years; BMI: 26.8 ± 2.8 kg/m^2) were measured twice on the same day, once with US and once with CT-scan to investigate the validity of US vs. CT. The following 25 patients (hence forward called 'group 2') (age: 68.6 ± 4.6 years; BMI: 26.3 ± 3.0 kg/m^2) were measured twice with US with a two day interval to assess the test-retest reliability of this measurement. The study was approved by the Biomedical Ethical Committee of the KU Leuven and written informed consent was obtained from all participants after full explanation of the aims and procedures.

Measurements

Rectus femoris ultrasound

All measurements were performed by a single experienced investigator (T.T). Rectus femoris diameter was measured by B-mode ultrasonography, wall tracking ultrasound system (Siemens Vivid 07 GE) with a 12 MHz linear array transducer (12 L transducer GE). The transducer was placed perpendicular to the long axis of the thigh with excessive use of contact gel and minimal pressure to avoid compression of the muscle [8,9]. The diameter of the RF was measured at the half point of the length between epicondylus lateralis and trochanter major of the femur. Measurements were taken on the patient's right leg with the patient lying in a supine position with both knees extended but relaxed and toes pointing the ceiling. A set of five consecutive pictures was taken and further analyzed offline. The vertical diameter of the RF muscle was measured on the inner edge of the muscle on the five pictures (Figure 1). The average of the five pictures was used as the RF diameter and further analyzed. Datasets from both US measurements were analyzed blind and at random.

Rectus femoris CT-scan

CT scans were performed using a Siemens Sensation 16®. Similarly, measurements of the RF were taken on the right leg at the half point of the length between epicondylus lateralis and trochanter major of the femur with the patient lying in a supine position with both knees extended but relaxed and toes pointing the ceiling. Half way point of the femur was determined using a scout view longitudinal scan of the femur with minimal radiation dose (< 0.05 milliSievert). Five adjacent slices of 0.5 cm thickness were taken (one at mid-point, two directly above and two directly below the midpoint).

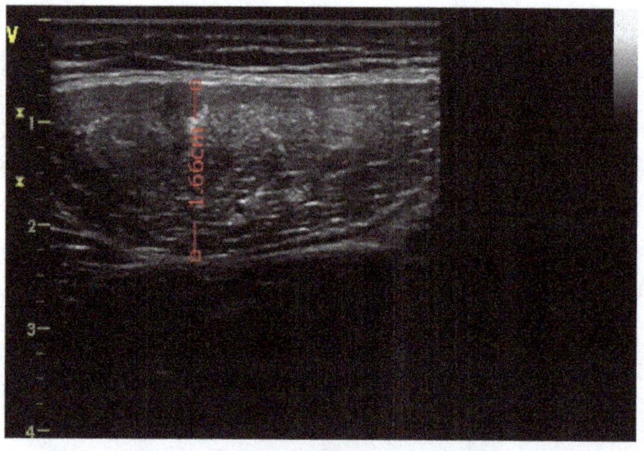

Figure 1 Image of the rectus femoris with indication of the diameter, obtained with ultrasound imaging.

Additionally femur length, local muscle volume and fat volume in a slice of 2.5 cm (sum of 5 slices) at the middle of the right upper leg were determined with CT (radiation dose < 0.05 milliSievert). Local muscle mass was defined as 0 to 100 Hounsfield Units found in the total leg CSA subtracted with the same densities found in bone marrow. Local fat mass was defined as 0 to -190 Hounsfield Units subtracted with the same densities found in bone marrow. All CT measurements were executed by the same experienced researcher (W.C)

Quadriceps strength and anthropometric characteristics

Muscle strength testing was only performed in group 1. After a warming up period of five minutes on a cycle ergometer, maximal voluntary muscle strength of the hamstrings and quadriceps muscles was tested on a BIODEX System 3 Pro (Biodex Medical Systems, 20 Ramsay Road, Shirley, New York, USA). Isometric strength of the quadriceps was measured at 60° (fully extended leg is zero°). Four attempts were given with 30 s interval. The highest peak torque was withheld as the maximal voluntary quadriceps strength. Isokinetic measurements of the quadriceps were measured at 60°/s and 180°/s. Patients performed four consecutive attempts at every speed. Resting interval between both measurements was one minute. Peak torque during both speeds was withheld for further analysis. Vocal encouragement was given by the investigator during the tests.

Finally, height, weight, skinfolds (Harpenden-caliper) and circumference of the mid-thigh and body fat percentage (Omron BF 300; OMRON, Matoukasa Co. Ltd, Japan) were assessed in this group to examine potential associations between anthropometric characteristics and muscle strength, RF diameter, local muscle and fat volume.

Statistical analyses

Data were analyzed using SAS statistical software version 9.2 for Windows (SAS Institute Inc, Cary, NC, USA). Data were reported as means ± standard deviation (SD) for anthropometric measurements, RF diameter and muscle strength measurements. The differences between both techniques were reported as means ± SD. The intraclass correlation coefficient ($ICC_{3,1}$) [10] values were computed to assess test-retest reliability of the US technique and the validity of US compared with CT-scan measurements. Additionally a Bland-Altman procedure was used to plot the difference between both techniques compared to the average for all participants and the data was checked for homoscedasticity by means of the correlation between the difference and average scores. Typical error of measurement (TEM) was calculated as the SD of the difference divided by the square root of 2. Zero order correlations (Pearson r) were calculated between anthropometric characteristics and muscle strength. The level of statistical significance was set at $p < 0.05$.

Results

A general overview of the descriptive characteristics of all included participants is shown in Table 1.

Ultrasound versus CT-measured rectus femoris diameter - validity

Baseline characteristics of group 1 are shown in Table 2. Diameter of the RF was 1.937 ± 0.31 cm with CT-scan and 1.925 ± 0.29 cm with US. The average difference (± SD) was non-significant (0.01 ± 0.12 cm, p = 0.66) resulting in a TEM of 0.08 cm or typical percentage error of 4.4%. The ICC between US and CT was 0.92 (95%CL: 0.81 - 0.97). The Bland-Altman plot presenting differences between both measurement procedures against average RF diameter is given in Figure 2. The limits of agreement (LOA) are (0.01 ± 0.24 cm). Only one score is out of the range of LOA. The correlation between the difference and average scores was -0.07 (p = 0.77) indicating homoscedasticity.

Results of the zero-order correlations between patient characteristics and muscle strength parameters are shown in Table 3. Highest correlations were found between muscle volume of the thigh and diameter of RF measured by CT with all muscle strength parameters. Correlations of diameter RF, measured by US, with strength parameters were lower than those of CT with strength. Muscle volume of the mid-thigh region correlated significantly with RF diameter measured with CT (r = 0.67, p = 0.001) and measured with US (r = 0.49, p < 0.05).

US RF diameter test-retest reliability

Table 4 shows the results of the two US measurements of the RF of 25 patients on two separate days. The

Table 1 Total group patient characteristics

	Mean ± SD or Number (%)
Gender (M/F)	44/1
Age (years)	68.4 ± 6.2
Height (cm)	171.7 ± 5.4
Weight (kg)	78.7 ± 11.3
BMI (kg/m^2)	26.6 ± 2.9
Time since last cardiac event (years)	6.0 ± 4.1
Past intervention	22 (49)
CABG (N patients)	
PCI (N patients)	22 (49)
Angina Pectoris (N patients)	1 (2)

BMI: Body mass index; CABG: Coronary artery bypass grafting; PCI: Percutaneous coronary intervention

Table 2 Rectus femoris diameter and patient characteristics in group 1 (N = 20)

	Mean	Std Dev
Height (cm)	172.2	4.5
Weight (kg)	78.1	11.1
Circumference thigh (cm)	50.5	3.4
Skinfold thigh (cm)	1.26	0.47
Body fat percentage (%)	29.0	4.1
Rectus Femoris Diameter with US (cm)	1.925	0.29
CT measurements		
Rectus Femoris Diameter (cm)	1.937	0.31
Femur Length (cm)	46.4	2.1
MuscleVolume (cm^3)	308	43.6
Fat Volume (cm^3)	116	40.8
Muscle strength		
Isometric extension 60° (Nm)	181	26
Isokinetic flexion 60°/s (Nm)	77.4	16.4
Isokinetic flexion 180°/s (Nm)	64.7	14.1
Isokinetic extension 60°/s (Nm)	129	21
Isokinetic extension 180°/s (Nm)	85.2	15

US: Ultrasound; CT: Computed tomography

difference between both measurements was non-significant (0.02 ± 0.10 cm, p = 0.4) with a TEM of 0.07 or a typical percentage error of 4.2%. The ICC was 0.97 (95% CL: 0.92 - 0.99) between the two measurements. The Bland-Altman plot presenting differences between both measurements against the average for both measurements is given in Figure 3. Two scores fall outside the boundaries of LOA. Minimal detectable difference (MDD) for this group of patients (N = 25) was 0.24 cm.

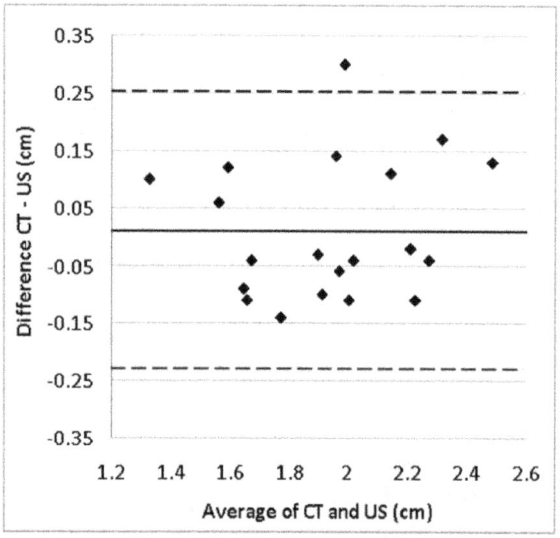

Figure 2 Bland-Altman plot for the difference between CT scan and Ultrasound for the rectus femoris diameter. CT: CT-Scan measurement, US: Ultrasound measurement of Rectus femoris. Full 'bold' line: average difference between CT and US. Broken line: limits of agreement.

Discussion

This study shows that US is a valid and reliable tool to measure the diameter of the RF in stable, elderly CAD patients. It further shows that the diameter of RF, measured with US, is significantly correlated with different muscle strength parameters.

We found a high ICC for both test-retest of the measurement of the RF with US (0.97) as for the comparison of RF measurements with US and CT (0.92) in these older cardiac patients. This is in line with the study of Seymour et al. [9] who reported in COPD patients an ICC of 0.97 for test-retest reliability of US measurement of rectus femoris CSA and of 0.88 for validity of the US measurement of rectus femoris CSA compared with CT. Also Bemben et al. [11] and Kanehisa et al. [12] reported an ICC of 0.72 and 0.99 respectively for test-retest reliability of the CSA measurements using B-mode US technique in various age groups. Bemben et al. tested US and MRI reliability for muscle CSA of the RF at 15 cm above the patella and found no significant differences between both techniques in young subjects (age: 26 years). Similar results were found for the reliability of the US measurement of the vastus lateralis muscle (ICC between 0.997 and 0.999) and for the validity compared with MRI scans (ICC between 0.998 and 0.999) [13].

All patients included in this study were CAD patients without cardiac event during the last 9 months, who participated in at least one session of exercise training per week under supervision of a physiotherapist, and could therefore be considered to be still fairly active elderly.

The observed diameter of RF in our sample of cardiac patients is comparable to earlier findings. That is, Delaney et al. [14] showed a RF depth of 2.3 cm in resting position in healthy young males (mean age 24.6 years). Arts et al. [15] found a quadriceps diameter (thickness of rectus femoris + vastus intermedius) in males of 4.16 ± 1.02 cm (age range 17-90 years) whereas Nogueira et al. [16] found a RF diameter of 1.86 cm in 20 older men (age 69-76 years).

In addition we investigated the relation between muscle diameter, muscle force and muscle volume in this cohort. We found strong correlations (0.61-0.75) between muscle volume and diameter assessed with CT and all the muscle strength parameters. Muscle diameter assessed with US also significantly correlated (0.45-0.61) with all strength measures, although the correlations where somewhat less as compared to CT. Muscle volume of the mid-thigh region correlated significantly (r = 0.67, p = 0.001) with RF diameter (CT-technique),

Table 3 Zero-order correlations between rectus femoris diameter, anthropometric characteristics and muscle strength parameters in group 1

	Isometric extension (Nm)	Isokinetic flexion 60°/s (Nm)	Isokinetic flexion 180°/s (Nm)	Isokinetic extension 60°/s (Nm)	Isokinetic extension 180°/s (Nm)
Age (years)	-0.18	-0.47*	-0.38	-0.18	-0.29
Weight (kg)	0.52*	0.31	0.38	0.42	0.42
Height (cm)	0.79**	0.12	0.30	0.50*	0.58**
Femur length (cm)	0.65**	0.06	0.05	0.51*	0.42
Fat volume thigh (cm^3)	-0.05	-0.30	-0.15	-0.11	-0.22
Body fat percentage (%)	-0.16	-0.28	-0.14	-0.12	-0.28
Skinfold thigh (cm)	-0.03	-0.13	-0.26	-0.08	-0.25
Circumference thigh (cm)	0.50*	0.39	0.45*	0.49*	0.46*
Muscle volume thigh (cm^3)	0.62**	0.75***	0.61**	0.68***	0.69***
RF diameter CT (cm)	0.69***	0.66**	0.67**	0.63**	0.74***
RF diameter US (cm)	0.52*	0.54*	0.61**	0.45*	0.59**

*p < 0.05, **p < 0.01,***p < 0.001

Table 4 Test - retest reliability of the ultrasound measurement in group 2

Patient	Measurement 1	Measurement 2	Difference
1	1.97	1.91	-0.06
2	1.4	1.39	-0.01
3	1.55	1.63	0.08
4	1.26	1.22	-0.04
5	1.77	1.99	0.22
6	2.01	2.09	0.08
7	2.02	1.94	-0.08
8	1.51	1.56	0.05
9	1.88	1.85	-0.03
10	1.51	1.82	0.31
11	1.31	1.3	-0.01
12	1.5	1.59	0.09
13	1.54	1.55	0.01
14	1.63	1.65	0.02
15	1.37	1.28	-0.09
16	1.64	1.65	0.01
17	1.9	2.02	0.12
18	1.74	1.67	-0.07
19	1.8	1.85	0.05
20	2.08	2.06	-0.02
21	1.94	1.84	-0.1
22	1.35	1.34	-0.01
23	1.66	1.63	-0.03
24	0.76	0.68	-0.08
25	0.72	0.72	0
Average	1.593	1.609	0.02 ± 0.10^{NS}

^{NS}: not significant

which was comparable to the results reported by Seymour et al. [9] in a healthy control group. RF diameter measured with US also significantly correlated with muscle volume ($r = 0.49$, $p < 0.05$). The reason for the less strong correlations when RF diameter was assessed by the US technique could be due to the higher variability of consecutive measurements in US (compression of the muscle tissue, deviation from perpendicular

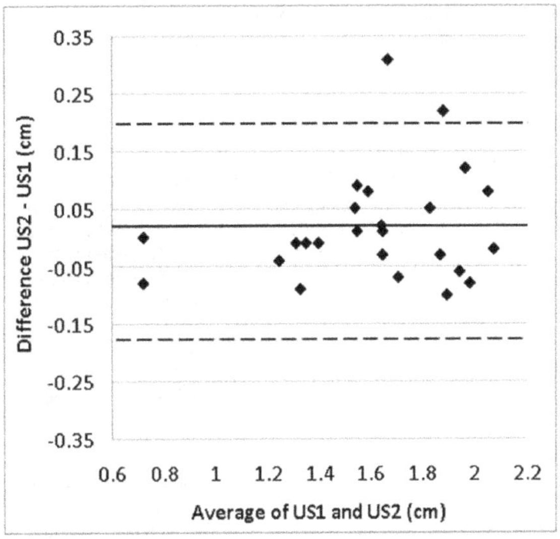

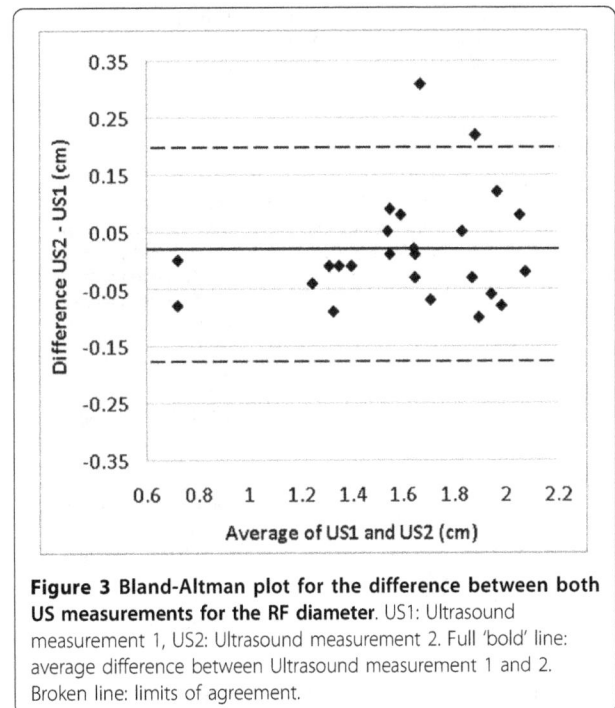

Figure 3 Bland-Altman plot for the difference between both US measurements for the RF diameter. US1: Ultrasound measurement 1, US2: Ultrasound measurement 2. Full 'bold' line: average difference between Ultrasound measurement 1 and 2. Broken line: limits of agreement.

viewing). The more accurate determination of the middle of the femur using CT (visualization of the bone structure by means of the scout view) compared with surface determination of bony landmarks in US could also be an important factor.

Earlier, the US technique has shown to be a valid and reliable alternative to CT or MRI in studies comparing muscle RF CSA of COPD patients with healthy controls [9] and in a study to determine the effects of resistance training on muscle thickness or muscle volume in older men [16]. In the latter study, an increase of 0.21 cm was found in the high velocity power training group, which is comparable with the MDD of 0.24 cm we found for test-retest reliability.

Conclusions

Nowadays, guidelines recommend the inclusion of resistance exercises in rehabilitation programs of cardiac patients. The observed validity and reliability make the use of an ultrasound device in cardiac rehabilitation an interesting tool to measure (changes in) muscle mass following exercise in all phases of cardiac rehabilitation.

Acknowledgements

This study was supported by grants from the Fund for Scientific Research -Flanders 'Fonds voor Wetenschappelijk Onderzoek - Vlaanderen', Belgium (F. W.O. grant G.0624.08 and G.0124.02) and from the Research Council of the University of Leuven 'Onderzoeksraad KU Leuven', Belgium (grant OT/07/064 and OT/01/046).

Author details

[1]Cardiovascular Rehabilitation Unit, Department of Rehabilitation Sciences, Katholieke Universiteit Leuven, Tervuursevest 101, 3001 Heverlee, Belgium. [2]Exercise and Health Research Group, Department of Kinesiology, Katholieke Universiteit Leuven, Tervuursevest 101, 3001 Heverlee, Belgium. [3]Radiology, University Hospital Leuven, Herestraat 49, 3000 Leuven, Belgium.

Authors' contributions

TT analyzed and interpreted the data, performed statistical analysis, and drafted the manuscript. MT performed statistical analyses, assisted with interpretation of the data. SO assisted with the collection and analyses of the data. WC acquired and interpreted the CT scan. VC assisted with interpretation of the data. LV conceived and designed the research. All authors read, approved and contributed to the manuscript.

Competing interests

The authors declare that they have no competing interests.

References

1. World Health Organization: **The top ten cause of death.**[http://www.who.int/mediacentre/factsheets/fs310_2008.pdf].
2. Metter EJ, Talbot LA, Schrager M, Conwit R: **Skeletal muscle strength as a predictor of all-cause mortality in healthy men.** *J Gerontol A Biol Sci Med Sci* 2002, **57**:B359-B365.
3. Rantanen T: **Muscle strength, disability and mortality.** *Scand J Med Sci Sports* 2003, **13**:3-8.
4. Rantanen T, Harris T, Leveille SG, Visser M, Foley D, Masaki K, Guralnik JM: **Muscle strength and body mass index as long-term predictors of mortality in initially healthy men.** *J Gerontol A Biol Sci Med Sci* 2000, **55**: M168-M173.
5. Ghroubi S, Chaari M, Elleuch H, Massmoudi K, Abdenadher M, Trabelssi I, Akrout M, Feki H, Frikha I, Dammak J, Kammoun S, Zouari N, Elleuch MH: **The isokinetic assessment of peripheral muscle function in patients with coronary artery disease: correlations with cardiorespiratory capacity.** *Ann Readapt Med Phys* 2007, **50**:295-301.
6. Sumide T, Shimada K, Ohmura H, Onishi T, Kawakami K, Masaki Y, Fukao K, Nishitani M, Kume A, Sato H, Sunayama S, Kawai S, Shimada A, Yamamoto T, Kikuchi K, Amano A, Daida H: **Relationship between exercise tolerance and muscle strength following cardiac rehabilitation: comparison of patients after cardiac surgery and patients with myocardial infarction.** *J Cardiol* 2009, **54**:273-281.
7. Kida K, Osada N, Akashi YJ, Sekizuka H, Omiya K, Miyake F: **The exercise training effects of skeletal muscle strength and muscle volume to improve functional capacity in patients with myocardial infarction.** *Int J Cardiol* 2008, **129**:180-186.
8. de Bruin PF, Ueki J, Watson A, Pride NB: **Size and strength of the respiratory and quadriceps muscles in patients with chronic asthma.** *Eur Respir J* 1997, **10**:59-64.
9. Seymour JM, Ward K, Sidhu PS, Puthucheary Z, Steier J, Jolley CJ, Rafferty G, Polkey MI, Moxham J: **Ultrasound measurement of rectus femoris cross-sectional area and the relationship with quadriceps strength in COPD.** *Thorax* 2009, **64**:418-423.
10. Shrout PE, Fleiss JL: **Intraclass correlations: usesin assessing rater reliability.** *Psych Bull* 1979, **86**:420-428.
11. Bemben MG: **Use of diagnostic ultrasound for assessing muscle size.** *J Strength Cond Res* 2002, **16**:103-108.
12. Kanehisa H, Ikegawa S, Tsunoda N, Fukunaga T: **Crosssectional areas of fat and muscles in limbs during growth and middle age.** *Int J Sports Med* 1994, **15**:420-425.
13. Reeves ND, Maganaris CN, Narici MV: **Ultrasonographic assessment of human skeletal muscle size.** *Eur J Appl Physiol* 2004, **91**:116-118.
14. Delaney S, Worsley P, Warner M, Taylor M, Stokes M: **Assessing contractile ability of the quadriceps muscle using ultrasound imaging.** *Muscle Nerve* 2010, **42**:530-538.
15. Arts IM, Pillen S, Schelhaas HJ, Overeem S, Zwarts MJ: **Normal values for quantitative muscle ultrasonography in adults.** *Muscle Nerve* 2010, **41**:32-41.
16. Nogueira W, Gentil P, Mello SN, Oliveira RJ, Bezerra AJ, Bottaro M: **Effects of power training on muscle thickness of older men.** *Int J Sports Med* 2009, **30**:200-204.

Ultrasonographic assessment of carpal tunnel syndrome of mild and moderate severity in diabetic patients by using an 8-point measurement of median nerve cross-sectional areas

Shu-Fang Chen[1,2†], Chi-Ren Huang[1†], Nai-Wen Tsai[1], Chiung-Chih Chang[1,2], Cheng-Hsien Lu[1], Yao-Chung Chuang[1] and Wen-Neng Chang[1*]

Abstract

Background: Using high-resolution ultrasonography (US) to measure the median nerve cross-sectional areas (CSAs) such as in the "inching test" conducted in nerve conduction studies is a valuable tool to assess carpal tunnel syndrome (CTS). However, using this US measurement method to assess the median nerve CSA in diabetic patients with CTS has rarely been reported. Therefore, we used this US measurement method in this study to measure median nerve CSAs and to compare the CSAs of idiopathic, diabetic and diabetic polyneuropathy (DPN) patients with CTS.

Methods: 124 hands belonging to 89 participants were included and assigned into four groups: control (32), idiopathic (38), diabetic (38) and DPN (16) CTS. In the latter two groups, only patients with mild and moderately severe CTS were included. The median nerve CSAs were measured at 8 points marked as *i*4, *i*3, *i*2, *i*1, *w*, *o*1, *o*2, and *o*3 in the inching test. The measured CSAs in each group of participants were compared.

Results: Compared with the CSAs of the control group, enlarged CSAs were found in the idiopathic, diabetic and DPN CTS groups. The CSAs were larger at *i*4, *i*3 and *i*2 in the diabetic CTS group compared to the idiopathic CTS group. The CSAs measured at the *i*1 and *w* levels of the DPN CTS group were smaller than those of the diabetic CTS group. In the diabetic CTS group, the cut-off values of CSAs measured at the inlet, wrist crease, and outlet were 15.3 mm^2, 13.4 mm^2 and 10.0 mm^2, respectively, and 14.0 mm^2, 12.5 mm^2 and 10.5 mm^2, respectively, in the DPN CTS group.

Conclusions: Compared with the median nerve CSAs of the control and idiopathic CTS groups, the median nerve CSAs of the diabetic patients with CTS were significantly enlarged. However, compared with the diabetic CTS group, the CSAs were significantly smaller in the DPN CTS group. This US 8-point measurement method can be of value as an important complementary tool for CTS studies and diagnosis among diabetic patients.

* Correspondence: cwenneng@ms19.hinet.net
†Equal contributors
[1]Department of Neurology, Kaohsiung Chang Gung Memorial Hospital and Chang Gung University College of Medicine, Tai-Pei road, Kaohsiung 833, Taiwan
Full list of author information is available at the end of the article

Background

Carpal tunnel syndrome (CTS) is a common entrapment neuropathy with prevalence rates of 2% in the general population, 14% in diabetic patients without diabetic polyneuropathy (DPN), and 30% in diabetic patients with DPN [1,2]. The diagnosis of CTS is usually based on clinical symptoms as well as the results of nerve conduction studies (NCS). However, because of diabetic hand syndromes, the diagnosis of CTS in patients with diabetes can be difficult if using clinical symptoms and NCS with various comparative tests [3-7] alone. Ultrasonography (US) is a non-invasive and easily performed procedure for median nerve morphology measurement. Based on the findings of median nerve cross-sectional area (CSA) enlargement in the carpal tunnel, US can be used to confirm CTS with a high degree of accuracy [8-10]. US has been used in clinical studies on diabetic neuropathy [11,12], however its use in the clinical evaluation of CTS in diabetic patients has not been reported in the literature. In our previous study, we reported the results of an US study [10] for the evaluation of idiopathic CTS using the same 8-point measurements of the median nerve CSAs from inlet to outlet as in the "inching test" of antidromic sensory studies using 1-cm increments of the median nerve [13]. Although there were some limitations to the study, the results showed the value of this US measurement method as an important complementary tool to confirm CTS. Therefore we used this US measurement method in this study to measure median nerve CSAs, and to compare the measured CSAs of idiopathic, diabetic and DPN patients with CTS.

Methods

Patients

This prospective case–control study was carried out over a period of four years (2006–2009), and was approved by the Ethics Committee of Chang Gung Memorial Hospital (IRB 100-1390B). In this study, the following procedures were used to enroll the study cases: first, those who had signs and symptoms fulfilling the clinical diagnostic criteria of CTS were referred by the authors to undergo NCS and US studies; then, those who fulfilled the inclusion criteria of idiopathic CTS, diabetic CTS or DPN CTS were further considered for enrollment, and finally, those who agreed to sign informed consent forms were enrolled into this study. Normal controls were also recruited.

In this study, diabetic patients were defined as those who had symptoms (polyuria, polydipsia, and unexplained weight loss) of diabetes mellitus (DM) plus a casual plasma glucose concentration ≥ 200 mg/dL, or a fasting plasma glucose level of ≥ 126 mg/dL on at least two occasions, or a plasma glucose level of ≥ 200 mg/dL at two hours for a 75-g oral glucose tolerance test (OGTT) [14]. In the control and idiopathic CTS groups, DM was excluded by a fasting serum glucose level < 100 mg/dl, or a two-hour postprandial serum glucose level < 110 mg/dl and no clinical symptoms of DM. Serum glycohemoglobin (HbA1C) levels of all enrolled participants were measured. Patients with other systemic diseases including gout, rheumatic arthritis, thyroid disease, renal disease, hepatic disease, abnormal serum cortisol levels or elevated serum antinuclear antibodies were excluded by blood tests and clinical history. None of the participants had a history of wrist surgery or fracture, and none had a history or any clinical evidence of neurologic disorders (e.g. ulnar neuropathy, radiculopathy, polyneuropathy (not DM related), myelopathy, or stroke) that may have resulted in numbness or paresthesia of the hand. Participants with a variant of carpal tunnel such as accessory muscles, bifid median nerve and persistent median artery found by US were also excluded. In addition, none of the female participants were pregnant at the time of the study.

Definition of clinical CTS

Clinical CTS was defined according to the criteria of The American Academy of Neurology practice parameters [15,16] as follows:

1. Paresthesia, pain, swelling, weakness, or clumsiness of the hand provoked or worsened by sleep, sustained hand or arm position, or repetitive action of the hand or wrist that is mitigated by changing posture or by hand shaking.
2. Sensory deficits in the median nerve innervated region of the hand.
3. Motor deficit or hypotrophy of the median nerve innervated thenar muscles.
4. Positive provocative clinical tests (positive Phalen's maneuver and/or Tinel's sign).

Clinical CTS was defined as the fulfillment of criterion 1 and one or more of the other criteria.

Clinical definition of polyneuropathy

The symptoms and signs of suspected DPN were examined according to the recommendations of the American Academy of Electrodiagnostic Medicine (AAEM) [17]. A combination of neuropathic symptoms, neuropathic signs and abnormal electrodiagnostic studies provides the diagnosis of distal symmetric polyneuropathy. In this study, an electrodiagnostic abnormality plus at least one sign and one symptom were sine qua non for the confirmation of the presence of polyneuropathy. The neuropathic symptoms included sensory symptoms (distal numbness, burning, prickling paresthesia, dysesthesia and allodynia) and/or motor symptoms (decreased sensibility on the distal lower extremity, distal muscle weakness or atrophy). The neuropathic signs included an absent or decreased ankle deep tendon reflex, distal sensory decrease or absence, and distal weakness and muscle atrophy. Abnormal electrodiagnostic studies included at least a sural, or peroneal and one median or ulnar nerve dysfunction, however entrapment lesions were excluded

Electrophysiologic methods

NCS was performed for all participants according to the recommended protocol of the AAEM [18] using a Nicolet Viking Select system (Nicolet Biomedical Inc. Madison, USA). The comparative tests and the cut-off points were as follows [19-23]: 1) median-ulnar sensory conduction between the wrist and ring finger; 2) median sensory nerve conduction comparison between the wrist and palm; 3) median-radial sensory conduction between the wrist and thumb; and 4) antidromic sensory test using 1-cm increments of the median nerve; 5) median nerve distal sensory latency < 3.4 ms; 6) median nerve distal motor latency over the thenar < 4.2 ms; 7) a difference between the median and ulnar nerve distal sensory latencies < 0.4 ms; 8) transcarpal median motor conduction velocity < 40.6 ms; and 9) antidromic sensory testing using 1-cm increments of the median nerve < 0.4 ms. The locations of the inching test were as shown in Figure 1, with the wrist crease as the zero reference point extending proximally by 3 cm and distally by 4 cm. In total, eight points (*i*4, *i*3, *i*2, i1, *w*, *o*1, *0*2, *0*3) were marked in the subsequent inching test. According to the results of the NCS, the CTS hands were categorized into six groups of severity [23]: negative, minimal, mild, moderate, severe and extreme. In this study, only those belonging to the mild (abnormal digit/wrist sensory nerve conduction velocity and normal distal motor latency) and moderate (abnormal digit/wrist sensory nerve conduction velocity and abnormal distal motor latency) NCS groups were included in the final analysis.

NCS for polyneuropathy detection was also performed according to the study protocol of the AAEM [17]. Sural, tibial, ulnar and peroneal nerves were also examined to determine whether or not the included participants fit the diagnostic criteria of polyneuropathy. The segmental tests (ulnar nerve at elbow and peroneal nerve at the fibula head) were also performed to exclude entrapment neuropathy.

The normal limits of NCS of the abovementioned nerves other than the median nerve were as follows: ulnar nerve (distal motor latency < 3.4 ms, motor conduction velocity > 52 m/s, sensory conduction velocity > 44 m/s, compound muscle action potential > 5.5 mV, sensory nerve action potential > 9 μV), peroneal (distal latency < 5.5 ms, conduction velocity > 42 m/s, compound motor action potential > 2.1 mV), tibial nerve (distal latency < 6.4 ms, conduction velocity > 41 m/s, compound motor action potential > 4.7 mV), and sural nerve (conduction velocity > 38 m/s, sensory nerve action potential > 5 μV).

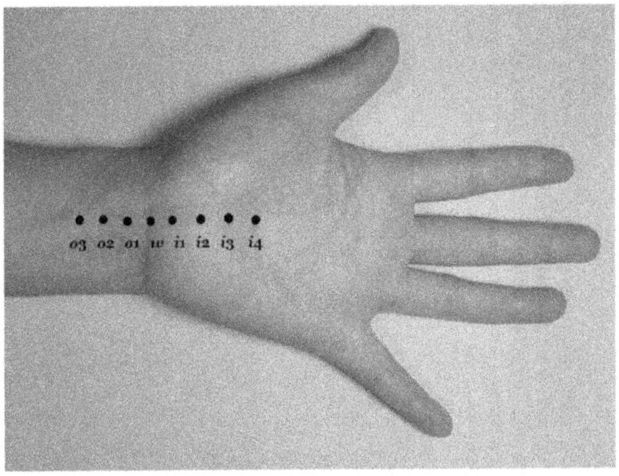

Figure 1 The 8 points (*i*4, *i*3, *i*2, *i*1, *w*, *o*1, *o*2, and *o*3) for recording in both the "inching test" and ultrasonography. *i*4, *i*3, *i*2, *i*1 represent levels at 4, 3, 2, and 1 cm distal to the wrist crease in the inlet of the carpal tunnel; *w* represents the level of the wrist crease and *o*1, *o*2, and *o*3 represent levels at 1, 2, and 3 cm proximal to the wrist crease in the outlet of the carpal tunnel.

Ultrasound assessment technique

The US assessment technique we used in this study has been previously described [10]. In brief, high-resolution US were performed using a scanner with a 12/5-MHz linear array transducer for the carpal tunnel study (Philips HDI 5000; Philips Medical Systems, Bothell, WA, USA). US examinations were performed on the same day as the NCS. During the examination, the patient sat in a comfortable position facing the examiner, with the measured forearm resting on the table, the palm supine, and fingers semi-extended in the neutral position [24]. The median nerve was imaged in a longitudinal scan first, placing the US probe at the midline between the radius and ulna with the center of the probe at the distal wrist crease, to obtain an initial general overview of the median nerve which was then used to assist the examiner in order to obtain optimal axial (cross-sectional) images. Then a transverse scan, keeping the probe directly perpendicular to the long axis of the median nerve in order to ensure that the area measured indeed reflected a CSA, was performed to record the CSA (calculated by continual tracing of the nerve circumference, excluding the hyperechoic epineurial rim) and elliptical (the transverse and the anteroposterior) diameters. The measurements were performed from the inlet of carpal

Table 1 Demographic data of the 89 participants (124 hands)

	Control hands	Idiopathic CTS hands	Diabetic CTS hands	DPN CTS hands	*p* value
Numbers	32	38	38	16	
Sex	9 M/23 F	9 M/29 F	9 M/29 F	4 M/12 F	0.971[+]
Age (yrs)	56.5 ± 8.0 (54.5, 48.0-76.0)	59.2 ± 9.3 (57.0, 44.0-83.0)	58.6 ± 9.4 (56.0, 38.0-76.0)	61.0 ± 7.8 (63.0, 50.0-73.0)	0.365
BH (cm)	160.6 ± 8.6 (159.0, 151.0-184.0)	157.0 ± 5.1 (157.0, 147.0-167.0)[※]	155.3 ± 5.3 (154.0, 146.0-170.0)	151.7 ± 4.8 (150.0, 143.0-160.0)	0.002[*]
BW (kg)	61.8 ± 9.6 (60.0, 51.3-96.0)	63.3 ± 9.5 (62.0, 47.0-82.0)	68.0 ± 12.0 (67.0, 45.0-92.0)	61.6 ± 10.9 (60.0, 50.0-88.0)	0.099
BMI kg/m^2	23.9 ± 2.3 (24.2, 19.7-28.4)	25.6 ± 3.2 (24.9, 20.3-31.6)	28.0 ± 4.5 (27.2, 19.7-35.9)	26.8 ± 4.8 (25.6, 21.4-39.1)	0.002[*]
HbA1c (%)	5.6 ± 0.4 (5.6, 5.0-6.2)	5.8 ± 0.3 (5.8, 5.3-6.3)	7.3 ± 1.0 (7.2, 5.7-9.5)	7.9 ± 3.0 (6.9, 6.1-18.9)	0.904

CTS = carpal tunnel syndrome; DPN = diabetic polyneuropathy; BH = body height; BW = body weight; BMI = body mass index; M = male; F = female.
The data shown are mean ± standard deviation (SD) (median, range).
[*] = $p < 0.05$ (significant difference among the normal control, idiopathic, diabetic and DPN CTS hands) by the Kruskal-Wallis test.
[+] = a comparison of the sex difference and symptom duration among the control, idiopathic, diabetic and DPN CTS hands by the Chi-Square test.
[※] = a comparison of the BH between the control and the idiopathic CTS hands by the Mann–Whitney U test showed no significant difference.

Table 2 The measured CSAs of the control, idiopathic, diabetic and DPN groups

	Control hands (n = 32)	Idiopathic CTS hands (n = 38)	Diabetic CTS hands (n = 38)	DPN CTS hands (n = 16)	*p* value^1	*p* value^2	*p* value^3
i4	12.6 ± 3.0 (12.0, 6.0-19.0)	17.5 ± 6.4 (16.5, 8.0-39.0)	20.4 ± 5.4 (19.5, 13.0-34.0)	20.9 ± 13.8(15.5, 8.4-62.0)	0.015*	0.109	0.000*
i3	12.2 ± 2.9 (12.0, 6.0-19.0)	16.3 ± 5.8 (15.5, 8.0-33.0)	19.3 ± 5.5 (19.0, 10.0-31.0)	19.0 ± 9.1 (15.5, 8.4-43.0)	0.015*	0.310	0.000*
i2	11.5 ± 2.5 (11.0, 7.0-18.0)	12.5 ± 3.7 (12.0, 6.0-29.0)	14.2 ± 3.9 (13.5, 9.0-24.0)	13.6 ± 5.9 (11.5, 9.0-34.0)	0.026*	0.242	0.010*
i1	10.8 ± 2.1 (10.2, 7.0-17.0)	14.0 ± 4.8 (13.0, 8.0-28.0)	15.5 ± 4.4 (14.8, 7.7-26.1)	12.7 ± 3.1 (13.0, 7.0-21.0)	0.105	0.043*	0.000*
w	11.8 ± 2.6 (11.0, 8.0-19.0)	16.2 ± 4.5 (15.0,11.0-31.0)	17.9 ± 6.6 (16.0, 8.1-45.8)	14.8 ± 4.7 (13.5, 8.0-28.0)	0.217	0.039*	0.000*
o1	10.6 ± 2.4 (10.0, 6.0-16.0)	14.0 ± 3.7 (13.4, 8.0-23.0)	15.4 ± 5.9 (14.0, 7.0-42.8)	14.3 ± 5.5 (13.0, 7.0-30.0)	0.237	0.458	0.000*
o2	11.0 ± 2.6 (10.5, 7.0-17.0)	12.2 ± 2.6 (12.0, 8.0-19.5)	13.8 ± 4.0 (13.0, 8.6-29.0)	12.8 ± 5.3 (12.5, 7.4-29.0)	0.090	0.181	0.006*
o3	10.0 ± 2.4 (9.5, 7.0-15.0)	10.8 ± 2.2 (10.4, 6.0-16.0)	12.4 ± 3.5 (11.7, 7.0-20.0)	12.2 ± 4.0 (10.5, 8.7-25.0)	0.060	0.601	0.017*

CTS = carpal tunnel syndrome; CSA = cross-sectional area; DPN = diabetic polyneuropathy.
The data shown are mean ± standard deviation (SD) (median, range).
Unit of CSA = mm^2.
i4, i3, *i2*, *i1*, *w*, *o1*, *o2*, and *o3* = the 8 points marked.
***p* value^1** = a comparison between the idiopathic and the diabetic CTS hands using the Mann–Whitney U test.
***p* value^2** = a comparison between the diabetic and the DPN CTS hands using the Mann–Whitney U test.
***p* value^3** = a comparison among control, idiopathic CTS, the diabetic and the DPN CTS hands using the Kruskal-Wallis test.
* = $p < 0.05$.

Table 3 The cut-off values of CSA of the idiopathic, diabetic and DPN CTS groups (compared with the control group)

Location	Idiopathic CTS group					Diabetic CTS group					DPN CTS group				
	Sen.	Spec.	Area	Cuff-off value of CSA	Sig.	Sen.	Spec.	Area	Cuff-off value of CSA	Sig.	Sen.	Spec.	Area	Cuff-off value of CSA	Sig.
i4	73.7	59.4	0.760	13.0	0.000*	84.2	84.4	0.921	15.3	0.000*	62.5	59.4	0.750	14.0	0.005*
i3	73.7	62.5	0.734	12.8	0.001*	76.3	93.7	0.889	15.3	0.000*	62.5	68.7	0.784	14.0	0.001*
i2	63.2	62.5	0.602	11.4	0.142	63.2	71.9	0.722	12.4	0.001*	50.0	62.5	0.620	11.5	0.179
i1	71.1	62.5	0.727	11.5	0.001*	76.3	62.5	0.813	11.4	0.000*	62.5	62.5	0.716	11.5	0.016*
w	78.9	68.7	0.824	12.5	0.000*	81.6	71.9	0.859	13.4	0.000*	62.5	68.7	0.731	12.5	0.010*
o1	68.4	65.6	0.777	11.5	0.000*	81.6	65.6	0.832	11.2	0.000*	75.0	65.6	0.757	11.7	0.004*
o2	60.5	65.6	0.647	11.5	0.035*	76.3	65.6	0.744	11.0	0.000*	56.3	65.6	0.600	11.5	0.265
o3	73.7	50.0	0.598	9.5	0.159	68.4	56.2	0.698	10.0	0.004*	50.0	56.2	0.688	10.5	0.035*

CSAs = cross-sectional areas; DPN = diabetic polyneuropathy; Sen. =sensitivity; Spec. =specificity; Sig. =significance; ROC = Receiver Operating Characteristic; CTS = carpal tunnel syndrome; NCS = nerve conduction study.
i4, i3, i2, i1, w, o1, o2, and *o3* = the 8 points marked.
Unit of CSA = mm^2; Sen. = %; Spec. = %.
* = Sig. < 0.05 (asymptotic significance under the ROC curve).

tunnel to the distal segment of the forearm, as shown in Figure 1, at the 8 points (*i4*, *i3*, *i2*, i1, *w*, *o1*, *02*, *03*) [10].

Study patient groups

In total, 124 hands belonging to 89 participants were enrolled in this study, and they were divided into four groups as follows:

1. Control group (22 participants, 32 hands): Healthy volunteers who had no clinical or electrophysiologic evidence of CTS or other neurologic disorders.
2. Idiopathic CTS group (30 participants, 38 hands): Those who had clinical and electrophysiologic evidence of CTS, but no other medical or neurologic disorders that may have resulted in numbness or paresthesia of the hands.
3. Diabetic CTS group (26 participants, 38 hands): Those who had clinical symptoms and findings of CTS, and also fulfilled the electrophysiologic criteria of CTS. They did not have clinical or electrophysiologic evidence of polyneuropathy, ulnar or radial neuropathy.
4. DPN CTS group (11 participants, 16 hands): Diabetic patients who had clinical symptoms and findings of CTS and also fulfilled the electrophysiologic criteria of CTS. They also had clinical and electrophysiologic evidence of polyneuropathy.

Among the enrolled CTS patients, bilateral hand involvement was noted in 11 patients of the idiopathic CTS group, 7 in the diabetic CTS group and 3 in the DPN CTS group.

Statistical analysis

The data were all presented as mean ± standard deviation (median, range) for statistical analysis. Comparisons between the demographic data of the control, idiopathic, diabetic CTS and DPN CTS groups were made using the Kruskal-Wallis test for continuous variables including age, body weight (BW), body height (BH), body mass index (BMI). The chi-square test was used for the categorical variables including sex. To evaluate the differences in CSA values measured at the 8 points between the idiopathic, diabetic and DPN CTS hands, the Mann–Whitney U test was used. Significance was set at $p < 0.05$ in the Mann–Whitney U test and Kruskal-Wallis test. The area under the receiver operating characteristic (ROC) curves and the cut-off-values of CSA were calculated for the idiopathic, diabetic and DPN CTS groups. The Statistical Package for Social Sciences software (SPSS Inc., version 13.0 for Windows) was used for all statistical analyses.

Results

The demographic data of the 89 participants (142 hands) are shown in Table 1. There were no significant differences in age, gender and BW among the control, idiopathic, diabetic and DPN CTS groups. Compared with the control group, the BH was shorter in the diabetic and DPN CTS groups; however the BMI was higher in the idiopathic, diabetic and DPN CTS groups. If the control group was not included for analysis, differences in MBI values among the idiopathic, diabetic and DPN CTS groups were not significant ($p = 0.165$). There were no significant differences in HbA1c values between the diabetic and DPN CTS groups.

The CSAs measured at the 8 points (*i4*, *i3*, *i2*, *i1*, *w*, *o1*, *o2*, *o3*) of the four groups of participants are listed in Table 2. The measured CSAs were larger at *i4*, *i3* and *i2* of the diabetic group than those of the idiopathic CTS group. Compared with the diabetic group, the CSAs measured at the *i1* and *w* levels of the DPN group were smaller.

Table 3 and Figure 2 show the cut-off values and corresponding sensitivities and specificities of CSAs in the diagnosis of CTS in the idiopathic, diabetic and DPN groups. These cut-off values were derived from a comparison with the CSAs of the control group. In the idiopathic group, the cut-off values of CSAs measured at the inlet, wrist crease, and outlet were 13.0 mm^2, 12.5 mm^2 and 9.5 mm^2, respectively; in the diabetic group 15.3 mm^2, 13.4 mm^2 and 10.0 mm^2, respectively; and 14.0 mm^2, 12.5 mm^2 and 10.5 mm^2, respectively, in the DPN group. The largest CSA cut-off value at the *w* level was in the diabetic group. At the outlet levels, there were no significant differences in cut-off values between the control and the idiopathic group, however there were statistically significant differences between the control (CSA cut-off value = 9.5 mm^2) and diabetic group (CSA cut-off value = 10.0 mm^2), and between the control and the DPN group (CSA cut-off value = 10.5 mm^2).

Discussion

In clinical practice, it is difficult to distinguish CTS from other neuropathic syndromes in diabetic patients, even when electrodiagnostic tests are also applied for such purposes [2,5,6]. An enlargement of median nerve CSA measured in CTS hands is a well established US finding [8-10], and with multiple-level CSA measurements, the complementary role of US in the diagnosis of CTS becomes more valuable [10]. The same US findings were also noted in the present study which showed enlarged CSAs in patients with idiopathic CTS as well as in those with diabetic CTS and DPN CTS. There are reports [11,12] of US studies of peripheral nerves in diabetic patients, however using US to measure the CSAs at 8

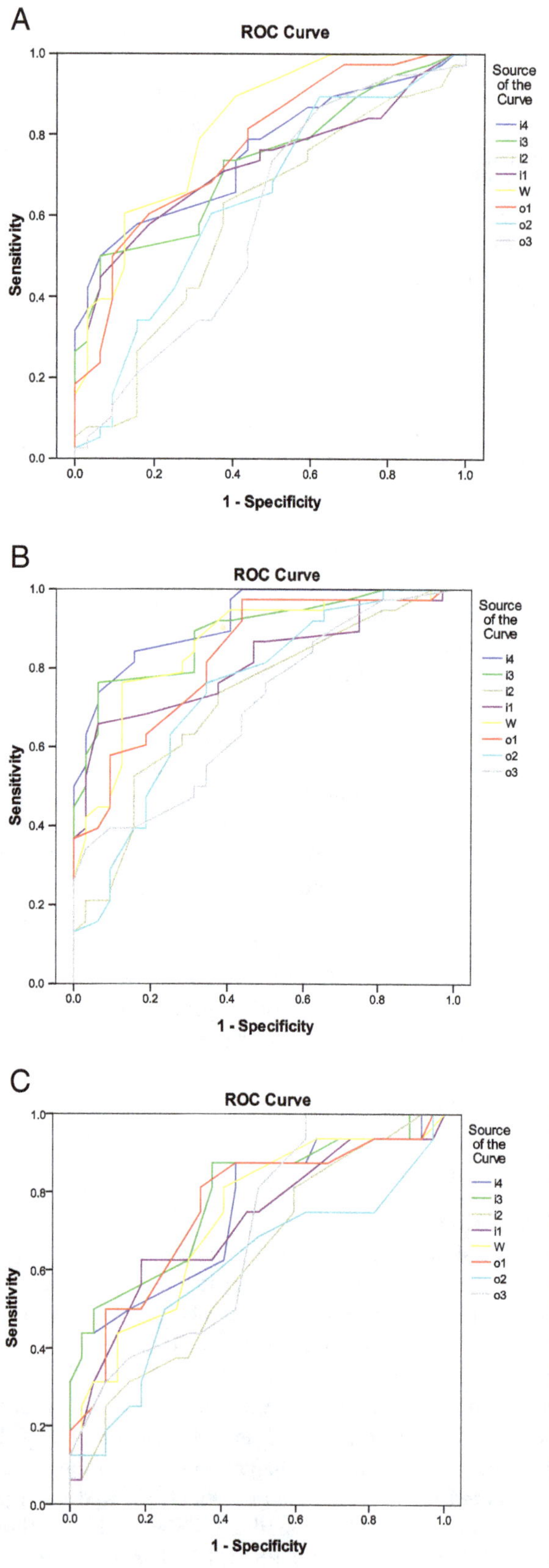

Figure 2 ROC curves of the cut-off values of cross-sectional areas (CSA) of the idiopathic (A), diabetic (B) and diabetic polyneuropathy (DPN) (C) carpal tunnel syndrome (C).

points such as in the "inching test" to assess CTS in diabetic patients has not been reported before.

The study results showed that the measured CSAs in both the diabetic and DPN groups were larger than those measured in the idiopathic and control groups. The BMIs of patients of the CTS groups were significantly larger than those of patients in the control group. It has been proposed that a higher BMI may increase the incidence of symptomatic CTS [3], however a significant correlation with median nerve CSA measured at the wrist level was not found in the study of Werner et al. [25]. It may deserve further investigations to demonstrate if a correlation exists between BMI and CSA in diabetic patients with CTS. BH was another statistically significant factor between the different groups. It has been proposed that a difference in BH may influence the result of nerve conduction velocity [26], however it is not a known factor to influence the median nerve CSA [27].

In US studies, different CSA cut-off values (9 mm^2 – 14 mm^2) at the entry level (inlet) of the carpal tunnel have been reported for CTS confirmation in idiopathic CTS patients [28]. In the present study, we revealed the cut-off values of CSAs measured at different levels of the patients with idiopathic, diabetic and DPN CTS. Although larger CSAs measured in the carpal tunnel 5 cm proximal to the wrist and elbow joint of the median nerve in diabetic and diabetic polyneuropathy patients were reported by Watanabe et al. [11,12], comparative results of measured CSAs at the inlet level of diabetic patients have not been reported before. In the present study, we measured the CSAs within the carpal tunnel in the hands of the diabetic patients with CTS, and the results also showed larger CSAs when compared with the CSAs measured in both the control and idiopathic groups. Several factors are known to be contributing factors to CTS, including mechanical and ischemic factors, external epineurial and perineurial thickening and fibrosis [29], and all of these factors may in-part explain the local enlargement of median nerve CSAs. However, as shown in this study, there may be additional factors contributing to the focal enlargement of median nerve CSAs in diabetic patients, and especially at the level of the inlet. In DM, the polyol pathway, glycation and proinflammatory reactions are known to contribute to the presence of diabetic peripheral nerve injuries [30], and a reduction in myelinated nerve fibers and capillary density may predispose DM patients to the development of CTS [31]. In addition, more ischemic and biochemical changes may further result in the enlargement of median nerve CSAs.

One peculiar finding of the present study is that the measured median nerve CSAs of the patients in the DPN group, especially at *i*1 and *w* levels, were smaller than those measured in the diabetic group. This finding has not been reported previously, but may be partially related to the loss of nerve regeneration capacity in advanced diabetic neuropathy [4,31,32]. This finding may also partially explain why the response to CTS treatment in diabetic patients varies greatly, especially when different intervention methods are used, when compared with the therapeutic results of idiopathic CTS [33-35].

There are limitations to this study. First, some of the patients may have been included twice if they had bilateral CTS symptoms. Second, the number of cases is limited; therefore, US findings in the different subgroups of CTS patients could not be fully analyzed. Further large-scale studies of US findings in CTS among diabetic patients are needed for a better delineation.

Conclusion

This is the first study to use US and an 8-point measurement method to assess and compare the median nerve CSAs of participants belonging to control, idiopathic, diabetic and DPN CTS groups. We suggest the cut-off values for CTS confirmation in each group, and also show the following: 1) Compared with the controls, the CSAs were significantly enlarged in patients with idiopathic CTS, diabetic CTS and DPN CTS; 2) Compared with the idiopathic group, the CSAs were significantly enlarged in patients with diabetic CTS and DPN CTS; and 3) Compared with the diabetic group, the CSAs were significantly smaller in patients in the DPN group. Several pathophysiologic mechanisms may, at least partially, explain the findings of the inter-group differences of median nerve CSAs. This US 8-point measurement method can be of value as an important complementary tool for the diagnosis of CTS among diabetic patients.

Competing interests

All of the authors declare no competing or conflicts of interests.

Authors' contributions

All authors have read and approved the submitted manuscript. SFC and CRH contributed to the conception and design, data acquisition and analysis, and drafting and revision of the manuscript; CHL, YCC, NWT, and CCC contributed to the conception and design, and clinical data analysis; and WNC contributed to the conception and design, data analysis, and critical revision and final approval of the manuscript.

Author details

[1]Department of Neurology, Kaohsiung Chang Gung Memorial Hospital and Chang Gung University College of Medicine, Tai-Pei road, Kaohsiung 833, Taiwan. [2]Department of Biological Science, National Sun Yat-Sen University, Kaohsiung, Taiwan.

References

1. Wilbourn AJ: **Diabetic entrapment and compression neuropathies.** In *Diabetic Neuropathy.* Edited by Dyck PJ, Thomas PK. Philadelphia: Saunders; 1999:481–508.
2. Perkins BA, Olaleye D, Bril V: **Carpal tunnel syndrome in patients with diabetic polyneuropathy.** *Diabetes Care* 2002, **25:**565–569.
3. Makepeace A, Davis WA, Bruce DG, Davis TM: **Incidence and determinants of carpal tunnel decompression surgery in type 2 diabetes: the Fremantle Diabetes Study.** *Diabetes Care* 2008, **31:**498–500.
4. Yasuda H, Terada M, Maeda K, Kogawa S, Sanada M, Haneda M, Kashiwagi A, Kikkawa R: **Diabetic neuropathy and nerve regeneration.** *Prog Neurobiol* 2003, **69:**229–285.
5. Gazioglu S, Boz C, Cakmak VA: **Electrodiagnosis of carpal tunnel syndrome in patients with diabetic polyneuropathy.** *Clin Neurophysiol* 2011, **122:**1463–1469.
6. Yagci I, Gunduz OH, Sancak S, Agirman M, Mesci E, Akyuz G: **Comparative electrophysiological techniques in the diagnosis of carpal tunnel syndrome in patients with diabetic polyneuropathy.** *Diabetes Res Clin Pract* 2010, **88:**157–163.
7. Imada M, Misawa S, Sawai S, Tamura N, Kanai K, Sakurai K, Sakamoto S, Nomura F, Hattori T, Kuwabara S: **Median-radial sensory nerve comparative studies in the detection of median neuropathy at the wrist in diabetic patients.** *Clin Neurophysiol* 2007, **118:**1405–1409.
8. Klauser AS, Halpem EJ, De Zordo T, Feuchtner GM, Arora R, Gruber J, Martinoli C, Loscher WN: **Carpal tunnel syndrome assessment with US: value of additional cross-sectional area measurements of the median nerve in patients versus healthy volunteers.** *Radiology* 2009, **250:**171–177.
9. Hobson-Webb LD, Massey JM, Juel VC, Sanders DB: **The ultrasononographic wrist-to-forearm median nerve area ratio in carpal tunnel syndrome.** *Clin Neurophysiol* 2008, **119:**1353–1357.
10. Chen SF, Lu CH, Huang CR, Chuang YC, Tsai NW, Chang CC, Chang WN: **Ultrasonographic median nerve cross-section areas measured by 8-point "inching test" for idiopathic carpal tunnel syndrome: a correlation of nerve conduction study severity and duration of clinical symptoms.** *BMC Med Imaging* 2012, **11:**22.
11. Watanabe T, Ito H, Morita A, Uno Y, Nishimura T, Kawase H, Kato Y, Matsuoka T, Takeda J, Seishima M: **Sonographic evaluation of the median nerve in diabetic patients: comparison with nerve conduction studies.** *J Ultrasound Med* 2009, **28:**727–734.
12. Watanabe T, Ito H, Sekine A, Katano Y, Nishimura T, Kato Y, Takeda J, Seishima M, Matsuoka T: **Sonographic evaluation of the peripheral nerve in diabetic patients: the relationship between nerve conduction studies, echo intensity, and cross-sectional area.** *J Ultrasound Med* 2010, **29:**697–708.
13. Nathan PA, Meadows KD, Doyle LS: **Sensory segmental latency values of the median nerve for a population of normal individuals.** *Arch Phys Med Rehabil* 1988, **69:**499–501.
14. American Diabetes Association: **Diagnosis and classification of diabetes mellitus.** *Diabetes Care* 2006, **29**(suppl 1):S43–S48.
15. Practice parameter for carpal tunnel syndrome (summary statement): **Report of the Quality Standards Subcommittee of the American Academy of Neurology.** *Neurology* 1993, **43:**2406–2409.
16. You H, Simmons Z, Freivalds A, Kothari MJ, Naidu SH: **Relationships between clinical symptom severity scales and nerve conduction measures in CTS.** *Muscle Nerve* 1999, **22:**497–501.
17. England JD, Gronseth GS, Franklin G, Millaer RG, Asbury AK, Carter GT, Cohen JA, Fisher MA, Howard JF, Kinsella LJ, Latov N, Lewis RA, Low PA, Sumner AJ: **American Academy of Neurology; American Association of Electrodiagnostic Medicine; American Academy of Physical Medicine and Rehabilitation. Distal symmetric polyneuropathy: a definition for clinical research: report of the American Academy of Neurology, the American Association of Electrodiagnostic Medicine, and the American Academy of Physical Medicine and Rehabilitation.** *Neurology* 2005, **64:**199–207.
18. Jablecki CK, Andary MT, Floeter RG, Miller CA, Quartly CA, Vennix MJ, Wilson JR: **American Association of Electrodiagnostic Medicine; American Academy of Neurology; American Academy of Physical Medicine and Rehabilitation: Practice parameter; Electrodiagnostic studies in carpal tunnel syndrome. Report of the American Association of Electrodiagnostic Medicine, American Academy of Neurology, and the American Academy of Physical Medicine and Rehabilitation.** *Neurology* 2002, **58:**1589 1592.

19. Jackson DA, Clifford JC: **Electrodiagnosis of mild carpal tunnel syndrome.** *Arch Phys Med Rehabil* 1989, **70:**199–204.
20. Uncini A, Lange DJ, Solomon M, Soliven B, Meer J, Lovelace RE: **Ring finger testing in CTS: a comparative study of diagnostic utility.** *Muscle Nerve* 1989, **12:**735–741.
21. Walters RJL, Murray NMF: **Transcarpal motor conduction velocity in carpal tunnel syndrome.** *Muscle Nerve* 2001, **24:**966–968.
22. Di Guglielmo G, Torrieri F, Repaci M, Uncini A: **Conduction block and segmental velocities in carpal tunnel syndrome.** *Electroencephalogr Clin Neurophysiol* 1997, **105:**321–327.
23. Padus L, LoMonaco M, Gregori B, Valente EM, Padua R, Tonali P: **Neurophysiological classification and sensitivity in 500 CTS hands.** *Acta Neurol Scand* 1997, **96:**211–217.
24. Kuo MH, Leong CP, Cheng YF, Chang HW: **Static wrist position associated with least median nerve compression: sonographic evaluation.** *Am J Phys Med Rehabil* 2001, **80:**256–260.
25. Werner RA, Jacobson JA, Jamadar DA: **Influence of body mass index on median nerve function, carpal canal pressure, and cross-sectional area of the median nerve.** *Muscle Nerve* 2004, **30:**481–485.
26. Bodofsky E, Tomaio A, Campellone J: **The mathematical relationship between height and nerve conduction velocity.** *Electromyogr Clin Neurophysiol* 2009, **49:**155–160.
27. Hunderfund AN, Boon AJ, Mandrekar JN, Sorenson EJ: **Sonography in carpal tunnel syndrome.** *Muscle Nerve* 2011, **44:**485–491.
28. Seror P: **Sonography and electrodiagnosis in carpal tunnel syndrome diagnosis, an analysis of the literature.** *Eur J Radiol* 2008, **67:**146–152.
29. Mackinnon SE: **Pathophysiology of nerve compression.** *Hand Clin* 2002, **18:**231–241.
30. Yagihashi S: **Recent advances in clinical practice and in basic research on diabetic neuropathy.** *Brain Nerve* 2011, **63:**571–582.
31. Thomsen NO, Mojaddidi M, Malik RA, Dahlin LB: **Reduced myelinated nerve fibre and endoneurial capillary densities in the forearm of diabetic and non-diabetic patients with carpal tunnel syndrome.** *Acta Neuropathol* 2009, **118:**785–791.
32. Kennedy JM, Zochodne DW: **Impaired peripheral nerve regeneration in diabetes mellitus.** *J Peripher Nerv Syst* 2005, **10:**144–157.
33. Nishimura T, Hirata H, Tsujii M, Iida R, Hoki Y, Iino T, Ogawa S, Uchida A: **Pathomechanism of entrapment neuropathy in diabetic and nondiabetic rats reared in wire cages.** *Histol Histopathol* 2008, **23:**157–166.
34. Ozkul Y, Sabuncu T, Kocabey Y, Nazligul Y: **Outcomes of carpal tunnel release in diabetic and non-diabetic patients.** *Acta Neurol Scand* 2002, **106:**168–172.
35. Kiylioglu N, Bicerol B, Ozkul A, Akyol A: **Natural course and treatment efficacy: one-year observation in diabetic and idiopathic carpal tunnel syndrome.** *J Clin Neurophysiol* 2009, **26:**446–453.

22

Ultrasound point shear wave elastography of the pancreas: comparison of patients with type 1 diabetes and healthy volunteers

Sophie Püttmann[1], Janina Koch[1], Jochen Paul Steinacker[2], Stefan Andreas Schmidt[2], Thomas Seufferlein[1], Wolfgang Kratzer[1*], Julian Schmidberger[1] and Burkhard Manfras[3]

Abstract

Background: The aims of this study were to establish shear wave elastography of the pancreas by comparing measurements in patients with type 1 diabetes (T1D) and healthy volunteers and to consider whether this method could contribute to the screening or prevention of T1D.

Methods: This pilot study included 15 patients with T1D (10 men, 5 women) and 15 healthy volunteers (10 men, 5 women) as controls. Measurements were performed with a Siemens Acuson S3000 (Siemens Healthcare, Erlangen, Germany) using a 6C1 convex transducer and the Virtual Touch™ tissue quantification (VTQ) method.

Results: The mean shear wave velocity of the head of the pancreas was 1.0 ± 0.2 m/s (median: 1.1 m/s) for the study group and likewise 1.0 ± 0.2 m/s (median: 0.9 m/s) for the control group. Velocities of 1.2 ± 0.2 m/s (median: 1.2 m/s) were measured in the body of the pancreas in both groups. There was a significant difference between the values obtained in the tail of the pancreas: patients 1.1 ± 0.1 m/s (median: 1.0 m/s) versus controls 0.9 ± 0.1 m/s (median: 0.8 m/s) ($p = 0.0474$). The mean value in the whole pancreas of the study group was not significantly above that of the control group: 1.1 ± 0.1 m/s (median: 1.0 m/s) versus 1.0 ± 0.1 m/s (median: 1.0 m/s) ($p = 0.2453$).

Conclusions: Sonoelastography of the pancreas revealed no overall difference between patients with T1D and healthy volunteers. Patients with T1D showed higher values only in the tail segment. Future studies need to determine whether specific regional differences can be found in a larger study population.

Keywords: Type 1 diabetes, Ultrasound p-shear wave elastography, Healthy volunteers, Pancreas

Background

Type 1 diabetes (T1D) is an autoimmune disease in which insulin-producing beta cells in the pancreas are destroyed. Comparative international figures show an annual increase of 3–4% in the global incidence rates of T1D [1]. Since there is a strong genetic contribution to T1D, further screening modalities could be of interest for patients at genetic risk [2]. Shear wave elastography presents a method for determining the elasticity of the target tissue, using ultrasound to determine the velocity of shear waves [3]. The procedure was originally developed as a non-invasive investigation for the early diagnosis and treatment of liver fibrosis [4]. D'Onofrio et al. and Kawada et al. described ductal adenocarcinoma as stiffened tissue with an increased shear wave velocity (Vs) due to the fibrotic process [3, 4]. Studies have also shown an increase in the Vs in patients with chronic pancreatitis [5]. Recent studies on type 2 diabetes (T2D) have demonstrated that elastographic examination of the pancreas shows an increased Vs in affected patients compared with healthy subjects [6]. Concerning type 1 diabetes, a recent study on children and adolescents did not show any increased values in those

* Correspondence: wolfgang.kratzer@uniklinik-ulm.de
[1]Department of Internal Medicine I, University Hospital Ulm, Albert-Einstein-Allee 23, 89081 Ulm, Germany
Full list of author information is available at the end of the article

with T1D. However, that study looked only at the body of the pancreas [7].

It is assumed that pathological mechanisms associated with fibrotic change cause the inflamed tissue to increase stiffness [3–5]. As inflammation in the islets of Langerhans (insulitis) and fibrosis also occur in T1D [8–10], questions arise as to whether the inflammatory process and the associated alteration in tissue consistency can be measured by shear wave elastography and whether changes can be detected even in the prediabetic phase, when an insulitic process is already taking place. As the results of the various elastographic studies show a certain lack of agreement regarding both examination precision and current clinical relevance [3, 5], this procedure has still to be established for the diagnostic investigation of pancreatic disease.

Although a growing understanding of the pancreatic pathology is allowing the development of novel immune intervention strategies to alter the course of insulitis, additional non-invasive diagnostic tools are still desirable for the early diagnosis of T1D and monitoring the course of disease [2].

The aims of this pilot study were therefore to establish shear wave elastography in the three anatomical regions of the pancreas (head, body, and tail) and evaluate possible alterations in stiffness due to the pathology of T1D by comparing elastographic measurements in patients with T1D and healthy controls.

Methods

Patients and healthy volunteers

The study population comprised 15 patients with T1D and 15 healthy volunteers as controls. Baseline characteristics are summarised in Table 1. We recruited the patients with type 1 diabetes from the hospital diabetes outpatient clinic and an endocrinology practice. Patients had been diagnosed previously with T1D in accordance with the guidelines and irrespective of the study [11]. The control group consisted of healthy volunteers selected to match the individual patients for age and sex. The following exclusion criteria were applied to the whole study population:

Table 1 Overview of the study population

	Mean ± SD median (min-max) IQR			
	Whole population	Patients with type 1 diabetes	Healthy volunteers	*p*-value
Sex				
Male	20 (66.7%)	10 (66.7%)	10 (66.7%)	1.0
Female	10 (33.3%)	5 (33.3%)	5 (33.3%)	
Age [years]	31.8 ± 9.6	32.1 ± 9.5	31.4 ± 10.1	0.9006
	30 (20.0–54.0)	30.0 (20.0–50.0)	28.0 (21.0–54.0)	
	17,0	17,0	17,0	
BMI [kg/m^2]	23.7 ± 2.7	24.3 ± 3.0	23.3 ± 2.4	0.3947
	22.9 (19.9–29.4)	24.8 (19.9–29.4)	22.3 (20.8–28.9)	
	3,7	5,1	3,0	
Duration of diabetes [months]		45.7 ± 42.3		
		25.0 (5.0–125.0)		
		61,0		
HbA_{1c} [%]		6.7 ± 0.9	5.2 ± 0.2	< 0.0001
		7.0 (5.4–8.0)	5.2 (4.8–5.6)	
		1,5	0,3	
Fasting glucose [mg/dl]		111.2 ± 37.0	90.0 ± 7.8	0.0777
		102.0 (66.0–191.0)	89.0 (73.0–104.0)	
		51,0	11,0	
C peptide[a] [μg/l]		0.9 ± 0.7	1.6 ± 0.5	0.0082
		0.7 (0.1–2.0)	1.6 (0.8–2.8)	
		1,1	0,4	
Basal insulin (IU/d]		13.9 ± 7.4		
		12.0 (2.0–30.0)		
		11,0		

SD Standard deviation, *min* Minimum, *max* Maximum, *IU* International unit, *level of significance* $P < 0.05$, *IQR* Inter quartile range
[a]C peptide was not measured in one female patient

- disease or surgery of the pancreas (acute or chronic pancreatitis, pancreatic cancer, partial or complete resection of the pancreas)
- disease of the liver or biliary tract (hepatitis, primary sclerosing cholangitis (PSC), primary biliary cirrhosis (PBC), alcoholic steatohepatitis (ASH), non-alcoholic steatohepatitis (NASH), cirrhosis of the liver, and portal hypertension)
- BMI > 30 kg/m^2
- fasting for < 6 h
- alcohol abuse (> 20 g alcohol for women, > 40 g alcohol for men)
- weight fluctuation +/– 10 kg in the last 3 months
- pregnancy.

Endocrine diseases were exclusion criteria in healthy volunteers but not in patients, since T1D is not uncommonly associated with other endocrine disorders.

Further exclusion criteria for the healthy volunteers were an HbA_{1c} of 5.7–6.4% (prediabetic range) or > 6.4%, as well as positive antibodies (IAA, IA2, GAD65). These parameters were measured in a venous blood sample from each participant. Data on the medical history were collected with a standardised questionnaire and we obtained additional information about the onset of the disease, duration, and treatment regimen from the patients. The study was conducted in conformity with the principles of the Helsinki Declaration and Good Clinical Practice and was approved by the local Ethics Committee (No. 331–15, 1 September 2015). All participants enrolled in the study gave their written informed consent.

Twenty-one patients with T1D and 17 healthy volunteers initially participated in our elastography study. Six patients and two healthy volunteers were subsequently excluded. One patient had no islet-cell autoantibodies. This patient and one other had a BMI over the limit of 30 kg/m^2. Two male patients were excluded because of high alcohol consumption > 40 g/d. A marked fluctuation in weight over the past 3 months led to the exclusion of two more patients. One patient had lost more than 10 kg in weight, while the other had gained more than 10 kg during this period.

Blood tests in one of the healthy volunteers revealed diabetes antibodies (GAD65 and IA2) leading to exclusion from the control group. Another healthy volunteer was excluded because of a fasting period less than 6 h.

Elastography

All p-shear wave elastographic measurements were carried out with Virtual Touch™ Quantification (VTQ) on a Siemens Acuson S3000 using a 6C1 convex transducer (Figs. 1, 2 and 3). VTQ is based on the technique of acoustic radiation force impulse (ARFI) imaging, using ultrasound waves to determine the tissue stiffness quantitatively and calculate the numerical Vs. At the start of each investigation, the pancreas was demonstrated in B-mode and the upper abdomen assessed to rule out any hepatic or cholestatic disease. In this study, a 10 × 5 mm region of interest (ROI) was selected for each pancreatic segment (head, body, and tail) and at least five elastographic measurements taken in each case. The confluence of the splenic and superior mesenteric veins was taken to mark the boundary between head and body. The tail of the pancreas was identified as the structure anterior to the left kidney, extending to the hilum of the spleen. It was particularly important to ensure that no blood vessels were located within the ROI, since pulsations (including those from the aorta) can interfere with ARFI [12]. Participants were positioned supine; they were asked

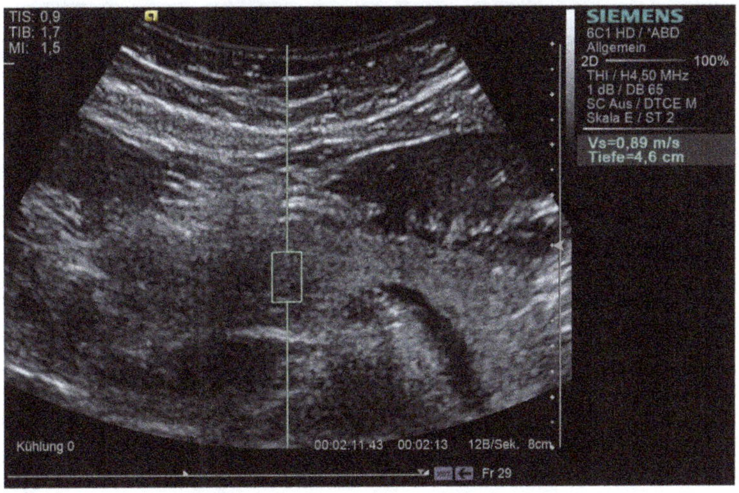

Fig. 1 Measurement of the shear wave velocity (Vs) of the head of the pancreas with VTQ

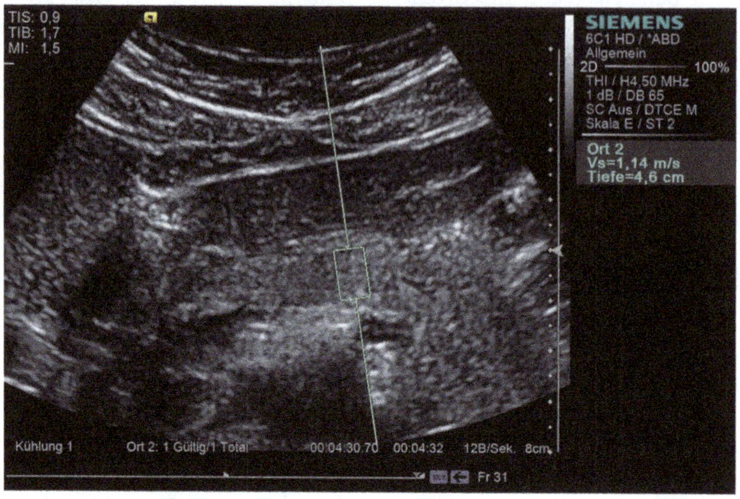

Fig. 2 Measurement of the shear wave velocity (Vs) of the body of the pancreas with VTQ

to exhale completely and hold their breath during each Vs measurement in order to reduce motion artefacts as much as possible. The mean and standard deviation were calculated for each pancreatic segment, and the median value also given in units of m/s. A single examiner, who was not blinded with respect to the diagnosis of diabetes, carried out all the measurements. The Vs measurements were also checked for correlation with the duration of diabetes and the BMI of both patients and healthy volunteers.

Statistical analysis

We used SAS 9.2 software (SAS Institute Inc., Cary, North Carolina, USA) for the statistical analysis. The mean, standard deviation, median, and the range (minimum-maximum) were calculated as continuous variables in each case. Discrete variables were given with absolute and relative frequencies. We used the Wilcoxon rank sum test to show any differences in continuous variables between two groups (e.g. patients and healthy volunteers or men and women) and chose the Wilcoxon signed rank test to compare two continuous variables. Correlation of parameters was calculated with Spearman's rank correlation coefficient. For all the statistical analyses, a p-value of less than 0.05 in two-tailed tests was considered to be significant. Gpower Version 3.1. was used for statistical power analysis and sample size analysis. Assuming a power of greater than 80% (1-β), the analysis yielded a total sample size of $n \geq 30$ for the statistical methods and the pilot study.

Results

Tissue elasticity was measured in the three pancreatic segments: head, body and tail. The mean overall

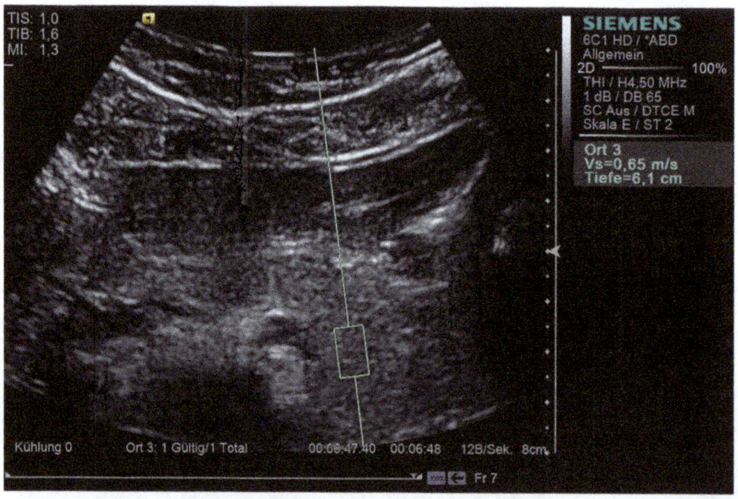

Fig. 3 Measurement of the shear wave velocity (Vs) of the tail of the pancreas with VTQ

velocity measured in the control group was 1.0 ± 0.1 m/s. The corresponding figure in the study group was 1.1 ± 0.1, showing no significant difference ($p = 0.2453$).

The shear wave velocity of the tail differed significantly between patients with T1D and healthy volunteers indicating a higher stiffness in T1D ($p = 0.0474$) (Table 2). In contrast, the Vs in the head and body was not significantly different between the two groups. With respect to the elastographic measurements, it was also of interest to establish the segment of the organ showing the highest and lowest velocity in each group. Comparing the means, we found the highest velocity in the body of the pancreas in both groups (1.2 ± 0.2).

In the control group of healthy volunteers, we found a positive correlation with age for the individual pancreatic segments of the head and body, as well as for the whole pancreas (head: $p = 0.0009$, $R = 0.76308$; body: $p = 0.0022$, $R = 0.72589$; whole pancreas: $p = 0.0012$, $R = 0.75430$) but established no such relationships in the patient group. There was no association between Vs and duration of diabetes in the study group for either of the individual pancreatic segments or the whole organ ($p = 0.7534$) nor was there any correlation between BMI and Vs in either group (patients: $p = 0.7129$; controls: $p = 0.5402$). The position of the pancreas in the abdomen meant that the maximum ultrasound penetration depth of 8 cm was insufficient in one patient and made it impossible to take any measurements in the deeper-lying segments. Large quantities of intestinal air can also make it more difficult or even impossible to measure the pancreas. For this reason, the tail segment could not be measured in two of our patients.

Table 2 Elastographic measurements in the head, body and tail of the pancreas of patients with type 1 diabetes and healthy volunteers

Vs in [m/s]	Mean ± SD median (min-max) IQR		
	Patients with type 1 diabetes	Healthy volunteers	*p*-value
Site 1 = head	1.0 ± 0.2[a]	1.0 ± 0.2	0.4193
	1.1 (0.7–1.5)	0.9 (0.6–1.3)	
	0,3	0,2	
Site 2 = body	1.2 ± 0.2	1.2 ± 0.2	0.9834
	1.2 (0.9–1.8)	1.2 (0.9–1.6)	
	0,18	0,4	
Site 3 = tail	1.0 ± 0.2[b]	0.9 ± 0.1	0.0474
	1.0 (0.8–1.3)	0.8 (0.7–1.2)	
	0,04	0,2	
Mean (1–3)	1.1 ± 0.1	1.0 ± 0.1	0.2453
	1.0 (0.9–1.4)	1.0 (0.8–1.2)	
	0,2	0,2	

Vs Shear wave velocity, *SD* Standard deviation, *min* Minimum, *max* Maximum, *IQR* Inter quartile range, *level of significance* $P < 0.05$
[a]1 Missing from 1 patient because a penetration depth > 8 cm not possible, only site 2 could be measured in this patient
[b]Missing from 2 patients

Discussion

Both ultrasound strain elastography and ultrasound shear wave elastography appear to play an increasing role in the diagnostic investigation of pancreatic disease [13, 14]. Despite the increasing importance of elastographic procedures in the diagnosis of pancreatic disease, we are aware of only a few studies on shear wave elastography of the pancreas in patients with diabetes [15, 16]. In our pilot study, we intended to demonstrate the feasibility of measuring all three anatomical parts of the pancreas and determine measurement limitations with respect to patient characteristics and examination conditions.

Our results (Table 2) show a significant difference between patients and healthy volunteers in the tail of the pancreas ($p = 0.0474$). The mean value for all segments showed only a trend towards a higher Vs in the patient group.

In a recent study, Saglam et al. did not find any significant differences between children and adolescents with T1D and healthy subjects, but the measurements were performed only on the body of the pancreas. This finding agrees with our results for that region. They reported Vs of 1.09 ± 0.22 m/s for the body of the pancreas in healthy control subjects and 0.99 ± 0.25 m/s for patients with type 1 diabetes – values slightly lower than we found in our patients [7].

Chronic inflammatory processes lead to fibrotic remodelling consistent with non-physiological wound healing not only in the islets of Langerhans (insulitis) but also in the exocrine tissue of the pancreas [17–19]. Pancreatic fibrosis particularly affects patients with longstanding disease [10, 20]. In our study, the longest duration of disease was about 10 years.

The higher velocities detected may not be due exclusively to fibrosis, as other histological changes may impact the physical properties of the tissue. But fibrotic changes are known to result from type 1 diabetes [17, 21, 22].

One possible explanation for our significant results from the tail could be a greater accumulation of inflammatory CD8+ T cells in this organ segment during insulitis. We can assume that these cells are not only responsible for considerable destruction of the beta cells but are also to be found in greater numbers in the exocrine tissue [19]. In the context of recurrent inflammation of the islets of Langerhans in T1D, Rajput et al. described a higher concentration of beta cells in the tail of the pancreas [10]. This would suggest that patients with T1D have stiffer tissue in the tail of the pancreas, giving higher Vs values in this segment.

Harada et al. used shear wave elastography with ultrasound to examine the body of the pancreas preoperatively in patients about to undergo pancreatic resection. They showed a strong correlation of Vs to the severity of pathological fibrosis in the pancreatic tissue [15].

Stumpf et al. found normal values for the head of the pancreas to be 1.44 ± 0.39 m/s for women and 1.19 ± 0.29 m/s for men. Values for the body were 1.49 ± 0.37 m/s for women and 1.26 ± 0.30 m/s for men, while the corresponding figures for the tail were 1.29 ± 0.36 m/s and 1.05 ± 0.30 m/s, respectively [14]. The values given by Harada et al., with 1.35 m/s for the body of the pancreas, are to a large extent in agreement with the values given by Stumpf et al. and our measurements [15]. Their results for male participants agree extremely well with our results. As the percentage of women in our healthy control group was only 30%, this may explain why the values in the literature for the two sexes combined are slightly higher than our results. Yashima et al. found mean values for head, body and tail of 1.23 m/s, 1.3 m/s and 1.24 m/s in healthy volunteers and of 1.65 m/s, 2.09 m/s and 1.68 m/s in patients with chronic pancreatitis [5]. Xie et al. reported mean values for the pancreatic head and body of 1.18 m/s and 1.21 m/s in healthy controls [23]. The data from Goertz et al. are in accordance with these measurements, with a mean of 1.2 m/s. The average for patients with chronic pancreatitis in that study was 2.21 m/s [24]. Mateen et al. reported results of 1.28 m/s, 1.25 m/s, and 3.28 m/s for healthy controls, patients with chronic pancreatitis, and patients with acute pancreatitis, respectively [25]. Llamoza-Torres et al. obtained figures of 1.27 m/s for healthy volunteers and 1.57 m/s for patients with chronic pancreatitis [26]. Further studies evaluate ARFI as a suitable and promising procedure for the non-invasive diagnostic investigation of chronic pancreatitis and other pancreatic conditions, both benign and malignant, such as cystic lesions and carcinomas [12, 26–29]. In the literature, the highest Vs was recorded in the body of the pancreas whenever the individual pancreatic segments were measured. Our results confirm these findings, as the Vs of the body of the pancreas was significantly higher in both groups.

In the healthy volunteers, we found a very strong relationship between the Vs and the age of the participant, confirming the observation of Stumpf et al. [14]. Nevertheless, in contrast to their study, we did not find any correlation between Vs and BMI. Nor did we determine a correlation between the Vs and the duration of diabetes ($p = 0.7534$), a finding which agrees with the results published by Saglam et al. [7].

Although our pilot study comprised only 30 participants and is therefore of limited statistical power, our results compare well with previously published data on pancreas elastography. Since one very experienced examiner carried out all the measurements, we eliminated any bias from different examiners. However, the ultrasound images were not checked by a second reader, which is a definite limitation of the study. Our examiner was not blinded to the participant being a healthy volunteer or a patient. In the present study, our findings were statistically significant in the tail of the pancreas: this part of the organ is the most difficult to examine with imaging techniques and might therefore also be the most inaccurate. The precision of Vs measurement by shear wave elastography may be affected by vascular pulsation and the maximum depth of shear wave detection may be a further limitation, especially in obese patients [12].

For such a detailed analysis of changes in pancreatic morphology in T1D, factors that would limit the measurement precision, as well as variations in the examination conditions, led to individuals being excluded from the study population. Furthermore, the average duration of diabetic disease in our patients was 45 months, which is not a very long time in the course of T1D. Results could be different in patients who have had the disease for a longer period.

Conclusion

In conclusion, we have presented the first elastographic measurements of all pancreatic segments in patients with T1D. We found no overall difference between patients and healthy volunteers. There is only a trend indicating that chronic inflammatory processes in T1D may lead to stiffer tissue in the tail of the pancreas. Elastography is a non-invasive, reliable, and rapidly available procedure offering additional information in the diagnostic investigation of pancreatic disease. Especially for patients at risk of T1D, it might represent a promising imaging modality for screening purposes. Additional studies need to clarify whether a higher Vs is associated with T1D-specific pancreatic changes and whether this finding is related to the duration of diabetes.

Abbreviations

ARFI: Acoustic radiation force impulse; ROI: Region of interest; T1D: Type 1 diabetes mellitus; Vs: Shear wave velocity; VTQ: Virtual Touch™ Quantification

Acknowledgements

The authors would like to thank the patients, the healthy volunteers, and everyone else who participated in the study.

Funding

No funding was received.

Authors' contributions

SP, JK, WK and BM conceived the study and participated in its design, data collection, statistical analysis and drafting of the manuscript. TS, JPS, SAS, JS participated in data collection and data analysis. All authors read and approved the final manuscript for publication.

Consent for publication

Not applicable.

Competing interests

The authors declare that they have no competing interests.

Author details

[1]Department of Internal Medicine I, University Hospital Ulm, Albert-Einstein-Allee 23, 89081 Ulm, Germany. [2]Department of Diagnostic and Interventional Radiology, University Hospital Ulm, Albert-Einstein-Allee 23, 89081 Ulm, Germany. [3]Medicover Medical Centre, Münsterplatz 6, 89073 Ulm, Germany.

References

1. Bendas A, Rothe U, Kiess W. Trends in incidence rates during 1999-2008 and prevalence in 2008 of childhood type 1 diabetes mellitus in Germany – model-based national estimates. PLoS One. 2015;10:1–12.
2. Noble JA. Genetics of the hla region in the prediction of type 1 diabetes. Curr Diab Rep. 2011;11:533–42.
3. D'Onofrio M, Crosara S, De Robertis R, Canestrini S, et al. Elastography of the pancreas. Eur J Radiol. 2014;83:415–9.
4. Kawada N, Tanaka S, Uehara H, Ohkawa K, et al. Potential use of point shear wave elastography for the pancreas: a single center prospective study. Eur J Radiol. 2014;83:620–4.
5. Yashima Y, Sasahira N, Isayama H, Kogure H, et al. Acoustic radiation force impulse elastography for noninvasive assessment of chronic pancreatitis. J Gastroenterol. 2012;47:427–32.
6. He Y, Wang H, Li XP, Zheng J-J, et al. Pancreatic elastography from acoustic radiation force impulse imaging for evaluation of diabetic microangiopathy. Am J Roentgenol. 2017;209:775–80.
7. Sağlam D, Bilgici MC, Kara C, Yılmaz GC, et al. Acoustic radiation force impulse elastography in determining the effects of type 1 diabetes on pancreas and kidney elasticity in children. Am J Roentgenol. 2017;209:1–7.
8. Bluestone J, Herold K, Eisenbarth G. Genetics, pathogenesis and clinical interventions in type 1 diabetes. Nature. 2010;464:1293–300.
9. Foulis A, Stewart J. The pancreas in recent-onset type 1 (insulin-dependent) diabetes mellitus: insulin content of islets, insulitis and associated changes in the exocrine acinar tissue. Diabetologia. 1984;26:456–61.
10. Rajput R, Ram M, Maheshwari S, Goyal RK, et al. Pancreatic imaging by ultrasonography in type 1 diabetes mellitus. Int J Diabetes Metab. 2001;9:75–80.
11. Kerner W, Brückel J. Definition, Klassifikation and Diagnostik des Diabetes mellitus. Diabetologie. 2014;9:96–9.
12. Kawada N, Tanaka S. Elastography for the pancreas: current status and future perspective. World J Gastroenterol. 2016;22:3712–24.
13. Chantarojanasiri T, Hirooka Y, Kawashima H, Ohno E, et al. Age-related changes in pancreatic elasticity: when should we be concerned about their effect on strain elastography? Ultrasonics. 2016;69:90–6.
14. Stumpf S, Jaeger H, Graeter T, Oeztuerk S, et al. Influence of age, sex, body mass index, alcohol, and smoking on shear wave velocity (p-swe) of the pancreas. Abdom Radiol. 2016;41:1310–6.
15. Harada N, Ishizawa T, Inoue Y, Aoki T, et al. Acoustic radiation force impulse imaging of the pancreas for estimation of pathologic fibrosis and risk of postoperative pancreatic fistula. J Am Coll Surg. 2014;219:887–94.
16. Roche EF, McKenna AM, Ryder KJ, Brennan AA, et al. Is the incidence of type 1 diabetes in children and adolescents stabilising? The first 6 years of a national register. Eur J Pediatr. 2016;175:1913–9.
17. Zechner D, Knapp N, Bobrowski A, Radecke T, et al. Diabetes increases pancreatic fibrosis during chronic inflammation. Exp Biol Med. 2014;239:670–6.
18. Ghosh AK, Quaggin SE, Vaughan DE. Molecular basis of organ fibrosis: potential therapeutic approaches. Exp Biol Med. 2013;238:461–81.
19. Rodriguez-Calvo T, Ekwall O, Amirian N, Zapardiel-Gonzalo J, et al. Increased immune cell infiltration of the exocrine pancreas: a possible contribution to the pathogenesis of type 1 diabetes. Diabetes. 2014;63:3880–90.
20. Gilbeau JP, Poncelet V, Libon E, Derue G, et al. The density, contour, and thickness of the pancreas in diabetics: ct findings in 57 patients. Am J Roentgenol. 1992;159:527–31.
21. Cecil RL. A study of the pathological anatomy of the pancreas in ninety cases of diabetes mellitus. J Exp Med. 1909;11:266–90.
22. Philippe M-F, Benabadji S, Barbot-Trystram L, Vadrot D, et al. Pancreatic volume and endocrine and exocrine functions in patients with diabetes. Pancreas. 2011;40:359–63.
23. Xie J, Zou L, Yao M, Xu G, et al. A preliminary investigation of normal pancreas and acute pancreatitis elasticity using virtual touch tissue quantification (vtq) imaging. Med Sci Monit. 2015;21:1693–9.
24. Goertz RS, Schuderer J, Strobel D, Pfeifer L, et al. Acoustic radiation force impulse shear wave elastography (arfi) of acute and chronic pancreatitis and pancreatic tumor. Eur J Radiol. 2016;85:2211–6.
25. Mateen MA, Muheet KA, Mohan RJ, Rao PN, et al. Evaluation of ultrasound based acoustic radiation force impulse (arfi) and esie touch sonoelastography for diagnosis of inflammatory pancreatic diseases. J Pancreas. 2012;13:36–44.
26. Llamoza-Torres C, Fuentes-Pardo M, Álvarez-Higueras F, Alberca-de-Las-Parras F, et al. Usefulness of percutaneous elastography by acoustic radiation force impulse for the non-invasive diagnosis of chronic pancreatitis. Rev Esp Enferm Dig. 2016;108:450–6.
27. D'Onofrio M, De Robertis R, Crosara S, Poli C, et al. Acoustic radiation force impulse with shear wave speed quantification of pancreatic masses: a prospective study. Pancreatology. 2016;16:106–9.
28. D'Onofrio M, Gallotti A, Martone E, Mucelli RP. Solid appearance of pancreatic serous cystatheoma diagnosed as cystic at ultrasound acoustic radiation force impulse imaging. J Pancreas. 2009;10:543–6.
29. Hirooka Y, Kuwahara T, Irisawa A, Itokawa F, et al. JSUM ultrasound elastography practice guidelines: pancreas. J Med Ultrason. 2015;42:151–74.

23

Ultrasonographic median nerve cross-section areas measured by 8-point "inching test" for idiopathic carpal tunnel syndrome: a correlation of nerve conduction study severity and duration of clinical symptoms

Shu-Fang Chen[1,2], Cheng-Hsien Lu[1], Chi-Ren Huang[1], Yao-Chung Chuang[1], Nai-Wen Tsai[1], Chiung-Chih Chang[1,2] and Wen-Neng Chang[1*]

Abstract

Background: Incremental palmar stimulation of the median nerve sensory conduction at the wrist, the "inching test", provides an assessment with reference to segments proximal and distal to the entrapment. This study used high-resolution ultrasonography (US) to measure the median nerve's cross-section areas (CSAs) like the "inching test" and to correlate with the nerve conduction study (NCS) severity and duration of carpal tunnel syndrome (CTS).

Methods: Two hundred and twelve (212) "CTS-hands" from 135 CTS patients and 50 asymptomatic hands ("A-hands") from 25 control individuals were enrolled. The median nerve CSAs were measured at the 8-point marked as *i4*, *i3*, *i2*, *i1*, *w*, *o1*, *o2*, and *03* in inching test. The NCS severities were classified into six groups based on motor and sensory responses (i.e., negative, minimal, mild, moderate, severe, and extreme). Results of US studies were compared in terms of NCS severity and duration of clinical CTS symptoms.

Results: There was significantly larger CSA of the NCS negative group of "CTS-hands" than of "A-hands". The cut-off values of the CSAs of the NCS negative CTS group were 12.5 mm^2, 11.5 mm^2 and 10.1 mm^2 at the inlet, wrist crease, and outlet, respectively. Of the 212 "CTS-hands", 32 were NCS negative while 40 had minimal, 43 mild, 85 moderate, 10 severe, and two extreme NCS severities. The CSAs of "CTS-hands" positively correlated with different NCS severities and with the duration of CTS symptoms. By duration of clinical symptoms, 12 of the 212 "CTS-hands" were in the 1 month group; 82 in >1 month and ≤12 months group, and 118 in >12 months group. In "inching test", segments *i4*-*i3* and *i3*-*i2* were the most common "positive-site". The corresponding CSAs measured at *i4* and *i3*, but not at *i2*, were significantly larger than those measured at points that were not "positive-site".

Conclusions: Using the 8-point measurement of the median nerve CSA from inlet to outlet similar to the "inching test" has positive correlations with NCS severity and duration of CTS clinical symptoms, and can provide more information on anatomic changes. Combined NCS and US studies using the 8-point measurement may have a higher positive rate than NCS alone for diagnosing CTS.

* Correspondence: cwenneng@ms19.hinet.net
[1]Department of Neurology, Kaohsiung Chang Gung Memorial Hospital and Chang Gung University College of Medicine, Kaohsiung, Taiwan
Full list of author information is available at the end of the article

Background

Carpal tunnel syndrome (CTS) is a common entrapment neuropathy of the median nerve [1]. Currently, nerve conduction study (NCS) is used to confirm the diagnosis and indicate the level of the lesion [2,3]. Among various NCS methods for evaluating CTS, incremental palmar stimulation of the median nerve sensory conduction at the wrist, the so-called "inching test", permits an assessment with reference to nerve segments proximal and distal to the entrapment [4]. Aside from NCS, peripheral nerve ultrasonography (US) is a promising complementary tool [3,5-9]. However, because of different US methods, the measured values of the median nerve in CTS also vary [7-10]. This study introduced an 8-point measurement of the median nerve's cross-sectional area (CSA) from inlet to outlet similar to those performed in the "inching test". The measured CSAs were also compared to NCS severity and duration of CTS symptoms.

Methods

This prospective case-control study conducted over a period of three years (2006-2008) enrolled 160 participants and 262 hands. Of the 160 participants, 135 with 212 hands had clinical symptoms of CTS ("CTS-hands") while the other 25 participants of 50 hands were asymptomatic ("A-hands") and acted as controls. Of the 135 symptomatic participants, 105 were women and 30 were men, aged 22-83 years (mean, 52.2 ± 11.7 years). Their body height ranged from 142 to 177 cm (mean, 158 ± 6.3 cm), body weight 40 to 86 kg (mean, 60.7 ± 8.7 kg), and body mass index 17.5 to 35.3 (mean, 24.1 ± 3.4). The basic information of the controls is listed in Table 1. The term "A-hands" was defined as a hand with normal NCS findings and not fulfilling any clinical definition of CTS.

In order to avoid other interfering factors, none of the 160 participants had diabetes mellitus, gout, rheumatoid arthritis, renal or liver disease, abnormal thyroid function, abnormal serum cortisol level, or elevated serum anti-nuclear antibody. None of the participants had a history of previous wrist surgery or fracture, or a history or clinical evidence of neurologic disorders (e.g. ulnar neuropathy, radiculopathy, polyneuropathy, myelopathy, or stroke) that might result in numbness or paresthesia. Participants with a variant of carpal tunnel, such as accessory muscles, bifid median nerve, and persistent median artery were also excluded. None of the female participants were pregnant at the time of the study. The hospital's Ethics Committee approved the study (IRB 100-1390B).

Two physicians (Drs CSF and TNW) previously trained by musculoskeletal radiologists and with more than three years of experience in patients with related disorders, especially those with clinical CTS, performed the US examinations. The clinical symptoms of each individual were recorded and the collected data were fully analyzed.

Clinical definition of "CTS-hands"

In this study, CTS was defined according to the criteria of the American Academy of Neurology practice parameters as follows [11,12]:

1. Paresthesia, pain, swelling, weakness, or clumsiness of the hand provoked or worsened by sleep, sustained hand or arm position, or repetitive action of the hand or wrist that is mitigated by a change in posture or by shaking of the hand;
2. Sensory deficits in the median nerve innervated regions of the hand;
3. Motor deficit or hypotrophy of the median nerve innervated thenar muscles; and
4. Positive provocative clinical tests (positive Phalen's maneuver and/or Tinel's sign)

The term "CTS-hand" was defined as criterion 1 and one or more of criteria 2-4 were fulfilled. For comparative analysis, the duration of CTS symptoms was classified into three groups, i.e. ≤1 month, >1 and ≤12 months, and > 12 months.

Neuro-physiologic assessment

The NCS was performed for all participants according to the recommended protocol of the American Association of Electrodiagnostic Medicine (AAEM) [2] using a

Table 1 Basic information of the control participants and the patients with NCS negative "CTS" hands

	"A-hands" (n = 50)	NCS negative "CTS hands" (n = 32)	*p* value
Sex	14 hands in man/36 hands in woman	4 hands in man/28 hands in woman	0.100
Age (yr)	44.2 ± 9.8 (46, 25-68)	48.6 ± 11.9 (49, 27-73)	0.135
BH (cm)	163 ± 7.2 (163, 148-174)	159 ± 6.9 (157.5, 150-177)	0.004*
BW (kg)	61.0 ± 8.1 (60, 46-76)	59.6 ± 10.8 (56, 46-86)	0.282
BMI	22.8 ± 3.0 (22.7, 17.5-28.3)	23.6 ± 4.4 (22.9, 17.5-35.3)	0.711

Abbreviations: A-hands, asymptomatic hands; CTS, carpal tunnel syndrome; NCS, nerve conduction study; BH, body heigh; BW, body weight; BMI, body mass index; Mean ± standard deviation (Median, minimum-maximus);

*$p < 0.01$ by Mann-Whitney U test

Nicolet Viking Select system (Nicolet Biomedical Inc. Madison, USA). All tests were done in the same room under similar temperature conditions. Skin temperature was maintained at ≥32°C. As regards NCS, the onset latency, amplitude, distance, and velocity of median, ulnar, and radial motor and sensory nerves were measured. The comparative tests included: 1) median-ulnar sensory conduction between the wrist and ring finger, 2) median sensory nerve conduction comparison between the wrist and palm, 3) median-radial sensory conduction between the wrist and thumb, and 4) antidromic sensory test using 1-cm increments of the median nerve with the wrist crease as the zero reference point extending proximally by 3 cm and distally by 4 cm. In total, eight points (Figure 1) were marked in the subsequent inching test.

The cut-off points used in the NCS were the following: 1) median nerve distal sensory latency <3.4 ms [13], 2) median nerve distal motor latency over the thenar <4.2 ms [13], 3) difference between the median and ulnar nerve distal sensory latencies <0.4 ms [14], 4) trans-carpal median motor conduction velocity <40.6 ms [15], and 5) antidromic sensory using 1-cm increments of the median nerve <0.4 ms [16]. Based on the NCS results, the CTS hands were categorized into six severity groups [17]: negative, for normal findings on all tests; minimal, for abnormal segmental or comparative tests only; mild, for abnormal digit/wrist sensory nerve conduction velocity and normal distal motor latency; moderate, for abnormal digit/wrist sensory nerve conduction velocity and abnormal distal motor latency; severe, for absence of sensory response and abnormal distal motor latency; and extreme, for the absence of motor and sensory response.

Ultrasound assessment technique

High-resolution US was performed using a scanner with a 12/5-MHz linear array transducer for the carpal tunnel study (Philips HDI 5000; Philips Medical Systems, Bothell, WA, USA) on the same day as the NCS. During the examination, the patient sat in a comfortable position facing the examiner, with the measured forearm resting on the table, the palm supine, and fingers semi-extended in the neutral position [18]. The median nerve was first imaged in a longitudinal scan, placing the US probe at the midline between the radius and ulna with the center of the probe at the distal wrist crease, to obtain an initial general overview of the median nerve. This was then used to assist the examiner in obtaining optimal axial (cross-sectional) images. The transducer was placed directly on the patient's skin with gel.

A transverse scan, keeping the probe directly perpendicular to the long axis of the median nerve in order to ensure that the area measured indeed reflected CSA, was then performed to record the CSA (calculated by continual tracing of the nerve circumference, excluding the hyper-echoic epineurial rim) and elliptical diameters (transverse and antero-posterior). Measurements were conducted from the tunnel inlet of the forearm (*i4*, *i3*, *i2*,

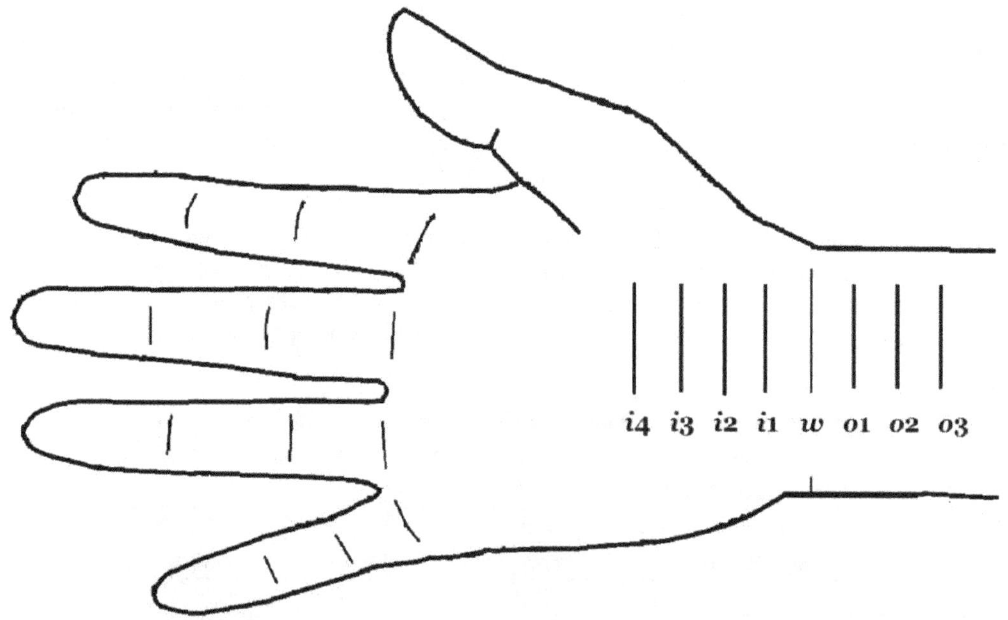

Figure 1 The 8-point for recording in both "inching test" and ultrasonography. The *i4*, *i3*, *i2*, *i1* represent levels at 4, 3, 2, and 1 cm distal to the wrist crease in the inlet of the carpal tunnel; *w* represents the level of the wrist crease and *o1*, *o2*, and *o3* represent levels at 1, 2, and 3 cm proximal to the wrist crease in the outlet of the carpal tunnel.

*i*1) to the wrist crease (*w*) and to the tunnel outlet (*o*1, *o*2, *o*3) (Figure 1).

Statistical analysis

Data were given as mean ± standard deviation. Subsequent ANOVA analysis followed by Scheffe's multiple comparison procedures were used to calculate the mean values of CSA among different symptom duration groups, NCS types, and inching sites. To evaluate differences in CSA value at the 8-point tested between asymptomatic and CTS hands in the NCS negative group, the Mann-Whitney U test was used for comparison, as a consequence of limited data. Significance was set at $p < 0.05$ in the ANOVA and $p < 0.01$ in the Mann-Whitney U tests. The area under the ROC (Receiver Operating Characteristic) curves and the CSA cut-off-values were calculated for the negative NCS CTS hands. The Statistical Package for Social Science (SPSS Inc., version 13.0 for Windows) was used for all statistical analyses.

Results

Based on the NCS severity classification, 32 of the 212 "CTS-hands" were in the negative group, 40 in the minimal group, 43 in the mild group, 85 in the moderate group, 10 in the severe group, and two in the extreme group. If classified according to the duration of clinical symptoms, 12 of the 212 "CTS-hands" were in the ≤1 month group, 82 in >1 month and ≤12 months group, and 118 in >12 months group.

Comparison of CSAs at the 8-point of A-hands and NCS negative CTS-hands

The comparative results revealed significantly larger CSA of the latter group of hands at six points (*i*4, *i*3, *i*2, *i*1, *w*, and *o*3). After comparison of the CSAs under the ROC, the cut-off-values of the significant sites were 12.5 mm^2, 11.5 mm^2, and 10.1 mm^2, respectively (Table 2).

Measured CSAs at the 8-point of CTS-hands with different NCS severities

The measured CSAs were compared. The NCS negative group and the mild to extreme NCS severity groups, except the minimal severity group, showed significantly larger CSA (Table 3). Because of limited case numbers, both severe and extreme groups were excluded from subsequent group comparisons; i.e. only the negative, minimal, mild, and moderate groups were included for further analysis. Mean CSAs of these four groups showed that the mean CSAs increased in accordance to severity, from negative to moderate (Figures 2 and 3).

Frequent positive sites of the "inching test" and their correspondence to the sizes of measured CSAs

The "positive-site" was defined as conduction delay (>0.4 ms) between the interval of the nearby marks in antidromic sensory test with 1 cm increments of the median nerve at the 8-point marks (Figure 4). Results showed that the most common "positive-site" were *i*4-*i*3 and *i*3-*i*2 (Table 4). The comparative results showed that CSAs corresponding to the "positive site" at *i*4-*i*3 were significantly larger than the CSAs of intervals that were not "positive-site" (Table 5). The CSAs measured at *i*2 did not show significant difference between the positive and the non-positive sites.

Comparison of CSAs of A-hands with those of CTS-hands by CTS symptom duration

The comparative results showed that CSAs of the "CTS-hands" with symptom duration >1 month and ≤12 months, and >12 months were significantly larger than the CSAs of "A-hands". The difference between the CSAs of the "A-hands" and the "CTS-hands" with symptom duration > 1 month was not significant. The "CTS-hands" with >12 months duration had significantly larger CSA than the "CTS-hands" with <1 month duration (Table 6).

Table 2 Comparison of CSAs measured at the 8-point of the A-hands and NCS negative CTS-hands

	CSAs		*p* value	Cut-off values of CSA	Sensitivity	Specificity
	A-hands (n = 50)	NCS negative CTS-hands(n = 32)				
*i*4	11.8 ± 2.4 (11, 8-19)	14.3 ± 4.6 (13, 7-28)	0.003*	12.5	0.688	0.720
*i*3	11.5 ± 2.3 (11, 8-19)	14.0 ± 4.3 (13, 8-28)	0.001*	12.5	0.688	0.760
*i*2	10.9 ± 1.9 (11, 8-16)	11.9 ± 2.1 (12, 8-17)	0.033*	11.5	0.563	0.660
*i*1	10.7 ± 1.7 (10.5, 8-15)	12.2 ± 2.7 (11.1, 7-20)	0.006*	11.1	0.500	0.680
w	10.7 ± 2.0 (10.5, 7-17)	12.2 ± 2.9 (12, 7-22)	0.002*	11.5	0.594	0.760
*o*1	10.1 ± 2.2 (10, 6-16)	11.0 ± 2.3 (10, 7-16)	0.082	10.5	0.469	0.600
*o*2	10.2 ± 2.1 (10, 7-17)	10.6 ± 2.0 (10.5, 6-15)	0.164	10.5	0.500	0.600
*o*3	9.4 ± 1.9 (9, 6-15)	10.6 ± 2.7 (11, 5-17)	0.031*	10.1	0.563	0.740

Abbreviations: CSAs, cross-section areas; A-hands, asymptomatic hands; CTS-hands, carpal tunnel syndrome hands; NCS, nerve conduction study

Markers of the 8-point: *i*4, *i*3, *i*2, *i*1, *w*, *o*1, *o*2, and *o*3 Unit of CSA = mm^2

*$p < 0.05$, by Mann-Whitney U test

Table 3 CSAs measured at the 8-point of the CTS-hands with different NCS severities (n = 212)

	Negative (n = 32)	Minimal (n = 40)	Mild (n = 43)	Moderate (n = 85)	Severe (n = 10)	Extreme (n = 2)
i4	14.3 ± 4.6 (7-28)	15.4 ± 4.7 (8-30)	17.3 ± 5.3 (8-34)*	19.8 ± 6.8 (8.9-41)*	17.3 ± 8.9 (8-40.8)	15.5 ± 3.5 (13-18)
i3	14.0 ± 4.3 (8-28)	15.0 ± 4.6 (8-27)	16.0 ± 4.6 (8-26)	18.4 ± 5.9 (8.9-42)*	17.3 ± 8.9 (8-40.8)	15.5 ± 3.5 (16-22)
i2	11.9 ± 2.1 (8-17)	12.0 ± 3.0 (7-21)	12.3 ± 2.4 (6-18)	13.8 ± 3.8 (7-29)	13.4 ± 4.7 (8-23.6)	17.0 ± 1.4 (16-18)
i1	12.2 ± 2.7 (7-20)	12.6 ± 3.1 (7-20)	14.8 ± 4.9 (8-28)	15.4 ± 5.0 (7-34.4)*	16.7 ± 6.7(11.1-34.3)*	14.5 ± 7.8 (9-20)
w	12.2 ± 2.9 (7-22)	12.9 ± 3.4 (7-22)	14.6 ± 3.4 (7-23) *	17.5 ± 5.8 (9-40.4)*	16.0 ± 5.7 (8.9-26)	26.5 ± 9.2 (20-33)*
o1	11.0 ± 2.3 (7-16)	12.2 ± 2.8 (8-20.7)	12.9 ± 3.0 (8-20) *	14.3 ± 3.2(8.7-27.4)*	13.9 ± 4.5 (7-20.3)	22.5 ± 4.9 (19-26)*
o2	10.6 ± 2.0 (6-15)	11.6 ± 2.6 (8-21)	12.0 ± 2.2 (8-17) *	12.8 ± 2.7 (7-21.3)*	13.9 ± 3.6 (9-19.9)	17.0 ± 0.0 (17-17)*
o3	10.6 ± 2.7 (5-17)	10.9 ± 2.0 (7-15)	11.2 ± 1.9 (7-15)	11.5 ± 2.5 (6-19)	12.0 ± 2.2 (9-16)	19.0 ± 0.0 (19-19)*

Abbreviations: CSAs, cross-section areas; CTS-hands, carpal tunnel syndrome hands; NCS, nerve conduction study Markers of the 8-point: *i4*, *i3*, *i2*, *i1*, *w*, *o1*, *o2*, and *o3*

Unit of CSA = mm^2

*$p < 0.01$, by Mann-Whitney U test (comparing CSAs of the minimal to extreme groups with the negative group)

Discussion

For CTS evaluation, several kinds of NCS measurement methods are used for confirmation. As to which measurement method is optimum remains the subject of, long-term debates [1-6,10-20]. In the meantime, although NCS in CTS diagnosis is highly specific [2], 10-25% of cases are unrecognized by classic NCS depending on the disease severity and the type of NCS technique used [2,21-23].

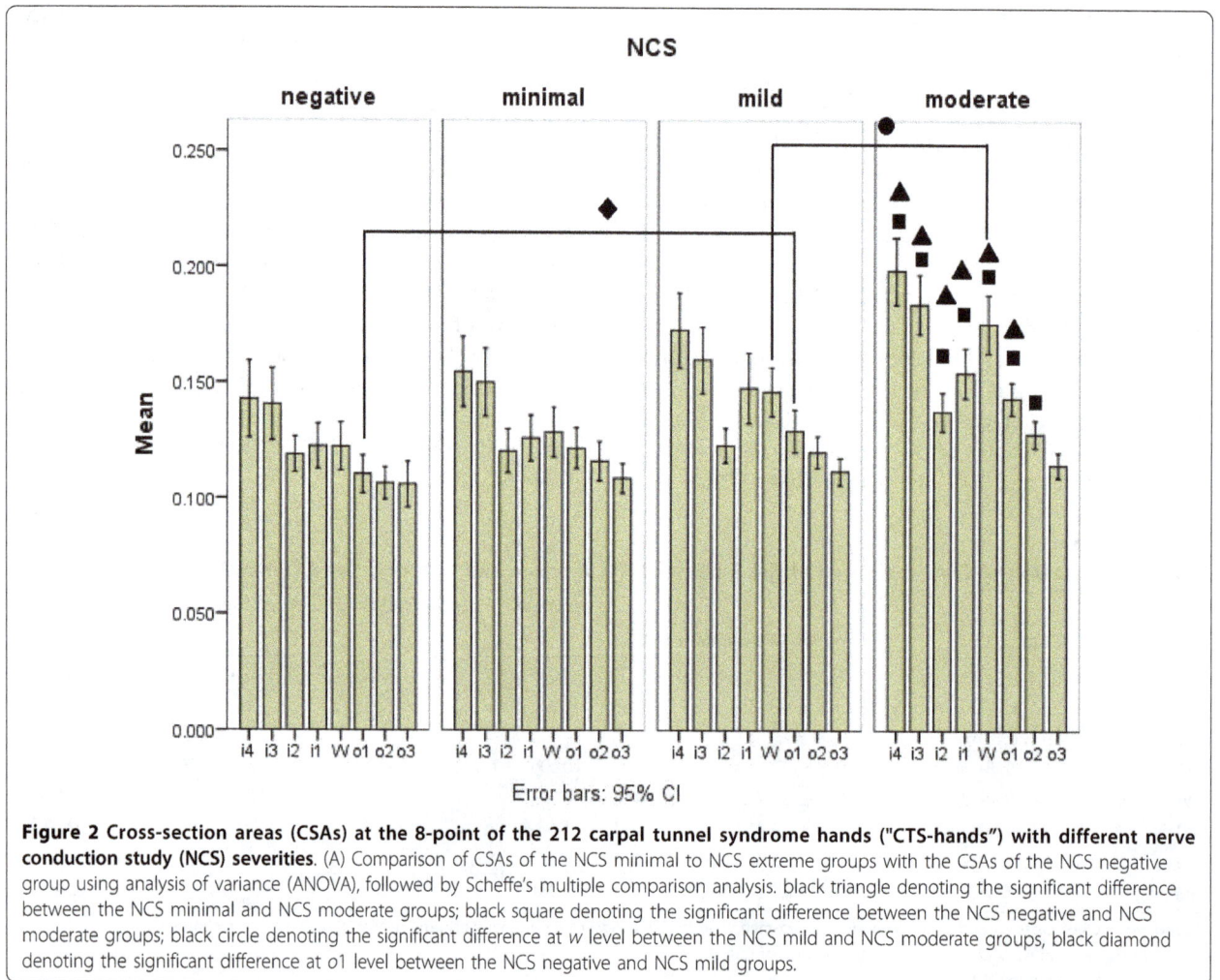

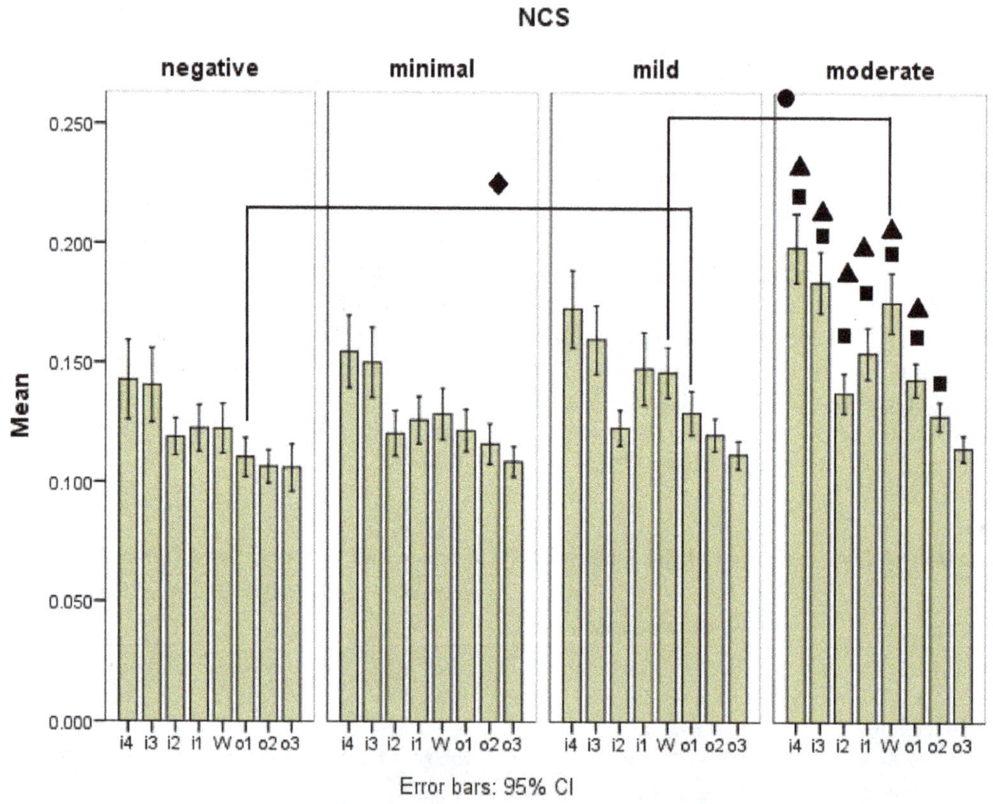

Figure 2 Cross-section areas (CSAs) at the 8-point of the 212 carpal tunnel syndrome hands ("CTS-hands") with different nerve conduction study (NCS) severities. (A) Comparison of CSAs of the NCS minimal to NCS extreme groups with the CSAs of the NCS negative group using analysis of variance (ANOVA), followed by Scheffe's multiple comparison analysis. black triangle denoting the significant difference between the NCS minimal and NCS moderate groups; black square denoting the significant difference between the NCS negative and NCS moderate groups; black circle denoting the significant difference at *w* level between the NCS mild and NCS moderate groups, black diamond denoting the significant difference at *o1* level between the NCS negative and NCS mild groups.

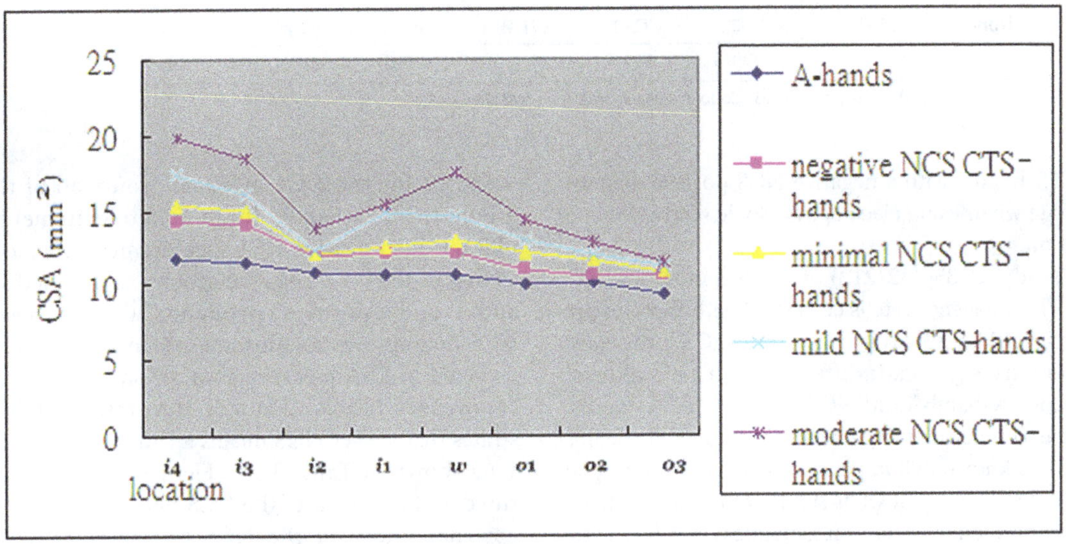

Figure 3 **The mean CSAs of "CTS-hands" with different NCS severities.**

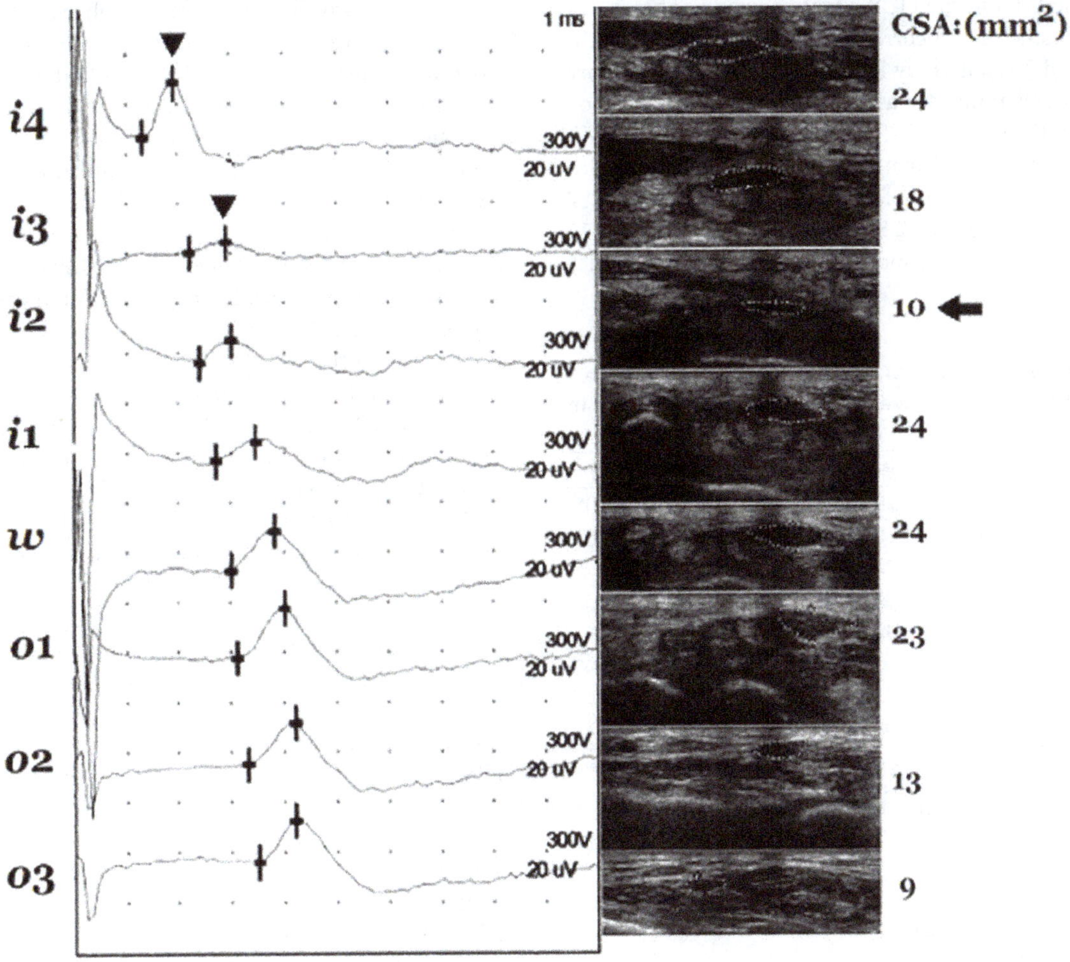

Figure 4 **An example of "positive-site" between *i*4 and *i*3 corresponding to the relatively smaller cross-section area (CSA) at *i*2**. The peak latencies (arrowhead) at *i*4 and *i*3 are 1.9 ms and 2.9 ms, respectively, and the difference between them is 1.0 ms, i.e. >0.4 ms. The CSA measured at *i*2 (arrow) is smaller than those measured at nearby levels. Markers of the 8-point: *i*4, *i*3, *i*2, *i*1, *w*, *o*1, *o*2, and *o*3.

Table 4 Distributions of the positive sites in inching test of all tested hands

Inching	None	*i*4-*i*3	*i*3-*i*2	*i*2-*i*1	*i*1-*W*	*W*-*o*1	*o*1-*o*2	*o*2-*o*3	double	Total
N (%)	119	37 (25.9)	55 (38.5)	6 (4.2)	10 (7.0)	8 (5.6)	2 (1.4)	0 (0)	25 (17.4)	262

Markers of the 8-point: *i*4, *i*3, *i*2, *i*1, *W*, *o*1, *o*2, and *o*3 "double" means more than two sites existed

Thus, "CTS-hands" with a negative NCS poses a diagnostic challenge when using electrophysiologic study alone for confirmation.

In this study, 15.3% (32/212) of "CTS-hands" are NCS negative. This incidence rate is consistent with those of previous reports [2,21-23]. With the 8-point CSA measurement, there are significant differences on several levels between the "A-hands" and NCS negative "CTS-hands". Most of the significant enlargements are located at the inlet (Table 2). It is known that in patients with a clinical diagnosis of CTS, the accuracy of US is similar to that of EMG but is probably preferable because it is painless, easily accessible, and favored by patients [24]. The findings of the present study further strengthen the importance of the complementary role of US in confirming the diagnosis of idiopathic CTS in the NCS negative group. This is also noted in a study of US correlation of CTS in NCS negative "CTS-hands" reported by Rahmani et al. [19]. Therefore, US can be recommended as a useful technique in diagnosing CTS patients when NCS results are not confirmatory in patients suspected of having median neuropathy. The present study also posits the following cut-off values of CSA for CTS confirmation: 12.5 mm^2 at the tunnel inlet, 11.5 mm^2 at the wrist crease, and 10.1 mm^2 at the tunnel outlet.

Table 5 Comparison of CSAs at the 8-points among the two most frequent positive sites and the negative site in the inching test

	none (n = 119)	i4-i3 (n = 37)	i3-i2 (n = 55)
*i*4	13.9 ± 4.8(7-40.8)	19.5 ± 6.9 (9-37)*	19.0 ± 6.9 (8-41)*
*i*3	13.6 ± 4.8 (8-40.8)	17.4 ± 5.0 (8-32) *	17.9 ± 6.3 (8-42)*
*i*2	12.0 ± 3.1 (8-29)	12.4 ± 3.1 (6-19)	13.2 ± 3.4 (8-25)
*i*1	12.4 ± 4.1 (7-34.4)	13.6 ± 4.5 (7-31)	14.6 ± 4.3 (7.4-25)*
w	12.5 ± 4.0 (7-31)	14.5 ± 4.6 (7-27)	15.6 ± 4.9 (7-33)*
*o*1	11.3 ± 2.8 (6-20.7)	13.1 ± 2.9 (9-20)	13.6 ± 3.6 (8-26)*
*o*2	11.0 ± 2.4 (6-18.5)	12.2 ± 2.4 (8-18)	12.8 ± 2.7 (8-21.3)*
*o*3	10.5 ± 2.6 (5-19)	10.5 ± 2.3 (6-16)	11.8 ± 2.4 (8-19)*

Note: CSA, cross-section area; none, no conductive delay >0.4 ms in median inching test in centimeter across the carpal tunnel; *i*4-*i*3, conductive delay >0.4 ms in inching test between 4 cm and 3 cm distal to the wrist crease; *i*3-*i*2, conductive delay >0.4 ms in inching test between 3 cm and 2 cm distal to the wrist crease

Markers of the 8-point: *i*4, *i*3, *i*2, *i*1, *w*, *o*1, *o*2, and *o*3

*i*4-*i*3 and *i*3-*i*2: the difference of latency measured between locations of *i*4 and *i*3, and *i*3 and *i*2 in the inching test

Unit of CSA = mm^2

*$p < 0.05$ in comparing the two most frequent positive sites and the negative one in inching test using analysis of variance (ANOVA) followed by Scheffe's multiple comparison procedure

Except for the NCS minimal group, all of the other groups of "CTS-hands" (from mild to extreme) have significant differences in CSA measurement when compared to that of the NCS negative group (Table 3 and Figures 2 and 3) and a positive correlation with the severities of NCS findings. Although some insignificant enlargements detected in CSA measurement are shown by inter-group comparison (Tables 2 and 3), the present study demonstrates that slower NCS means a larger CSA by US study.

As shown in Table 3 and Figures 2 and 3, CSAs measured at the 8-point of the NCS minimal group are all larger than those of the NCS negative group, but this difference is not statistically significant. This insignificance can be explained partly by the trivial difference in NCS and measured CSAs in these two groups of "CTS-hands". However, this study does not offer enough evidence to sufficiently explain the difference. Further large-scale study is needed for better delineation of the US findings between the NCS negative and NCS minimal groups. Nevertheless, with a measurement of CSA at the 8-point, US remains an important complementary tool for confirming clinical CTS.

As shown in Table 4, the segments between *i*4 and *i*3, and *i*3 and *i*2 are the most frequent "positive sites", and their respective CSAs are larger than those measured at "non-positive sites" (Table 5). This suggests a positive correlation in NCS severities and measured areas of CSA in the CTS study, a correlation also noted in other studies [10,20,25,26]. The present study (Tables 4 and 5) also reveals that most of the "positive sites" detected in the "inching test" involve the distal part (*i*2-*I*4) of the inlet, and the CSA measured at *i*2 is the smallest. These show that the area around *i*2 is the most possible site of nerve entrapment in idiopathic CTS, which may provide additional guidance for a more precise location for treatment.

As shown in Table 6, there is a positive correlation between the measured CSA with the symptom duration of clinical idiopathic CTS such that the longer the duration of symptoms correlated to larger measured CSA. This finding has not been previously reported. Nonetheless, US provides reproducible median nerve measurements [27]. As such, it can be used to assess changes in median nerve characteristics during follow-up studies of idiopathic CTS.

This study has several limitations. First, although 212 "CTS-hands" were included for examination, further large-scale study is warranted for a more even distribution of the case number in the different sub-groups of "CTS-hands". Second, the limitations of accuracy in

Table 6 Comparison of CSAs at the 8-point of the 'A-hands' with the "CTS-hands" of different symptom durations

	A-hands	CTS-hands		
	(n = 50)	1 month(n = 12)	> 1 month and 12 months (n = 82)	>12 months (n = 118)
i4	11.8 ± 2.4 (8-19)	14.1 ± 4.7 (8-24)	16.6 ± 5.1 (7-34)*	18.5 ± 6.9 (8-41)*
i3	11.5 ± 2.3 (8-19)	12.7 ± 2.9 (8-17)	16.0 ± 5.0 (8-28) *	17.3 ± 6.0 (8-42)*,#
i2	10.9 ± 1.9 (8-16)	11.2 ± 2.6 (7-17)	12.8 ± 2.8 (7-20) *	13.1 ± 3.7 (6-29)*
i1	10.7 ± 1.7 (8-15)	12.8 ± 2.0 (10-16)	13.6 ± 4.1 (7-24) *	15.0 ± 5.1 (7-34.4)*
w	10.7 ± 2.0 (7-17)	11.7 ± 3.3 (7-18)	14.8 ± 5.2 (7-40.4) *	16.0 ± 5.2 (7-33)*#
*o*1	10.1 ± 2.2 (6-16)	11.2 ± 2.9 (7-16)	12.8 ± 3.2 (7-23) *	13.7 ± 3.4 (8-27.4)*
*o*2	10.2 ± 2.1 (7-17)	10.8 ± 2.0 (8-15)	11.6 ± 2.3 (6-19) *	12.7 ± 2.8 (7-21.3)*
*o*3	9.4 ± 1.9 (6-15)	10.5 ± 2.6 (7-17)	11.1 ± 2.2 (5-16) *	11.4 ± 2.6 (6-19)*

Abbreviations: A-hand, asymptomatic hands; CTS-hands, carpal tunnel syndrome hand; CSAs, cross section areas Markers of the 8-point: *i4*, *i3*, *i2*, i1, *w*, *o*1, *o*2, and *o*3. Unit of CSA = mm^2

*$p < 0.05$ (a comparison of CSAs of the 'A-hands' with the CSAs of the 'CTS-hands' of different symptom durations using analysis of variance (ANOVA) followed by Scheffe's multiple comparison procedure)

#$p < 0.05$ (a comparison of CSAs of the CTS-hands with <1 month duration with the CSAs of the 'CTS-hands' with >12 months duration using analysis of variance (ANOVA) followed by Scheffe's multiple comparison procedure)

inching techniques need to be taken into consideration. This limitation is also noted in other studies [28,29]. Third, there is difficulty in accurately obtaining a chronology of the length of symptom duration. Fourth, there is a lack of using neuroimaging studies such as computed tomography and/or magnetic resonance imaging to test the accuracy of CSA measurement at varying levels and to delineate the local change of carpal tunnel. Fifth, besides CSA measurement, there are other useful, additional measurements of the median nerve with US such as the measurement of width and circumference of the wrist [30]. In this study we did not perform these additional measurements for CSA correlation. Lastly, there is a discrepancy of median nerve length between the conventional surface measurement and US measurement [31].

Conclusions

More than 15% of "CTS-hands" have negative NCS. The 8-point measurement of the median nerve CSA from inlet to outlet similar to the "inching test" provides more information on anatomic changes. This US finding has positive correlation with NCS severity and the duration of CTS clinical symptom. A combination of NCS and US studies, especially the 8-point measurement, may have a higher positive rate than NCS alone for diagnosing CTS

Author details

[1]Department of Neurology, Kaohsiung Chang Gung Memorial Hospital and Chang Gung University College of Medicine, Kaohsiung, Taiwan.
[2]Department of Biological Science, National Sun Yat-Sen University, Kaohsiung, Taiwan.

Authors' contributions

All authors have read and approved the submitted manuscript.
SFC contributed to the conception and design, data acquisition and analysis, and drafting and revision of the manuscript; CHL, CRH, YCC, NWT, and CCC contributed to the conception and design, and clinical data analysis; and WNC contributed to the conception and design, data analysis, and critical revision and final approval of the manuscript.

Competing interests

The authors declare that they have no competing interests.

References

1. Phalen GS: **The carpal-tunnel syndrome. Clinical evaluation of 598 hands.** *Clin Ortho Relat Res* 1972, **83**:29-40.
2. Jablecki CK, Andary MT, Floeter RG, Miller CA, Quartly CA, Vennix MJ, Wilson JR, American Association of Electro-diagnostic Medicine; American Academy of Neurology; American Academy of Physical Medicine and Rehabilitation: **Practice parameter; Electro-diagnostic studies in carpal tunnel syndrome. Report of the American Association of Electro-diagnostic Medicine, American Academy of Neurology, and the American Academy of Physical Medicine and Rehabilitation.** *Neurology* 2002, **58**:1589-1592.
3. Hobson-Webb LD, Massey JM, Juel VC, Sanders DB: **The ultrasonographic wrist-to-forearm median nerve area ratio in carpal tunnel syndrome.** *ClinNeurophysiol* 2008, **119**:1353-1357.
4. Kimura J: **The carpal tunnel syndrome: localization of conduction abnormalities within the distal segment of median nerve.** *Brain* 1979, **102**:619-635.
5. Wong SM, Griffith JF, Hui ACF, Lo SK, Fu M, Wong KS: **Carpal tunnel srndrome: diagnostic usefulness of ultrasonography.** *Radiology* 2004, **232**:93-99.
6. Ziswiler HR, Reichenbach S, Vogelin E, Bachmann LM, Villiger PM, Juni P: **Diagnostic value of sonography in patients with suspected carpal tunnel syndrome: a prospective study.** *Arthritis Rheum* 2005, **52**:304-311.
7. Beekman R, Visser LH: **Sonography in the diagnosis of carpal tunnel syndrome: a critical review of the literature.** *Muscle Nerve* 2003, **27**:26-33.
8. Koyuncuoglu HR, Kutluhan S, Oyar O, Guler K, Ozden A: **The value of ultrasonographic measurement in carpal tunnel syndrome in patients with negative electro-diagnostic tests.** *Eur J Radiol* 2005, **56**:365-369.
9. Mondelli M, Filippou G, Gallo A, Frediani B: **Diagnostic utility of ultrasonography versus nerve conduction studies in mild carpal tunnel syndrome.** *Arthritis Rheum* 2008, **59**:357-366.
10. Padua L, Pazzaglia C, Caliandro P, Granata G, Foschini M, Briani C, Martinoli C: **Carpal tunnel syndrome: ultrasound, neurophysiology, clinical and patient-oriented assessment.** *Clin Neurophysiol* 2008, **119**:2064-2069.
11. Practice parameter for carpal tunnel syndrome (summary statement): **Report of the Quality Standards Subcommittee of the American Academy of Neurology.** *Neurology* 1993, **43**:2406-2409.

12. You H, Simmons Z, Freivalds A, Kothari MJ, Naidu SH: **Relationships between clinical symptom severity scales and nerve conduction measures in CTS.** *Muscle Nerve* 1999, **22**:497-501.
13. Jackson DA, Clifford JC: **Electro-diagnosis of mild carpal tunnel syndrome.** *Arch Phys Med Rehabil* 1989, **70**:199-204.
14. Uncini A, Lange DJ, Solomon M, Soliven B, Meer J, Lovelace RE: **Ring finger testing in CTS: a comparative study of diagnostic utility.** *Muscle Nerve* 1989, **12**:735-741.
15. Walters RJL, Murray NMF: **Trans-carpal motor conduction velocity in carpal tunnel syndrome.** *Muscle Nerve* 2001, **24**:966-968.
16. Nathan PA, Meadows KD, Doyle LS: **Sensory segmental latency values of the median nerve for a population of normal individuals.** *Arch Phys Med Rehabil* 1988, **69**:499-501.
17. Padua L, LoMonaco M, Gregori B, Valente EM, Padua R, Tonali P: **Neurophysiologic classification and sensitivity in 500 CTS hands.** *Acta Neurol Scand* 1997, **96**:211-217.
18. Kuo MH, Leong CP, Cheng YF, Chang HW: **Static wrist position associated with least median nerve compression: sonographic evaluation.** *Am J Phys Med Rehabil* 2001, **80**:256-260.
19. Rahmani M, Ghasemi Esfe AR, Bozorg SM, Mazloumi M, Khalilzadeh O, Kahnouji H: **The ultrasonographic correlates of carpal tunnel syndrome in patients with normal electro-diagnostic tests.** *Radiol Med* 2011, **116**:489-496.
20. Lee CH, Kim TK, Yoon ES, Dhong ES: **Correlation of high-resolution ultrasonographic findings with the clinical symptoms and electro-diagnostic data in carpal tunnel syndrome.** *Ann Plast Sur* 2005, **54**:20-23.
21. Seror P: **Sensitivity of the various tests for diagnosis of carpal tunnel syndrome.** *J Hand Surg Br* 1994, **19**:725-728.
22. Preston DC: **Compressive and entrapment neuropathies of the upper extremity.** In *Neuromuscular Disorders in Clinical Practice.* Edited by: Katirji B et al. Boston: Butterworth-Heinemann; 2002:744-773.
23. Witt JC, Hentz JG, Stevens JC: **Carpal tunnel syndrome with normal nerve conduction studies.** *Muscle Nerve* 2004, **29**:515-522.
24. Karadag YS, Karadag O, Cicekli E, Ozturk S, Kiraz S, Ozbakir S, Filippucci E, Grassi W: **Severity of carpal tunnel syndrome assessed with high frequency ultrasonography.** *Rheumatol Int* 2010, **30**:761-765.
25. Mohammadi A, Afshar A, Etemadi A, Masoudi S, Baghizadeh A: **Diagnostic value of cross-sectional area of median nerve in grading severity of carpal tunnel syndrome.** *Arch Iran Med* 2010, **13**:516-521.
26. Visser LH, Smidt MH, Lee ML: **High-resolution sonography versus EMG in the diagnosis of carpal tunnel syndrome.** *J Neurol Neurosurg Psychiatry* 2008, **79**:63-67.
27. Impink BG, Gagnon D, Collinger JL, Boninger ML: **Repeatability of ultrasonographic median nerve measures.** *Muscle Nerve* 2010, **41**:767-773.
28. Kimura J: **Principles and pitfalls of nerve conduction studies.** *Ann Neurol* 1984, **16**:415-429.
29. Geiringer SR: **Inching Techniques are of limited usage.** *Muscle Nerve* 1998, **21**:1557-1561.
30. Claes F, Meulstee J, Claessen-Oude Luttikhuis TT, Huygen PL, Verhagen WI: **Usefulness of additional measurements of the median nerve with ultrasonography.** *Neurol Sci* 2010, **31**:721-725.
31. Rha DW, Im SH, Kim SK, Chang WH, Kim KJ, Lee SC: **Median nerve conduction study through the carpal tunnel using segmental nerve length measured by ultrasonographic and conventional tape method.** *Arch Phys Med Rehabil* 2011, **92**:1-6.

Permissions

All chapters in this book were first published in MI, by BioMed Central; hereby published with permission under the Creative Commons Attribution License or equivalent. Every chapter published in this book has been scrutinized by our experts. Their significance has been extensively debated. The topics covered herein carry significant findings which will fuel the growth of the discipline. They may even be implemented as practical applications or may be referred to as a beginning point for another development.

The contributors of this book come from diverse backgrounds, making this book a truly international effort. This book will bring forth new frontiers with its revolutionizing research information and detailed analysis of the nascent developments around the world.

We would like to thank all the contributing authors for lending their expertise to make the book truly unique. They have played a crucial role in the development of this book. Without their invaluable contributions this book wouldn't have been possible. They have made vital efforts to compile up to date information on the varied aspects of this subject to make this book a valuable addition to the collection of many professionals and students.

This book was conceptualized with the vision of imparting up-to-date information and advanced data in this field. To ensure the same, a matchless editorial board was set up. Every individual on the board went through rigorous rounds of assessment to prove their worth. After which they invested a large part of their time researching and compiling the most relevant data for our readers.

The editorial board has been involved in producing this book since its inception. They have spent rigorous hours researching and exploring the diverse topics which have resulted in the successful publishing of this book. They have passed on their knowledge of decades through this book. To expedite this challenging task, the publisher supported the team at every step. A small team of assistant editors was also appointed to further simplify the editing procedure and attain best results for the readers.

Apart from the editorial board, the designing team has also invested a significant amount of their time in understanding the subject and creating the most relevant covers. They scrutinized every image to scout for the most suitable representation of the subject and create an appropriate cover for the book.

The publishing team has been an ardent support to the editorial, designing and production team. Their endless efforts to recruit the best for this project, has resulted in the accomplishment of this book. They are a veteran in the field of academics and their pool of knowledge is as vast as their experience in printing. Their expertise and guidance has proved useful at every step. Their uncompromising quality standards have made this book an exceptional effort. Their encouragement from time to time has been an inspiration for everyone.

The publisher and the editorial board hope that this book will prove to be a valuable piece of knowledge for researchers, students, practitioners and scholars across the globe.

List of Contributors

Afshin Mohammadi
Radiology Department, Urmia University of Medical Sciences, Urmia, Iran

Mohammad Ghasemi-Rad
Student research committee, School of Medicine, Urmia University of Medical Sciences, Urmia, Iran

Maryam Khodabakhsh
School of Medicine, Urmia University of Medical Sciences, Urmia, Iran

Matthew W Urban, Randall R Kinnick, James F Greenleaf and Mostafa Fatemi
Department of Physiology and Biomedical Engineering, Mayo Clinic, 200 First Street SW, Rochester, MN 55905, USA

Azra Alizad
Department of Internal Medicine, Mayo Clinic, 200 First Street SW, Rochester, MN 55905, USA

John C Morris
Division of Endocrinology, Department of Internal Medicine, Mayo Clinic, 200 First Street SW, Rochester, MN 55905, USA

Carl C Reading
Department of Radiology, Mayo Clinic, 200 First Street SW, Rochester, MN 55905, USA

Yangyang Zhou and Jiang Wu
Department of Neurology, The First Norman Bethune Hospital of Jilin University, Xinmin Street 71#, 130021, Chang Chun, China

Yan Li, Yang Bai, Xiaofeng Sun and Yingqiao Zhu
Center for Abdominal Ultrasound, The First Norman Bethune Hospital of Jilin University, Chang Chun, China

Ying Chen and Yingqi Xing
Center for Neurovascular Ultrasound, The First Norman Bethune Hospital of Jilin University, Chang Chun, China

Frida Lindberg, Mattias Mårtensson and Lars-Åke Brodin
School of Technology and Health, Royal Institute of Technology (KTH), Huddinge, Sweden

Christer Grönlund
Department of Biomedical Engineering - R&D, Radiation science, Umeå University, Umeå, Sweden

Roberto Marci Giuseppe Lo Monte
Department of Morphology, Surgery and Experimental medicine, University of Ferrara, Via Aldo Moro 8, Ferrara, Cona 44124, Italy

Rocco Rago, Pietro Salacone, Immacolata Marcucci, Aurelio Aniceto Marcucci, Nicolina Pacini, Annalisa Sebastianelli and Luisa Caponecchia
Department of Andrology and Pathophysiology of Reproduction, S. Maria Goretti Hospital, Latina, Italy

Tommy Löfstedt, Olof Ahnlund, Michael Peolsson and Johan Trygg
Computational Life Science Cluster (CLiC), Department of Chemistry, Umeå University, Umeå, Sweden

Nicola Ingram, Gemma Marston, Ian M Carr, Alexander F Markham and P Louise Coletta
School of Medicine, University of Leeds Brenner Building, St James's University Hospital, Leeds LS9 7TF, UK

Stuart A Macnab and Adrian Whitehouse
School of Molecular and Cellular Biology, Faculty of Biological Sciences and Astbury Centre for Structural Molecular Biology, University of Leeds, Leeds LS2 9JT, UK

Nigel Scott
Department of Histopathology, Bexley Wing, St James's University Hospital, Leeds LS9 7TF, UK

Antonio I Cuesta-Vargas
School of Clinical Sciences, Faculty of Health, Queensland University of Technology (QUT), Victoria Park Road, Kelvin Grove QLD 4059, Australia

Manuel Gonzalez-Sanchez
Department of Physiotherapy, Faculty of Health Sciences, University of Malaga, 29071, Málaga, Spain

Valentin C Dones III, Karen Grimmer and Julie Luker
International Centre for Allied Health Evidence, University of South Australia, Adelaide, South Australia

Kerry Thoirs
Division of Health Sciences, University of South Australia, C8-26, Centenary Building, Adelaide, SA 5001, Australia

Consuelo G Suarez
Department of Rehabilitation Medicine, Faculty of Medicine and Surgery, University of Santo Tomas, Manila, Philippines

Ole Solheim and Geirmund Unsgård
Department of Neurosurgery, St.Olavs University Hospital, N-7006 Trondheim, Norway
National Competence Centre for Ultrasound and Image-guided Therapy, Trondheim, Norway
Faculty of Medicine, Norwegian University of Science and Technology, Olav Kyrres gate 9, Trondheim, Norway

Asgeir S Jakola
MI Lab, Norwegian University of Science and Technology, Trondheim, Norway
Department of Neuroscience, Norwegian University of Science and Technology, Trondheim, Norway
Department of Neurosurgery, St.Olavs University Hospital, N-7006 Trondheim, Norway
National Competence Centre for Ultrasound and Image-guided Therapy, Trondheim, Norway

Lisa M Sagberg and Tormod Selbekk
National Competence Centre for Ultrasound and Image-guided Therapy, Trondheim, Norway

Arve Jørgensen and Petter Aadahl
Department of Diagnostic Imaging, St.Olavs University Hospital, Trondheim, Norway

Tormod Selbekk
Department of Medical Technology, SINTEF, Trondheim, Norway

Ralf-Peter Michler
Department of Neurology and Clinical Neurophysiology, St. Olavs University Hospital, Trondheim, Norway

Sverre H Torp
Department of Laboratory Medicine, Children's and Women's Health, Norwegian University of Science and Technology, Trondheim, Norway
Department of Pathology and Medical Genetics, St.Olavs University Hospital, Trondheim, Norway

Eric Hildebrand Tomas Gottvall and Marie Blomberg
Department of Obstetrics and Gynaecology, and Department of Clinical and Experimental Medicine, Linköping University, Linköping, Sweden

Madeleine Abrandt Dahlgren
Department of Medicine and Health Sciences, Faculty of Health Sciences, Linköping University, Linköping, Sweden

Birgitta Janerot-Sjoberg
Department of Clinical Physiology and Nuclear Medicine, University Hospital, Linköping, Sweden

Catarina Sved
Department of Medicine & Health, Division of Cardiovascular medicine, Faculty of Health Sciences, Linköping University, Linköping, Sweden
Department of Clinical Physiology and Nuclear Medicine, University Hospital, Linköping, Sweden

Birgitta Janerot-Sjoberg
Department Biomedical Engineering, Linköping University, Linköping, Sweden
Department of Clinical Physiology, Karolinska University Hospital, Stockholm, Sweden
Department of Clinical Science, Division of Medical Imaging and Technology, Intervention and Technology, Karolinska Institutet, Stockholm, Sweden

Jouni K. Kuusisto and Juha P. Sinisalo
Division of Cardiology, Heart and Lung Center, Helsinki University Central Hospital, Meilahti Tower Hospital, FIN-00029 HUS Helsinki, Finland

Vesa M. Järvinen
Department of Clinical Physiology, Medical Imaging Center, Hospital District Helsinki and Uusimaa, Hyvinkää Hospital, Hyvinkää, Finland

Junko Sato, Yoshinori Ishii and Hideo Noguchi
Ishii Orthopaedic and Rehabilitation Clinic, 1089 Shimo-Oshi, Gyoda, Saitama 361-0037, Japan

Shin-ichi Toyabe
Division of Information Science and Biostatistics, Niigata University Graduate School of Medical and Dental Sciences, 1 Asahimachi Dori, Niigata, Niigata 951-8520, Japan

Ning Bi
School of Mathematics and Computational Science, Sun Yat-sen University, Guangzhou, P. R. China

Changxiu Song
Faculty of Applied Mathematics, Guangdong University of Technology, Guangzhou, P.R. China

Zhenyou Wang
Faculty of Applied Mathematics, Guangdong University of Technology, Guangzhou, P.R. China
School of Mathematics and Computational Science, Sun Yat-sen University, Guangzhou, P. R. China

Yanmei Xue
The School of Mathematics & Statistics, Nanjing University of Information Science Technology, Nanjing, Jiangsu, P.R. China

Jiang Zhu
Department of Ultrasound, Sir Run Shaw Hospital, College of Medicine ZheJiang University, Hangzhou, P.R. China

Héloïse Bleton and Ervin Sejdić
Department of Electrical and Computer Engineering, University of Pittsburgh, Pittsburgh, PA, USA
Department of Electrical and Computer Engineering, University of Pittsburgh, Pittsburgh, PA, USA

Subashan Perera
Division of Geriatric Medicine, University of Pittsburgh, Pittsburgh, PA, USA

Raffaele Liuzzi
Institute of Biostructure and Bioimaging, Italian National Research Council (CNR), Naples, Italy

Marcello Mancini
SDN Foundation IRCCS, Naples, Italy

Marco Salvatore and Emilia Vergara
Dipartimento di Scienze Biomediche Avanzate, Università degli Studi di Napoli "Federico II", 80131 Naples, Italy

Giuliana Salvatore
Dipartimento di Studi delle Istituzioni e dei Sistemi Territoriali, Università degli Studi di Napoli "Parthenope", Naples, Italy

Adelaide Greco and Arturo Brunetti
CEINGE-Biotecnologie Avanzate s.c.a.\r.l., Naples, Italy

Gennaro Di Maro
Dipartimento di Biologia e Patologia Cellulare e Molecolare, Università degli Studi di Napoli "Federico II", 80131 Naples, Italy

Gennaro Chiappetta and Rosa Pasquinelli
Functional Genomic Unit, Istituto Nazionale Tumori G. Pascale, Naples, Italy

Erwei Nie
College of Information and Control Engineering, Liaoning Shihua University, Fushun, People's Republic of China

Yanying Zhu and Jiao Yu
College of Science, Liaoning Shihua University, Fushun, People's Republic of China

Debaditya Dutta
Sensing and Computer Vision, Union Pacific Railroad, Omaha, USA

Li-Da Chen, Fu-Shun Pan, Lu-Yao Zhou, Jian-Yao Lv, Ming Xu, Xiao-Yan Xie, Ming-De Lu and Zhu Wang and Wei Wang
Department of Medical Ultrasonics, Institute of Diagnostic and Interventional Ultrasound, The First Affiliated Hospital of Sun Yat-Sen University, 58 Zhongshan Road 2, Guangzhou 510080, People's Republic of China

Yu-Bo Liu
Department of Ultrasound, State Key Laboratory of Oncology in South China, Sun Yat-Sen University Cancer Center, Guangzhou, China

Ming-De Lu
Department of Hepatobiliary Surgery, The First Affiliated Hospital of Sun Yat-Sen University, Guangzhou, China

Carlos Menendez-Castro, Maren Zapke, Fabian Fahlbusch, Heiko von Goessel, Wolfgang Rascher and Jörg Jüngert
Department of Pediatrics and Adolescent Medicine, University Hospital of Erlangen, Loschgestrasse 15, D-91054 Erlangen, Germany

Tormod Selbekk and Reidar Brekken
Department of Medical Technology, SINTEF, Olav Kyrres gate 9, Trondheim, Norway

Marit Indergaard, Tormod Selbekk and Reidar Brekken
Faculty of Medicine, Norwegian University of Science and Technology, Olav Kyrres gate 9, Trondheim, Norway

Tom Thomaes, Steven Onkelinx, Véronique Cornelissen and Luc Vanhees
Cardiovascular Rehabilitation Unit, Department of Rehabilitation Sciences, Katholieke Universiteit Leuven, Tervuursevest 101, 3001 Heverlee, Belgium

Martine Thomis
Exercise and Health Research Group, Department of Kinesiology, Katholieke Universiteit Leuven, Tervuursevest 101, 3001 Heverlee, Belgium

Walter Coudyzer
Radiology, University Hospital Leuven, Herestraat 49, 3000 Leuven, Belgium

Sophie Püttmann, Janina Koch, Thomas Seufferlein, Wolfgang Kratzer and Julian Schmidberger
Department of Internal Medicine I, University Hospital Ulm, Albert-Einstein-Allee 23, 89081 Ulm, Germany

Jochen Paul Steinacker and Stefan Andreas Schmidt
Department of Diagnostic and Interventional Radiology, University Hospital Ulm, Albert-Einstein-Allee 23, 89081 Ulm, Germany

Burkhard Manfras
Medicover Medical Centre, Münsterplatz 6, 89073 Ulm, Germany

Chi-Ren Huang, Nai-Wen Tsai, Cheng-Hsien Lu, Yao-Chung Chuang and Wen-Neng Chang
Department of Neurology, Kaohsiung Chang Gung Memorial Hospital and Chang Gung University College of Medicine, Tai-Pei road, Kaohsiung 833, Taiwan

Chiung-Chih Chang and Shu-Fang Chen
Department of Biological Science, National Sun Yat-Sen University, Kaohsiung, Taiwan
Department of Neurology, Kaohsiung Chang Gung Memorial Hospital and Chang Gung University College of Medicine, Tai-Pei road, Kaohsiung 833, Taiwan
Department of Biological Science, National Sun Yat-Sen University, Kaohsiung, Taiwan
Department of Neurology, Kaohsiung Chang Gung Memorial Hospital and Chang Gung University College of Medicine, Kaohsiung, Taiwan

Index

www.ingramcontent.com/pod-product-compliance
Lightning Source LLC
Chambersburg PA
CBHW082015190326
41458CB00010B/3198
9781639270842